Cosmetic Surgery

a Lange medical book

Cosmetic Surgery

Robert T. Grant, MD, MSc, FACS
Plastic Surgeon-in-Chief
New York-Presbyterian Hospital, the University Hospital of Columbia and Cornell
Associate Clinical Professor of Surgery
College of Physicians and Surgeon, Columbia University
Adjunct Associate Professor of Surgery (Plastic Surgery)
Weill Medical College of Cornell University
New York

Constance M. Chen, MD, MPH
Plastic & Reconstructive Surgery
Lenox Hill Hospital
New York Eye & Ear Infirmary
New York

McGraw Hill Medical

New York Chicago San Francisco Lisbon London Madrid Mexico City
New Delhi San Juan Seoul Singapore Sydney Toronto

The McGraw·Hill Companies

Cosmetic Surgery

1 2 3 4 5 6 7 8 9 0 CTP/CTP 14 13 12 11 10

ISBN 978-0-07-147079-7
MHID 0-07-147079-4

This book was set in Garamond light by Glyph International Limited.
The editors were Marsha Gelber and Harriet Lebowitz.
The production supervisor was Sherri Souffrance.
The illustration manager was Armen Ovsepyan.
The cover designer was Aimee Davis.
The illustrator was Catherine Delphia.
Cover photo: Helen McArdle/Photo Researchers, Inc
China Printing and Translation Services, Ltd. was the printer and binder.

This book is printed on acid-free paper.

Library of Congress Cataloging-in-Publication Data

Cosmetic surgery / [edited by] Robert T. Grant, Constance M. Chen.
p. ; cm.
"A Lange medical book."
Includes bibliographical references and index.
ISBN-13: 978-0-07-147079-7 (pbk. : alk. paper)
ISBN-10: 0-07-147079-4 (pbk. : alk. paper)
1. Surgery, Plastic. I. Grant, Robert T. II. Chen, Constance M.
[DNLM: 1. Reconstructive Surgical Procedures. 2. Cosmetic Techniques.
WO 600 C83414 2010]
RD119.C6815 2010
617.9′5—dc22

2010018802

CONTENTS

AUTHORS

Jeffrey Ascherman, MD, FACS
Site Chief, Division of Plastic Surgery
Associate Professor of Clinical Surgery
New York-Presbyterian Hospital/Columbia University Medical Center
Jaa7@columbia.edu
Chapter 12

Sophie Bartisch, MD
Plastic Surgery Resident
New York-Presbyterian Hospital
sophie.bartisch@hotmail.com
Chapter 16

Brooke Burkey, MD
Plastic Surgery Resident
New York-Presbyterian Hospital
brooke_burkey@yahoo.com
Chapter 5

Nicholas Clavin, MD
General Surgery Resident
New York-Presbyterian Hospital/Weill Cornell Medical center
nicholasclavin@yahoo.com
Chapter 5

Brian D. Cohen, MD
Plastic Surgery Resident
New York-Presbyterian Hospital
Bc2152@columbia.edu
Chapter 13

Kevin J. Cross, MD
Plastic Surgery Resident
New York-Presbyterian Hospital
kevinjaycross@gmail.com
Chapter 17, 19

Melissa A. Doft, MD
Plastic Surgery Resident
New York-Presbyterian Hospital
Mk2593@columbia.edu
Chapter 11

Jessica Erdmann-Sager, MD
General Surgery Resident
New York-Presbyterian Hospital-Columbia University Medical Center
jessixoh@hotmail.com
Chapter 10

Roy Foo, MD
Plastic Surgery Resident
New York-Presbyterian Hospital
rf2056@columbia.edu
Chapter 9

Kenneth R. Francis, MD
Assistant Clinical Professor of Surgery (Plastic Surgery)
New York-Presbyterian Hospital/Weill Cornell Medical center
KFRANMD@aol.com
Chapter 2

Vikisha Fripp, MD
Plastic Surgery Resident
New York-Presbyterian Hospital
vikisha@yahoo.com
Chapters 3, 4, 5

Lloyd B. Gayle, MD
Site Chief, Division of Plastic Surgery
New York-Presbyterian Hospital/Weill Cornell Medical College
Associate Clinical Professor of Surgery (Plastic Surgery)
lloydbgayle@msn.com
Chapter 14

Robert T. Grant, MD, MSc, FACS
Plastic Surgeon-in-Chief
New York-Presbyterian Hospital
Associate Clinical Professor of Surgery College of Physicians and Surgeons, Columbia University
Adjunct Associate Professor of Surgery, Weill Medical College of Cornell University
Introduction, Chapters 1, 7

Katherine Heiden, MD
General Surgery Resident
New York-Presbyterian Hospital/Weill Cornell Medical Center
katycarpizo@gmail.com
Chapter 15

Jeffrey D. Hoefflin, MD
Plastic Surgery Resident
New York-Presbyterian Hospital
jeff@hoefflin.com
Chapter 9

Lloyd A. Hoffman, MD
Associate Clinical Professor of Surgery (Plastic Surgery)
New York-Presbyterian Hospital/Weill Cornell Medical Center
Deepdale50@aol.com
Chapter 13

John G. Hunter, MD, MMM, FACS
Assistant Clinical Professor of Surgery (Plastic Surgery)
New York-Presbyterian Hospital/Weill Cornell Medical Center
jghmd@aol.com
Chapter 19

Tara L. Huston, MD
Plastic Surgery Resident
New York-Presbyterian Hospital
Taa9002@nyp.org
Chapter 2

Joshua B. Hyman, MD
Assitant Professor of Surgery (Plastic Surgery)
Weill Medical College of Cornell University
joshuahyman@hotmail.com
Chapters 1, 18

Gerald Imber, MD
Assistant Clinical Professor of Surgery (Plastic Surgery)
New York-Presbyterian Hospital/Weill Cornell Medical Center
drimber@aol.com
Chapters 7, 8

Mehul Kamdar, MD
Plastic Surgery Resident
New York-Presbyterian Hospital
mrk34@columbia.edu
Chapter 8

Peter Korn, MD
Plastic Surgery Resident
New York-Presbyterian Hospital
pkornmd@gmail.com
Chapter 14

Anthony N. LaBruna, MD, FACS
Associate Professor of Surgery (Plastic Surgery)
Associate Professor of Otolaryngology
New York-Presbyterian Hospital/Weill Cornell Medical Center
alabruna@aol.com
Chapter 11

Gregory S. LaTrenta, MD, FACS
Associate Clinical Professor of Surgery (Plastic Surgery)
New York-Presbyterian Hospital/Weill Cornell Medical Center
glatrenta@aol.com
Chapter 7, 10

Ferdinand Ofodile, MD
Clinical Professor of Surgery
College of Physician and Surgeons, Columbia University
Division Chief, Plastic Surgery
Harlem Hospital Center
fao1@columbia.edu
Chapter 12

Juliet C. Park, MD
Plastic Surgery Resident
New York-Presbyterian Hospital
jcp7@columbia.edu
Chapter 12

Beth Aviva Preminger, MD, MPH
Plastic Surgery Resident
New York-Presbyterian Hospital
aviva_beth@yahoo.com
Chapter 1

P. Pravin Reddy, MD
pravinreddymd@gmail.com
Chapter 7

Lawrence S. Reed, MD
Assistant Clinical Professor of Surgery (Plastic Surgery)
New York-Presbyterian Hospital/Weill Cornell Medical Center
lreed@the-reed-center.com
Chapters 3, 4, 5, 18

Christine Rohde, MD
Assistant Professor of Surgery
New York-Presbyterian Hospital/Columbia University Medical Center
crohde@gmail.com
Chapter 14

Kenneth O. Rothaus, MD
Associate Clinical Professor of Surgery (Plastic Surgery)
New York-Presbyterian Hospital/Weil Cornell Medical Center
kor@rothausmd.com
Chapter 6

Tal T. Roudner, MD
Plastic Surgery Resident
New York-Presbyterian Hospital
troudnermd@comcast.net
Chapters 13, 15

Mark Schwartz, MD
Assistant Clinical Professor of Surgery (Plastic Surgery)
New York-Presbyterian Hospital/Weill Cornell Medical Center
mhs33@aol.com
Chapter 16

John E. Sherman, MD, FACS
Assistant Clinical Professor of Surgery (Plastic Surgery)
New York-Presbyterian Hospital/Weill Cornell Medical Center
jesmd@nyplasticsurg.com
Chapter 17

Robert C. Silich, MD, FACS
Assistant Clinical Professor of Surgery (Plastic Surgery)
New York-Presbyterian Hospital/Weill Cornell Medical Center
rsilichmd@aol.com
Chapters 7, 8

Jason A. Spector, MD
Assistant Professor of Surgery (Plastic Surgery)
New York-Presbyterian Hospital/Weill Cornell Medical Center
jas2037@med.cornell.edu
Chapter 15

Henry M. Spinelli, MD
Clinical Professor of Surgery (Plastic Surgery)
New York-Presbyterian Hospital/Weill Cornell Medical Center
hmspinelli@aol.com
Chapter 9

Mia Talmor, MD
Associate Clinical Professor of Surgery (Plastic Surgery)
New York-Presbyterian Hospital/Weill Cornell Medical Center
MiaTMD@aol.com
Chapter 5

Nicholas Vendemia, MD
Plastic Surgery Resident
New York-Presbyterian Hospital
nicholas.vendemia@mac.com
Chapter 13

PREFACE

According to the American Society of Aesthetic Plastic Surgery (ASAPS), almost 10 million cosmetic surgical and nonsurgical procedures were performed in the United States in 2009. The tremendous interest in life-enhancing procedures has continued as technological advancements make cosmetic surgery safer and more affordable than ever before. More and more people are putting a high priority on their appearance, and are willing to make an investment to improve their quality of life. The purpose of this textbook is to teach clinicians how to perform the latest and most sought-after surgical and nonsurgical procedures in cosmetic surgery.

Cosmetic Surgery features a consistent, step-by-step approach to facilitate learning of common cosmetic surgical procedures. There are 600 full-color illustrations and photos to clarify each technique, and many diagrams have been created specifically for this volume. Each chapter covers patient selection and preparation, surgical technique, complications, and outcomes assessments. Key references are also provided. Topics addressed include facial surgeries such as facelift, browlift, blepharoplasty, otoplasty, rhinoplasty, and chin implants; breast surgery and body contouring; and nonsurgical procedures such as Botox, injectable fillers, chemical peels, dermabrasion, and laser surgery.

A unique feature of this book is that virtually all of the authors have a current or previous affiliation with the Division of Plastic and Reconstructive Surgery at New York-Presbyterian Hospital either at Columbia University Medical Center or Weill Cornell Medical Center. Importantly, it has been possible for the editors to work closely with all the authors to assure uniformity of presentation as well as clarity and relevance. As a result, the chapters are comprehensive and have been written by some of the leading plastic surgeons in the country. The intended audience for this textbook includes plastic surgeons, otolaryngologists, dermatologists, and other clinicians at various stages of training, all of whom can derive benefit from the easily accessible, up-to-date information that this book offers on diagnosis and treatment in cosmetic plastic surgery.

Robert T. Grant, MD, MSc, FACS
Constance M. Chen, MD, MPH

INTRODUCTION

Public Perceptions & the Business of Cosmetic Surgery

Beth Aviva Preminger, MD, MPH & Robert T. Grant, MD, MSc, FACS

The Sneetches,[1] one of the many stories written by Dr. Seuss, is a tale of two groups of Dr. Seuss characters who populate the beaches—the Plain-bellied Sneetches and the Star-bellied Sneetches. The Star-bellied Sneetches have stars on their bellies and though they are only little stars, they think these stars make all the difference. Compared with the Plain-bellied Sneetches, the Star-bellied Sneetches are sure that they are the best of the Sneetches. As they strut and stroll on the beaches with their noses in the air, they ignore the Sneetches with the plain bellies.

The Plain-bellied Sneetches are sullen and sad. They can not help but brood over the absence of stars on their bellies as they look with envy at the bellies of the Star-bellied Sneetches—until the arrival of Sylvester McMonkey McBean.

When Sylvester McMonkey McBean arrives on the scene, he announces that he has a remedy for the unhappiness of the Plain-bellied Sneetches. Although this remedy is not free, it is guaranteed. He knows what to do to solve their problem and make them content.

In this children's story, Dr. Seuss simplistically captures what is, in essence, the relationship between the cosmetic surgeon and the cosmetic surgery patient. The Sneetches, dissatisfied with their appearances, are consumers of aesthetic change; Mr. McMonkey McBean has the tools to alter their appearances. He offers his services at a price.

Clearly, the appeal of cosmetic surgery is not new. It is linked to an underlying desire to appear beautiful. From a very early age, even children notice physical differences in appearance. We begin to grapple with ideas of beauty, ugliness, and difference in tales such as "The Star Bellied Sneetches," and "The Ugly Duckling." Eventually, however, what begins as merely an awareness of difference often escalates into mocking, causing the subject of derision significant emotional discomfort.

Unfortunately, these feelings may carry well into adulthood. Plato wrote, "The three wishes of every man: to be healthy, to be rich by honest means, and to be beautiful." Even some of the most respected historical figures have lamented their appearances. When Eleanor Roosevelt was asked if she had any regrets, she responded that she wished she had been prettier.[2] President Andrew Jackson suffered throughout his life from permanent facial scarring inflicted by a British soldier. He must have been self-conscious of this deformity because he is always featured with his head turned askance in portraits and renderings. Aware of the importance of one's perception of one's own beauty, Leo Tolstoy wrote, "Nothing has such a striking impact on a man's development as his appearance, and not so much his actual appearance as a conviction that it is either attractive or unattractive."[3]

Amazingly, this physical attractiveness phenomenon impacts every individual, regardless of race, ethnicity, class, or nationality. While definitions of beauty may vary, each society possesses its own beauty canon; hence, the international appeal of cosmetic surgery. In the United States, people spend millions of dollars each year on tanning creams, while people in the Far East buy skin-whitening products. In some regions of the world, buttock augmentation is common, while in other regions, women seek liposuction to reduce these areas.

The appeal of cosmetic surgery can be linked to a century-old desire to be beautiful. In the Old Testament, Jacob was so taken with Rachel's looks that he was willing to be a servant of her household for 7 years in order to have her as his wife. The Greeks were clearly obsessed with ideas of beauty; Helen of Troy's pulchritude "launched a thousand ships, and burnt the topless towers of Ilium." In 1715, riots broke out in France when the use of flour on the hair of aristocrats led to a food shortage that was ended only by the French Revolution. Today, in Brazil, there are more Avon ladies than members of the army, and, in the United States, more money is spent on beauty than on education and social services.[4]

The size of this beauty premium is also economically significant and comparable to the race and gender gaps in the U.S. labor market. Workers of above-average beauty earn 10% to 15% more than workers of below-average beauty. Economists even performed an experiment to uncover the root causes of this so-called beauty premium. They found that employers tend to assume that more beautiful people will be more productive employees.[5] This was linked to an underlying feeling that more attractive individuals are likely to be more self-confident and better communicators.

Cosmetic procedures are no longer reserved only for movie stars and society's elite but have been marketed to consumers by television programs, such as *Extreme Makeover*, *Dr. 90210*, and *The Swan*. In an effort to facilitate payment for cosmetic procedures, some financial firms have even begun to offer several options for financing cosmetic procedures.[6] Most recently, a Lebanese bank began offering a new line of loans for people who want cosmetic improvements. Clients can borrow up to $5000 to cover plastic surgery, orthodontic procedures, and other nips and tucks. So far, the bank has received more than 200 phone calls a day about the loan.[7]

A growing number of Americans seek cosmetic procedures. According to the American Society of Plastic Surgeons, Americans spent $10.3 billion on cosmetic procedures in 2008. Some 12.1 million surgical and nonsurgical cosmetic procedures were performed, including 245,138 liposuctions, 279,218 rhinoplasties, 307,230 breast augmentations, and 221,398 eyelid procedures. Approximately 5 million injections of Botox were administered.[8] The American Society for Aesthetic Plastic Surgery points to an almost 400% increase in the total number of cosmetic procedures since 1997. Most of these patients were between the ages of 35 and 50.[9]

The cosmetic surgery market has been shown to follow standard laws of economics.[10] This results from the fact that consumers pay for cosmetic surgery directly, without interference from third party payers. Because buyers are price-sensitive and willing to shop around, they have bargaining power over cosmetic surgeons. Appealing substitutes exist in the form of alternative procedures that are often offered by competing specialties, and plastic surgeons face an ever-increasing entrance of cosmetologists into the workforce. To compete in this market, plastic surgeons have struggled to distinguish themselves.[11] A recent *New York Times* article entitled, "More doctors turning to the business of beauty," described these trends. One dermatologist remarked, "Everyone wants to be a plasticologist." An obstetrician-gynecologist wanting to enter this market added, "I know core physicians don't want noncore physicians like me in it, but dermatologists and plastic surgeons can't own aesthetic medicine by themselves."[12] Economic theory predicts that increasing the supply of cosmetic surgeons results in lower fees for services.

Conflict and contradiction about physical attractiveness and the decision to actively pursue such attractiveness through surgery persists. Many express disapproval or even disdain for those who take innovative steps to achieve greater physical attractiveness. Undeniably, however, more and more people are seeking cosmetic procedures. Nevertheless, cosmetic surgery remains "a most unusual medical practice." This is largely due to the fact that, unlike other surgeons, cosmetic surgeons have the privilege of operating on people who are largely "normal." Certain bioethicists have even accused cosmetic surgeons of threatening the professional integrity of medicine.[13]

In this context, cosmetic surgeons must continuously determine the limits of which cosmetic procedures they consider acceptable and what constitutes a breach of professional norms. Mr. McMonkey McBean faced no such dilemma. He continued to place and remove stars on the Sneetches. "Then, when every last cent of their money was spent, the Fix-It-Up-Chappie packed up and he went."[1] Education is what distinguishes plastic surgeons from so called "beauty quacks." It allows plastic surgeons not merely to cater to market demands but to rise above and perform ethically. It is our hope that this book will contribute to this effort.

REFERENCES

1. Dr. Seuss. *The Sneetches and Other Stories*. New York: Random House, Inc.; 1961.
2. Steinem G. *Revolution from Within, A Book of Self Esteem*. Boston: Little Brown; 1992:216.
3. Tolstoy L. *Childhood, Boyhood, Youth*. Scammel M, trans. New York: McGraw-Hill; 1964:145.
4. Etcoff N. *Survival of the Prettiest: The Science of Beauty*. New York: Anchor Books; 1999:6.
5. Mobius MM, Rosenblat TS. Why beauty matters. *American Economic Review*. March 2006.
6. Knight V. Facing costs of plastic surgery. *The Wall Street Journal*. March 7, 2007:B3H.
7. Plastic surgery loans a hit for Lebanese bank. *National Public Radio*. April 23, 2007.
8. American Society of Plastic Surgeons. Web site available at: http://www.plasticsurgery.org/media/stats/2008-US-cosmetic-reconstructive-plastic-surgery-minimally-invasive-statistics.pdf. Accessed June 1, 2009.
9. The American Society for Aesthetic Plastic Surgery. Web site available at: http://www.surgery.org/download/2008stats.pdf. Accessed June 1, 2009.
10. Krieger LM et al. Aesthetic surgery economics: lessons from corporate boardrooms to plastic surgery practices. *Plast Reconstr Surg*. 2000 Mar;105(3):1205–10. [PMID: 10724282]
11. Krieger LM. Discount cosmetic surgery: Industry trends and strategies for success. *Plast Reconstr Surg*. 2002 Aug;110(2):614–9. [PMID: 12142686]
12. Singer N. More doctors turning to the business of beauty. *New York Times*. November 20, 2006:A1.
13. Miller FG et al. Cosmetic surgery and the internal morality of medicine. *Camb Q Healthc Ethics*. 2000 Summer;9:353–64. [PMID: 10858884]

CHAPTER 1

Evaluation of the Patient for Cosmetic Surgery

Joshua B. Hyman, MD & Robert T. Grant, MD, MSc, FACS

PATIENT SELECTION

Patient selection in cosmetic surgery is a difficult and arduous task that is unique to the specialty. Because the patient is electing to have surgery, surgeons have the luxury of refusing to participate in the patient's care if he or she is not an appropriate candidate for cosmetic surgery. Although some patients may not realize, the surgeon ultimately selects the patient and not vice versa. Plastic surgeons have often tried to categorize patient characteristics preoperatively that could help predict behavior postoperatively, which is a difficult if not impossible task. Perhaps some day a battery of behavior examinations will accurately define a patient's personality so that surgeons can more objectively and definitively determine which patients will be pleased with the results of cosmetic surgery and which patients have unrealistic expectations. For now, however, good communication is the best method.

The patient's dissatisfaction with his or her physical appearance may range from a healthy self-concern to a preoccupation with one's appearance that impairs daily functioning. **Body dysmorphic disorder** is defined as a preoccupation with an imagined or slight defect in appearance that leads to markedly excessive concern. This disorder was initially called dysmorphophobia when it first appeared in the European medical literature in 1886. In other early descriptions, body dysmorphic disorder was termed "l'obsession de la honte du corps" (obsession with shame of the body) or dysmorphophobic syndrome. Body dysmorphic disorder is the only diagnostic category directly addressing body image concerns in the *Diagnostic and Statistical Manual of Mental Disorders* (*DSM-IV*). The preoccupation must cause significant distress or impairment in social, occupational, or other areas of functioning. Although any area of the body may be the focus, the most common areas seem to be the skin, face, and nose. Men may become preoccupied with their genitals, height, hair, and body build, whereas women typically report concerns with their weight, hips, legs, and breasts. Body dysmorphic disorder appears to affect men and women with equal frequency. Patients with body dysmorphic disorder may report preoccupation with five to seven body parts over the course of the disease. Following are some questions to ask the patient in the preoperative visit:

- Do you worry about the appearance of your face or body?
- If so, what is your concern? How bad do you think your face or body part appears?
- How much time do you spend worrying about the appearance of your face or body part?
- Have you done anything to hide the problem or rid yourself of the problem?
- Does this concern with your appearance affect any aspect of your life (eg, school, job, or social life)?

THE INITIAL PHONE CALL

The cosmetic surgery consultation often begins with a telephone call or e-mail. This contact leaves a lasting impression on both the patient and surgeon. Proper telephone etiquette is important for both parties involved. The office receptionist is often the first person in contact with the patient, and this person needs to be instructed on how much or little involvement they should have with the patient. At a minimum, the receptionist should inform the patient of available times for appointments, consultation fees, and the various procedures the surgeon performs. It is disheartening for the patient to hear such template responses as the surgeon is booked for the next 3 months or he or she specializes in all aspects of cosmetic surgery. Although the surgeon cannot always accommodate every convenient appointment time for the patient, the surgeon should try to see the patient within a reasonable time frame. The receptionist should also be aware of the surgeon's credentials, hospital affiliations, as well as specialties within cosmetic surgery. It is usually not appropriate for the receptionist to give prospective patients surgical fees and clinical information.

The scheduler should obtain some basic patient information such as the caller's name, address, and contact information as well as the reason for the consultation. It is also helpful to find out who referred the patient so that the person can be contacted ahead of the consultation if needed.

Some cosmetic surgery practices may want to send the patient an information package prior to the appointment with information about the office and surgeon, maps and directions, and local hotels (if the patient is from out of town). Information about the operating room and its accreditation (ie, The Joint Commission on the Accreditation of Healthcare Organization [JCAHO] or American Association for Accreditation of Ambulatory Surgery Facilities [AAAASF]) may also be included.

A patient who is uncooperative, abusive, or rude to the receptionist will often prove difficult to communicate with effectively. Another red flag that may indicate patients have unrealistic expectations about their treatment course is applying extraordinary pressure to get an early appointment or to be seen at inconvenient times. In some instances, a patient will call the office and declare themselves "VIPs." In addition, some patients refuse to give any basic information to the receptionist, which can also be seen as an early sign of incompliance.

THE CONSULTATION

Upon arrival, the patient should be greeted by the receptionist in a warm, friendly manner. The necessary forms, which include the hospital intake form (Figure 1–1) as well as privacy statements, should be given to the patient.

The Health Insurance Portability and Accountability Act (HIPAA) of 1996 mandates

PERSONAL/FAMILY MEDICAL HISTORY AND EVALUATION

(Please fill out completely; a staff member can help with any questions you may be uncertain about.)

PATIENT NAME:________________________ Date________________________

Age______ Sex: M___ / F_____

HABITS:

1. Are you a smoker? If so, please tell us how much and for how long. If you have recently quit, please tell us how long ago:________________________
2. Are you a regular coffee, tea or caffeinated soda drinker?: Yes or No (circle one)
3. Do you consume alcohol on a regular or social basis? Yes or No (circle one)
4. Do you exercise regularly? Yes or No (circle one)

PHYSICIANS REGULARLY SEEN: If you are presently under the care of any type of doctor- whether an internist, primary care physician or specialist- for a current, chronic or long term medical condition, please list the doctors' names, phone numbers and area of expertise. If you do not have an internist or primary care physician, please indicate that.
(Please note: we will not contact any physician **without** your expressed permission.)

DOCTOR	PHONE NUMBER	SPECIALTY	DATE LAST SEEN

ALLERGIES AND SENSITIVITIES: Is there a history of skin or any other untoward reaction or sickness following injection, oral administration or exposure to any of the following?
If you answer yes, please the explain nature of reaction/sickness

	Circle one		Explanation
A. Penicillin or other antibiotics	yes	no	
B. Morphine, codeine, Demerol or other narcotics	yes	no	
C. Novocaine or other local anesthetics	yes	no	
D. Sodium Pentothal or other anesthetics	yes	no	
E. Sulfa drugs	yes	no	
F. Tetanus antitoxin or other serums	yes	no	
G. Adhesive tape	yes	no	
H. Iodine or Merthiolate, Phisohex or other antiseptics	yes	no	
I. Any other drug or medication	yes	no	
J. Any foods such as eggs, milk, or chocolate	yes	no	
K. Do you have a latex allergy?	yes	no	
L. Do you have a surgical tape allergy?	yes	no	
M. Any reactions to puffers or inhalers	yes	no	

DRUGS RECENTLY TAKEN: Please inform us of any of the following drugs you have taken within the past six months (unless another time frame is specified)

A. Cortisone/steroids (taken within the past 2 years)	yes	no	
B. Antidepressants (including MAO inhibitors)	yes	no	
C. Anticoagulants (blood thinners)	yes	no	
D. Tranquilizers	yes	no	
E. Hypotensives (high blood pressure medication)	yes	no	
F. Cardiac drugs (Pronestyl, digitalis, etc.)	yes	no	

Figure 1–1. Hospital intake form. (Reproduced, with permission, from Davison SP et al. Prevention of venous thromboembolism in the plastic surgery patient. *Plast Reconstr Surg.* 2004 Sep1;114(3):43E–51E.)

MEDICAL HISTORY AND EVALUATION

DRUGS RECENTLY TAKEN(cont'd from previous page)

G. Inderal yes no ____________________
H. Accutane(within the past year) yes no ____________________
I. Diuretics (water pills) yes no ____________________
J. Anti-diabetic drugs yes no ____________________
K. Any other prescribed or non-prescribed medications(if none, please write none)
____

L. Any homeopathic, herbal or vitamin preparations(if none, please write none)
____

In the following space, please provide a complete list of all drugs/preparations/medications which you **currently** take, including those listed above. This list is helpful in avoiding possible cross-drug reactions:____
____
____
____
____

DETAILED MEDICAL HISTORY: Do you or a family member have a history of:

	Circle one	Who/What
1. Diabetes(high blood sugar)	yes no	____________
2. High blood pressure	yes no	____________
3. Low blood sugar	yes no	____________
4. Heart disease(if mitral valve prolapse, please specify)	yes no	____________
5. Rheumatic heart disease	yes no	____________
6. Heart pacemaker	yes no	____________
7. Lung disease	yes no	____________
8. Kidney disease	yes no	____________
9. Pulmonary embolus	yes no	____________
10. Neurological disorders	yes no	____________
11. Thyroid, pancreatic or other endocrine disorders such as hypoglycemia(low blood sugar)	yes no	____________
12. Phlebitis	yes no	____________
13. Migraine headaches	yes no	____________
14. Abnormal bleeding	yes no	____________
15. Anormal clotting	yes no	____________
16. Anesthetic problems	yes no	____________
17. Cancer(including skin cancer)	yes no	____________
18. Coronary surgery	yes no	____________
19. Tuberculosis	yes no	____________
20. Other serious illnesse	yes no	____________
21. Mitral valve prolapse	yes no	____________
22. Anemia	yes no	____________
23. Atrial fibrillation	yes no	____________
24. Asthma	yes no	____________
25. Hepatitis	yes no	____________
26. Prostate disorders	yes no	____________
27. Acid regurgitation(heartburn)	yes no	____________
28. Angina	yes no	____________
29. Rheumatic fever	yes no	____________
30. Emphysema	yes no	____________

Figure 1–1. (Continued)

MEDICAL HISTORY AND EVALUATION

ADDITIONAL PERSONAL INFORMATION:

1. Any weight change past 12 months? yes no ______
2. Stomach problems yes no ______
3. Ulcers yes no ______
4. Urination problems yes no ______
5. Other serious illness or medical problem yes no ______
6. Any previous surgery yes no ______
7. Ever received a blood transfusion (if yes: what year) yes no ______
8. Do you use contact lenses yes no ______
9. Do you wear glasses yes no ______
10. Do you use dentures yes no ______
11. Do you use a hearing aid yes no ______
12. Do you form keloids? yes no ______
13. Do you form thick, red or raised scars? yes no ______
14. Do you have any thick, red, raised keloidal scars on your body? yes no ______
15. Have you ever undergone scar revisions or treatment for improving scarring? yes no ______

Female patients:

16. number of pregnancies: ______ number of children:______
    did you breast feed: yes:______ no:______
    last menstrual period:______

BLEEDING PROFILE:

1. Do you have any problems with bleeding
   - in general yes no ______
   - after a razor cut yes no ______
   - after a tooth extraction yes no ______
   - after a previous surgery yes no ______
   - after a delivery yes no ______
2. Do you bruise easily or remain bruised for long periods of time yes no ______
3. Have you ever received blood transfusions or blood products (plasma, platelets, etc.) yes no ______
4. Is there a family history of bleeding problems yes no ______
5. Do you use aspirin regularly yes no ______
6. NSAIDs such as Advil, Motrin, Ibuprofen Aleve, Naproxen etc. yes no ______
7. Do you take Vitamin E yes no ______
8. Do you take blood thinners yes no ______

Please indicate whether or not you regularly use the following drugs which contain aspirin:

Darvon	yes:__	no:____	Empirin	yes:__	no:____
Midol	yes:__	no:____	Alka Seltzer	yes:__	no:____
Percodan	yes:__	no:____	Alka Seltzer Plus	yes:__	no:____
Fluorinal	yes:__	no:____	Coricidin	yes:__	no:____
Bufferin	yes:__	no:____	Excedrin	yes:__	no:____
Ascriptin	yes:__	no:____			

Figure 1–1. (Continued)

MEDICAL HISTORY AND EVALUATION

BLEEDING PROFILE (cont'd from previous page)
Please see separate accompanying list of drugs and foods known to cause bleeding and list any you take regularly. Also please list any other foods or drugs you feel make you bruise easily:

____

____

Please list any other medical problem(s) not included above:

____

____

PREVIOUS PERSONAL AND FAMILY SURGICAL HISTORY

1. Have you had previous surgery?______________________________

____

2. If so, please indicate the type(s) of anesthesia used as well as any **complications** or **reactions** you experienced.
   - Local anesthesia______________________________
   - General anesthesia______________________________
   - Spinal/epidural______________________________
   - Sedation______________________________
   - Twilight sleep______________________________
3. Have there been unexpected deaths or complications from anesthesia (including in the dental office) in any members of your family?______________________________

____

____

4. Is there a personal or family history of unexplained high fevers (known as malignant hyperthermia) following drug administration or general anesthesia?______________________________

____

5. Is there a personal or family history of unexplained high fever following surgery?

____

6. Is there a personal or family history of dark or cola-colored urine following anesthesia?______________________________
7. Is there a personal or family history of masseter muscle rigidity (MMR)? This is a severe, sustained contracture of the jawbone muscle.______________________________

____

8. Do you have a personal or family history of the following:
   - a) scoliosis or kyphosis (hunched back)______________________________
   - b) muscle disorder______________________________
   - c) spontaneous muscle cramps______________________________
   - d) squint______________________________
   - e) any other problems with muscle function______________________________

____

Please **sign** your name and indicate the date on the line below:

______________________________ name ______________ date

Figure 1–1. (Continued)

significant changes in the legal and regulatory environments governing the provision of health benefits, the delivery and payment of healthcare services, and the security and confidentiality of individually identifiable, protected health information.

HIPAA makes it easier for individuals and small businesses to get and keep health insurance. To reduce the cost of health insurance, HIPAA also includes an administrative simplification section to encourage electronic transactions. Due to the electronic transactions, HIPAA also has a host of new regulations to ensure the security and privacy of electronically stored medical data. The regulations set standards for electronic transactions, the privacy of all medical records and all identifiable health information, and the security of electronically stored information.

To be compliant, the surgeon's practice must implement procedures to provide patients access to their medical information including providing copies at their request, an ability to make amendments to their records, and accountings of any and all disclosures made of their medical information for any use other than treatment, payment, and firm operations.

To be compliant with HIPAA regulations, sign-in lists where patients can see other patients' names should be avoided. Also, the receptionist should sit in an enclosed space. The receptionist or nurse should avoid announcing the patients name loudly in the waiting room or elsewhere. The reason for the consultation should also never be announced or spoken loud enough for other patients to hear.

A cosmetic surgery practice must notify each patient of these rights with a "Notice of Privacy Practices" (Figure 1–2). This notice must include the patient's rights, the practice's HIPAA policies, and the address of where to complain.

Fines, penalties, and possible jail time can be imposed for noncompliance. The office intake form should be accompanied by the form shown in Figure 1–2.

A. Discussion of Expectations

Before proceeding with any cosmetic surgical procedure, it is absolutely necessary to completely evaluate the patient not only physically, but also psychologically. In other words, cosmetic surgery is a unique form of surgery that requires the surgeon to explore the patient's psychological status to help determine whether the patient is a good candidate for the particular procedure. Günter and Gorney have both written about identifying "danger signs" that may be exhibited by certain cosmetic surgery patients and recommended that these patients be approached

RECEIPT OF NOTICE OF PRIVACY PRACTICES

I ______________________________ have been given the opportunity to read and keep a copy of ________________________ center's Notice of Privacy Practices.

________________________ ________________

Patient Signature *Date*

Figure 1–2. Patients must acknowledge receipt of HIPAA policies, which include HIPAA regulations, explanation of patient's rights, and the address of where to complain.

with caution. Günter identified the following 13 danger signs that may signify underlying psychological issues:

1. Minimal disfigurement.
2. Delusional distortion of body image.
3. Problems of sexual ambivalence.
4. Confused motives for wanting surgery.
5. Unrealistic expectations of change in life situation as a result of surgery.
6. History of poorly established social and emotional relationships.
7. Unresolved grief or current crisis situation.
8. Present misfortunes blamed on physical appearance.
9. Older neurotic man who is overly concerned with aging.
10. Sudden dislike for one's anatomy, especially in an older man.
11. A hostile, blaming attitude toward authority figures.
12. A history of seeing physicians and being dissatisfied with them.
13. Indication of paranoid thoughts.

Gorney described systems to help identify potential problem patients. The patient may be described using the acronym SIMON (**s**ingle **i**mmature **m**ales **o**verly expectant, **n**arcissistic).

In addition to the above characteristics, other behaviors that may indicate the patient has unrealistic expectations include bringing in magazine photos of Brad Pitt or Angelina Jolie, obtaining multiple opinions (excessive shopping around), and starting the consultation by asking the cost of the procedure without allowing for an opening dialog; these patients are not good candidates for surgery and will likely be poorly compliant.

Patients who choose to tell the surgeon about a friend who had a similar procedure and was "maimed" or "butchered" by the plastic surgeon are usually difficult to treat. It is acceptable for a patient to want to discuss complications if done appropriately. Surgeons need to remember that they are selecting the patients who are candidates for surgery.

B. Physical Examination

The patient should change into a gown to expose the areas that need to be examined. Robes that make the patient feel more like he or she is at a spa than a medical office are preferable. Do not make patients wait in examination rooms. If the physician is delayed, the patient should be informed of the delay and given the opportunity to reschedule prior to being corralled in an examination room. If the patient cannot wait for the surgeon, then reschedule a free consultation as a good will gesture. If a medical student, resident, or fellow is going to evaluate the patient with the surgeon, it is prudent to ask the patient's permission.

If the patient is going to have surgery, a detailed physical examination is needed. The patient should be evaluated in a private clinical examination room. The surgeon should only expose those areas of the body that are the focus of the procedure. Avoid exposing areas of the body that are not pertinent to the examination in efforts to avoid making the patient feel vulnerable or uncomfortable. The surgeon should always have an assistant in the room during examinations for medical-legal considerations. Patients with any chronic medical conditions should be examined and cleared by their internist prior to the cosmetic procedure.

PREOPERATIVE LABORATORY TESTS

Internists are generally asked to assess preoperative risk in most patients who are to undergo cosmetic surgery. Despite a low risk of perioperative complications, the use of laboratory tests before surgery has become ingrained in clinical practice in the United States. Clinicians think it reasonable to order tests to detect abnormalities that might lead to increased morbidity or mortality in the perioperative period. Routine laboratory tests are often necessary at most ambulatory surgery centers and hospitals despite the fact they are neither helpful nor cost-effective.

If the laboratory test results were normal within the 4 months prior to surgery and if no change in the patient's clinical status has occurred, there should be no need to repeat these tests. Finally, this strategy applies only to healthy, asymptomatic patients undergoing elective surgery. Patients with suspected pulmonary or cardiac disease or those undergoing urgent operation require additional evaluation that is beyond the scope of this section.

A. CBC Count

Most guidelines recommend preoperative hemoglobin testing if the history is suggestive of underlying anemia or if a significant blood loss is anticipated during the operation.

B. Electrolytes

Electrolyte determination is not routinely recommended for elective surgery in healthy individuals. Unanticipated electrolyte abnormality (sodium, potassium, bicarbonate, chloride) ranges from 0.2% to 8.0% among surgery patients. A recent, systemic literature review reported that unsuspected electrolyte abnormality is 1.4% among healthy elective surgery patients. Although hypokalemia is considered a minor risk factor for perioperative cardiac complications based on the Goldman risk index, no study has shown a relation between hypokalemia and perioperative morbidity and mortality.

C. Creatinine

Testing kidney function with serum creatinine level is recommended for all patients older than 40 years, especially if hypotension or use of nephrotoxic medications is anticipated.

The prevalence of elevated creatinine levels in asymptomatic patients ranges from 0.2% to 2.4% and increases with age. Approximately 9.8% of patients aged between 46 to 60 years have elevated creatinine levels.

Patients with mild-to-moderate renal insufficiency are usually asymptomatic but have an increased risk of perioperative morbidity and mortality.

D. Blood Sugar

Only in certain operations, such as vascular surgery and coronary artery bypass grafting, is diabetes associated with higher perioperative risks; hence, routine blood sugar determination is not recommended unless the patient is at high risk for diabetes (eg, obesity, strong family history, and use of corticosteroids) or will be undergoing vascular or bypass surgery.

The frequency of abnormal glucose laboratory results in asymptomatic patients ranges from 1.8% to 5.5%. The frequency increases with age, so that nearly 25% of patients older than 60 years have a fasting blood sugar level above 120 mg/dL.

E. Liver Enzymes

Routine preoperative screening is not recommended for healthy individuals. The frequency of a hepatic aminotransferase enzyme (aspartate aminotransferase [AST], alanine aminotransferase [ALT]) abnormality is estimated to be approximately 0.3%. Although Powell-Jackson and colleagues showed that severe liver test abnormalities may lead to an increase in surgical morbidity and mortality risk, no evidence confirms that mild elevation in liver enzymes is associated with such an increased risk.

F. Hemostasis

Prothrombin time (PT), activated partial thromboplastin time (aPTT), and bleeding time are not recommended for routine screening.

In the absence of a history of bleeding diathesis in elective surgery patients, abnormal bleeding time, PT, and aPTT results are estimated to be less than 1%.

aPTT does not predict the risk of perioperative bleeding. Similarly, the bleeding time has no predictive value on the incidence of perioperative bleeding in healthy elective surgery patients.

G. Urinalysis

The primary rationale for ordering urinalysis preoperatively is to detect either asymptomatic kidney disease or underlying urinary tract infection (UTI). To detect unsuspected kidney disease, serum creatinine measurement is recommended for any elective surgery patient older than 40 years, although it is unclear if any correlation exists between asymptomatic UTI and surgical wound infection.

One study that included 200 patients undergoing orthopedic procedures showed that physicians addressed only 5 of 27 abnormal urine test results. A further economic analysis showed that in order to prevent a single wound infection, approximately $1.5 million must be spent on urinalysis; therefore, urinalysis is not recommended routinely for asymptomatic patients.

H. Fecal Occult Blood

Insufficient evidence exists to support routine screening for fecal occult blood.

The prevalence of positive fecal occult blood findings among healthy individuals undergoing elective surgery is unknown. In addition, the benefits of routine screening are unclear.

I. Pregnancy Testing

Testing to rule out pregnancy should be done in any premenopausal female for whom there is a suspicion or possibility of pregnancy. If this test is done, it should be performed within 24 hours of surgery (the morning of surgery is recommended).

J. ECG

Routine ECG is recommended for all patients older than 40 years undergoing elective surgery. The prevalence of abnormal ECG findings among healthy elective surgery patients ranges from 14% to 53% and increases with age in a continuous fashion.

The rationale for obtaining ECG preoperatively is to identify high-risk patients with prior myocardial infarction or arrhythmia.

K. Chest Radiograph

Chest radiography should be done routinely in patients older than 60 years. The frequency of abnormal chest radiograph findings increases with age.

ROLE OF PREOPERATIVE MAMMOGRAPHY

Mammography is a sensitive, noninvasive diagnostic and screening modality that is used to supplement breast self-examination and clinician examination. Large, prospective clinical trials have demonstrated its capability to reduce the mortality of breast cancer. Mammography has the ability to detect approximately 85% to 90% of breast cancers when properly utilized. The use of mammography routinely in cosmetic breast surgery patients is somewhat controversial due to the young age of most of the patients in this group. The routine use of a baseline preoperative mammography in women aged 30 years and older undergoing aesthetic breast surgery as well as a routine postoperative follow-up that includes annual clinical examinations is a safe recommendation.

Some plastic surgeons have proposed that because of the critical importance of the lower abdomen to women considering breast reconstruction, it would seem appropriate to perform preoperative mammography routinely on women considering abdominoplasty, particularly if they are of appropriate age (30–65 years).

AGENTS TO AVOID BEFORE & AFTER SURGERY

Table 1–1 lists the medications that should be avoided before and after surgery. Table 1–2 lists the ointments that should be avoided postoperatively.

▶ TABLE 1–1. MEDICATIONS TO AVOID BEFORE AND AFTER SURGERY

Aspirin and aspirin containing compounds

Alka-seltzer	Florinal
Anacin	Midol
Bo	Percodan
Bufferin	Robaxisal
Cheracol	Sine-aid
Cope	Sine-off
Coricidin	Sinu-tab
Darvon comp.	Stenion
Dristin	Synalgod-dc
Empirin	Triminicin
Excedrin	Vanquish

Anorexant (reacts with adrenaline)
Tenuate dospan

Antispasmodic
Tenuate

Antibiotics
Flagyl
Rysteclin F
Tetracycline
Tobramycin

Anticoagulants
Antihistamines
Ru-tuss

Analgescis (non-narcotic)
Talfon

Zyloprimin (allopurinol)

Non-steriodals, anti-inflammatories
Clinoril
Kutapressin
Indocin
Motrin (Advil, Nuprin)
Naprosyn/Aleve (5 days off)
Tolectin
Tolectin D S
Zomax
Butazoline
Anaprox

Tricyclic antidepressants (reacts with adrenaline)
Elavil
Pamalor
Triavil
Surmontil
Endep
Tofranil

Phenothaizine derivatives
Sparine
Mellaril
Trilafon
Compazine
Stelzine

Additional drugs/vitamins
Persantine (coronary vasodilator)
Vitamin E
Nardil

Herbal remedies

St. John's wort	Kava
Yohimbe	Black kohosh
Ginko Biloba	Valerin
Ginger, garlic, cayenne	Fish oil
Ginseng	
Melatonin	

TABLE 1–2. OINTMENTS TO AVOID BEFORE AND AFTER SURGERY[1]

Topical medications containing salicylate derivatives	
Absorbent rubs	Mentholatum deep heating
Absorbine arthritic	Mineral ice
Absorbine Jr.	Musterole regular
Act-on rub	Musterole childrens strength
Analbalm	Musterole extra
Analgesic balm	Neurabalm
Antiphlogistine	Oil-o-sol
Arthralgen	Omega oil
Aspercreme	Panalgesic
Benaig	Rid-A-Pain
Baumodyne	Rumarub
Ben Gay	Sloan's
Ben Gay extra strength	Soltice Hi-Therm
Ben Gay greaseless/stainless original	Soltice quick rub
Ben Gay original	SPO
Counterpain rub	Stimurub
Doan's rub	Sorin
End-ake rub	Uni-balm
Exocaine plus	Yaker's ointment
Exocaine tube rub heat	Zemo liquid
Icy hot	Zemo liquid extra strength
Infra-rub	Zemo ointment
All MAO inhibitors must be stopped 14 days before surgery	

[1]Please check all other topical ointments, lotions, medications with staff

INFORMED CONSENT

In elective surgery situations, the surgeon has plenty of time and opportunity to discuss the risks, benefits as well as alternatives of the planned procedure. Informed consent has become the most important aspect of any preoperative consultation. Mark Gorney has described six elements of informed consent that fulfill what the law requires:

1. The diagnosis or suspected diagnosis.
2. The nature and purpose of the proposed treatment or procedure and its anticipated benefits.
3. The risks, complications, or side effects.
4. The probability of success, based on the patient's condition.
5. Reasonable available alternatives.
6. The possible consequences if advice is not followed.

REFERENCES

Gorney M. Claims prevention for the aesthetic surgeon: preparing for the less-than-perfect outcome. *Facial Plast Surg.* 2002;18(2):135–42. [PMID: 12063661]

Powell-Jackson P et al. Adverse effects of exploratory laparotomy in patients with unsuspected liver disease. *Br J Surg.* 1982 Aug;69(8):449–51. [PMID: 7104630]

Turnbull JM et al. The value of preoperative screening investigations in otherwise healthy individuals. *Arch Intern Med.* 1987 Jun;147(6):1101–5. [PMID: 3592875]

CHAPTER 2

Patient Safety & Preparation

Tara L. Huston, MD & Kenneth R. Francis, MD

PATIENT EVALUATION & SELECTION

Providing safe care to the patient who is undergoing plastic surgery is traditionally composed of two components: establishing quality of care and preparing the patient for the clinical procedure. This chapter will be separated based on that distinction. Establishing quality of care involves ensuring the safety of the facility, obtaining certification, retaining necessary equipment and personnel, as well as, being able to expeditiously transfer a patient to the next level of care for extended or emergency needs. Preparing the patient for the procedure involves preoperative testing, thorough medical evaluation, prophylactic therapies when indicated, and a comprehensive drug history that includes use of herbal agents and cosmeceuticals. The guidelines provided in this chapter are not rules but suggestions about how to maintain the highest level of patient safety. Only a small number of states have laws governing the practice of plastic surgery. The onus remains on the physician to uphold the Hippocratic oath to maintain patient safety as the first priority.

A. Facility and Procedure Selection

When deciding the location at which surgery can be performed safely, plastic surgeons need to consider the risk factors associated with each patient and each plastic surgery procedure. The American Society of Anesthesiologists (ASA) has developed a classification system to help categorize patients for surgery; it is useful in determining the appropriate facility setting for a cosmetic surgical intervention. This grading system was designed to categorize physiologic status of patients in order to create a uniform system of patient classification. Although not fully predictive of perioperative risk of complication, the classification helps define a level of systemic physiologic disease that may impact surgical morbidity. ASA category 1 defines patients as normal and healthy. ASA category 2 classifies patients as having mild systemic disease with no functional limitations. These two groups of patients are the preferred candidates for ambulatory cosmetic surgery and can safely undergo office-based procedures. Patients in ASA category 3 have moderate systemic disease with functional limitations and are acceptable candidates for local anesthesia with some level of moderate sedation. They may undergo office-based cosmetic surgery in an accredited facility. Patients in ASA category 4 have severe systemic disease that is a constant threat to life; these patients cannot be given anything more potent than local anesthesia in the office-based setting. More complex procedures in this group of patients must be done in a hospital setting.

When considering the number and type of cosmetic procedures to be performed on a patient, procedure morbidity must be assessed. Blood loss, potential for hypothermia, potential for circulatory stasis, and procedure duration may add to the risk of complications. Adding liposuction to other procedures results in prolonging hypothermia and anesthesia time, increasing operative morbidity.

There is significant risk of hypothermia when performing ambulatory surgery. Risk factors include a cold operating room, unclothed patient, intravenous fluids at room temperature, and the impairment of a patient's thermoregulatory system with anesthesia. To combat hypothermia, the operating environment and the patient may be pre-warmed prior to the induction of anesthesia. Intravenous fluids can be warmed, and the patient's exposure should be limited as much as possible. Forced air warming devices should be available. If the above warming devices are not readily available, all procedures should be limited to less than 2 hours and no more than 20% of the body surface area should be exposed at a time.

If it is possible that the intraoperative blood loss could be greater than 7 mL/kg (about 500 mL for a 70-kg patient), then the procedure should be performed in a setting where adequate blood components are immediately available.

The overall duration of an ambulatory procedure should be limited to 6 hours. Longer procedures ending no later than 3 PM allow an adequate postoperative recovery time. Extended procedures are more likely to result in high incidences of postoperative nausea, vomiting, inflammation, and bleeding, all of which may require an overnight stay. Postoperative nausea, vomiting, pain, and dizziness are responsible for up to 10% of unplanned hospital admissions. Increased operative times may result in higher rates of unexpected hospital admission.

Liposuction, especially large volume and when combined with other procedures such as abdominoplasty, can cause serious complications. The mortality rate for isolated liposuction is 0.0021% (1/47,415) but jumps to 0.0137% (1/7314) when coupled with non-abdominoplasty procedures and 0.0305% (1/3281) when combined with abdominoplasty. Regardless of the additional procedures performed, it is unsafe to aspirate more than 5000 mL in total in the ambulatory setting.

B. Preoperative Counseling and Recommendations

During the initial patient visit, a comprehensive history and a targeted physical examination should be obtained (Figure 2–1). The patient's goals and actual needs are determined. The surgeon assesses the likelihood of achieving these goals and needs, and the proposed procedure is discussed with the patient. Risks and complications of the proposed procedures, alternatives to the proposed procedures, expected recovery from the proposed procedures, and a realistic expectation of the results should all be openly discussed in accordance with informed consent. Printed literature, photographs, videos, and image-altering software may be used to aid in the patient education process.

A second consultation can be beneficial to the patient education process and may serve as a preoperative visit approximately 1 week prior to surgery to confirm goals, finalize the

Name: ______________________________ **Date:** ______________

SOCIAL

Age: __________ Sex: M ❑ F ❑ Married: Y ❑ N ❑ Occupation: ______________

Responsible adult available to assist during recovery period: Y ❑ N ❑ Relationship: ______________

HABITS

Smoke: Y ❑ N ❑ Amount: ______________ Coffee/Tea/Cola: Y ❑ N ❑ Amount: ______________

Alcohol: Y ❑ N ❑ Amount: ______________ Daily Exercise: Y ❑ N ❑ Amount: ______________

MEDICATIONS: List dose or number of pills per day

Prescription Drugs

____

____

____

____

Non Prescription (Vitamins; Herbs)

____

____

____

____

Regular Aspirin Use: Y ❑ N ❑ Dosage & frequency: ______________

NSA (Advil, Motrin, Ibuprofen): Y ❑ N ❑ Dosage & frequency: ______________

Cortisone Injections Past Year: Y ❑ N ❑ Date(s) and injection location: ______________

Drug Allergy: Y ❑ N ❑ List drug(s) and type of reaction: ______________

____

Latex Allergy: Y ❑ N ❑ Tape Allergy: Y ❑ N ❑

FAMILY HISTORY: Have any blood relatives every had the following problems:

Abnormal Bleeding: Y ❑ N ❑ Coronary Surgery: Y ❑ N ❑ Kidney Disease Y ❑ N ❑

Abnormal Clotting: Y ❑ N ❑ Diabetes: Y ❑ N ❑ Tuberculosis: Y ❑ N ❑

Anesthetic Problems: Y ❑ N ❑ Heart Attack: Y ❑ N ❑ Other Serious Illness: Y ❑ N ❑

Cancer: Y ❑ N ❑ Hypertension: Y ❑ N ❑

Please describe questions with a "Yes" answer: ______________

____

PERSONAL PAST HISTORY: Have you ever had:

Abnormal Bleeding: Y ❑ N ❑ Asthma: Y ❑ N ❑ Hypertension: Y ❑ N ❑

Abnormal Clotting: Y ❑ N ❑ Diabetes: Y ❑ N ❑ Sleep Apnea: Y ❑ N ❑

Acid Regurgitation: Y ❑ N ❑ Fainting Spell: Y ❑ N ❑ Snoring: Y ❑ N ❑

Anemia: Y ❑ N ❑ Heart Attack: Y ❑ N ❑ Weight Change Past 12 Mo.: Y ❑ N ❑

Angina: Y ❑ N ❑ Hepatitis: Y ❑ N ❑ Other Serious Illness: Y ❑ N ❑

Please describe questions with a "Yes" answer: ______________

____

Have you ever received a transfusion? Y ❑ N ❑ If yes, what year? ______________

Have you been tested for HIV? Y ❑ N ❑ If yes, what year?__________ Test results: ❑ Positive ❑ Negative

Do you wear: Contact lenses: Y ❑ N ❑ Eye glasses: Y ❑ N ❑ Hearing aid: Y ❑ N ❑ Dentures: Y ❑ N ❑

Previous Surgery, year and type of procedure: ______________

____

Indicate the type(s) of anesthesia received in the past, list any complications/reactions you experienced:

❑ Local anesthesia - (complications/reactions): ______________

❑ General anesthesia - (complications/reactions): ______________

❑ Spinal/Epidural - (complications/reactions): ______________

Date last seen by Primary Care Physician: ______________

Primary Care Physician (name) ______________ (telephone) (________)______________

(address) ______________

WOMEN PATIENTS ONLY:

Number of pregnancies __________ Number of children __________ Last menstrual period __________ Did you breast feed? Yes No

Figure 2–1. History and physical examination forms. (Reproduced, with permission, from Iverson RE et al; ASPS Task Force on Patient Safety in Office-Based Surgery Facilities. Patient safety in office-based surgery facilities: II. Patient selection. *Plast Reconstr Surg.* 2000. Dec;110(7):1785–90.)

Name: ____________________ **MRN:** ____________________ **Date:** __________

Completed by Physician

REVIEW OF SYSTEMS

Loose Dental Devices:	Y ❑	N ❑	Chest Pain:	Y ❑	N ❑
Neck Mobility problem:	Y ❑	N ❑	Irregular Heart Beat:	Y ❑	N ❑
Short Neck:	Y ❑	N ❑	Vomiting:	Y ❑	N ❑
Cough:	Y ❑	N ❑	Difficult Voiding:	Y ❑	N ❑
Shortness of Breath:	Y ❑	N ❑	Seizure:	Y ❑	N ❑
Recent Upper Respiratory Infection:	Y ❑	N ❑	Current Pregnancy:	Y ❑	N ❑
Normal Menstrual Period:	Y ❑	N ❑	Black Out:	Y ❑	N ❑
Stroke:	Y ❑	N ❑	Obesity:	Y ❑	N ❑

Comments: ____________________

PHYSICAL EXAMINATION

Height: __________ Weight: __________ Blood Pressure: __________ Pulse: ______ Temp: ______

GENERAL STATUS COMMENT

HEENT: ______ Vision: ______ Pharynx: ______ Dental Devices: ______
Pulmonary: ____________________
Heart: ____________________
Abdomen: ____________________
Extremity: ____________________
Neurologic (if applicable): ____________________

Comments: ____________________

LABORATORY (if applicable)

H/H: __________
PT: __________
Mammogram: __________
Pregnancy Test: __________
Potassiurn: __________
BUN: __________

WBC: __________
Chest X-Ray: __________
EKG (Pt over 40): __________
Sodium Chloride: __________
CO_2: __________
Creatinine: __________

Comments: ____________________

DIAGNOSES

1. __________
2. __________
3. __________

ASA CLASSIFICATION

- ❑ P1 A normal healthy patient
- ❑ P2 A patient with mild systemic disease
- ❑ P3 A patient with severe systemic disease
- ❑ P4 A patient with severe systemic disease that is a constant threat to life

FACILITY SELECTED

- ❑ Office-based Surgical Facility
- ❑ Ambulatory Surgery Center
- ❑ Hospital

Figure 2–1. (Continued)

▶ **TABLE 2-1. INSTRUCTIONS FOR PATIENTS PREPARING FOR SURGERY**

Starting immediately

- Stop smoking: Smoking reduces circulation to skin and impedes healing. It is best to avoid smoking; second-hand smoke; and cigarette replacements, including nicotine patches or gums.
- Take multivitamins: Start taking multivitamins twice daily to improve general health.
- Take vitamin C: Begin taking 500 mg of vitamin C twice daily to promote wound healing.
- Do not take ibuprofen or aspirin: Stop taking medications containing ibuprofen or aspirin. Such drugs can cause bleeding problems during and after surgery. Instead, use medicines containing acetaminophen.
- Limit vitamin E: Limit intake to no more than 400 mg/d.
- Fill prescriptions: Prescriptions for medications will be given during the final preoperative visit. Please have them filled before the surgery and bring them on the day of the surgery.

The day before surgery

- Confirm surgery time: Someone from the surgeon's office will call you to confirm the time of your procedure. If you will not be available, please call the office to confirm.
- Prescriptions: Make sure that the prescriptions you were given for antibiotics and pain control have been filled. Bring this medication on the day of surgery.
- Cleansing: At night, shower and wash the surgical site with a mild soap.
- Eating and drinking: Do not eat or drink anything—including water—past 12 midnight.

The morning of surgery

- Special information: Do not eat or drink anything! If you take a daily medication, you may take with a sip of water in the morning.
- Oral hygiene: You may brush your teeth but do not swallow water.
- Cleansing: Shower and wash the surgical site again with a mild soap.
- Make-up: Please refrain from using moisturizer, cream, lotion, or make-up.
- Clothing: Wear only comfortable, loose-fitting clothing that does not go over your head, but zips or buttons up the front or back. Remove hairpins, wigs, and jewelry. Please do not bring valuables with you.

operative plan, obtain objective measurements, and preoperative photographs as well as give preoperative instructions (Table 2–1). Several examples of forms are available for use, or each physician may construct forms specific to their preferences and practices.

Table 2–2 outlines the fasting recommendations made by the ASA. Patients should refrain from clear liquids (including water, pulp-free fruit juices, carbonated beverages, tea and black coffee) for at least 2 hours prior to the induction of general anesthesia or monitored sedation. The volume ingested is less important than the consistency. For infants and young children, breast milk should be given no more than 4 hours prior to the induction

▶ **TABLE 2-2. FASTING RECOMMENDATIONS TO REDUCE THE RISK OF PULMONARY ASPIRATION**

Ingested Material	Minimum Fasting Period
Clear liquids	2 hours
Breast milk	4 hours
Infant formula	6 hours
Non-human milk	6 hours
Light meal	6 hours

Souce: American Society of Anesthesiologists Task Force on Sedation and Analgesia by Non-Anesthesiologists. Practice guidelines for sedation and analgesia by non-anesthesiologists. *Anesthesiology.* 2002 Apr;96(4):1004–17.

of general anesthesia or monitored sedation. Since formula is digested more slowly, it should be stopped 6 hours prior to the induction of anesthesia. For solids and non-human milk, it is appropriate to fast for 6 or more hours preoperatively. In addition, fried or fatty foods may prolong gastric emptying time and require a preoperative fast greater than 6 hours.

PATIENT SAFETY: QUALITY OF CARE

A. Administrative

The first level of quality assessment lies at the administrative level. The physician who is responsible for the operation of the facility must be certified by the American Board of Medical Specialties, American Osteopathic Association, or an approved state medical board. The surgeon should only perform procedures within the scope of their training, licensing, and board certification. The surgeon in charge should develop a system of quality assessment with regular reporting of outcomes and errors in order to identify and minimize preventable errors. Ideally, this is in the form of written policy/guidelines for employee obligations, accountabilities, and supervision, with quality health care and patient safety as the primary focus. Every facility should have a patient bill of rights emphasizing respect, privacy, and confidentiality. The facility in addition to the personnel should be state licensed or accredited by an organized and recognized accrediting body, such as the Accreditation Association for Ambulatory Health Care, the American Association for the Accreditation of Ambulatory Surgical Facilities, The Joint Commission, or the Healthcare Facilities Accreditation Program of the American Osteopathic Association. Facilities should comply with all applicable federal, state, and local laws; codes and regulations pertaining to fire prevention; building construction and occupancy; accommodations for the disabled; occupational safety and health; and disposal of medical waste and hazardous waste. Policies and procedures should comply with laws and regulations pertaining to controlled drug supply, storage, and administration.

In the event of unforeseen complications or natural disasters, emergency protocols need to be in place. The facility should have medications, equipment, and written protocols available to treat malignant hyperthermia when triggering agents are used. The facility should have a written protocol in place for the safe and timely transfer of patients to a prespecified alternate care facility when extended or emergency services are needed to protect the health or well being of the patient. In order to properly care for patients, and obviate preventable injury, personnel with advanced training, such as advanced cardiac life support and pediatric advanced life support, should be available until all patients are discharged from the facility. Discharge criteria should be written and include vital signs, level of alertness and orientation, voluntary movement, pain control, level of nausea/emesis, and ability to tolerate liquids according to the ASA guidelines for recovery and discharge (Table 2–3).

Accrediting bodies, in general, maintain requirements for governance of facility, equipment, quality assurance reporting or peer review, and clinical standards. Accreditation by one of these bodies ensures that standards for patient care and safety have been met. Subcategory certifications may be obtained based on level of anesthesia administered.

B. Informed Consent

Informed consent must be obtained from all patients. Information necessary for the patient to give informed consent includes details of the surgery; benefits, possible consequences, and side effects of the operation; potential risks and adverse outcomes as well as their probability

TABLE 2–3. RECOVERY AND DISCHARGE CRITERIA AFTER SEDATION AND ANALGESIA[1]

General principles

1. Medical supervision of recovery and discharge after moderate or deep sedation is the responsibility of the operating practitioner or a licensed physician.
2. The recovery area should be equipped with, or have direct access to, appropriate monitoring and resuscitation equipment.
3. Patients receiving moderate or deep sedation should be monitored until appropriate discharge criteria are satisfied. The duration and frequency of monitoring should be individualized depending on the level of sedation achieved, the overall condition of the patient, and the nature of the intervention for which sedation/analgesia was administered. Oxygenation should be monitored until patients are no longer at risk for respiratory depression.
4. Level of consciousness, vital signs, and oxygenation (when indicated) should be recorded at regular intervals.
5. A nurse or other individual trained to monitor patients and recognize complications should be in attendance until discharge criteria are fulfilled.
6. An individual capable of managing complications (eg, capable of establishing a patent airway and providing positive pressure ventilation) should be immediately available until discharge criteria are met.

Guidelines for discharge

1. Patients should be alert and oriented; infants and patients whose mental status was initially abnormal should have returned to their baseline status. Practitioners and patients must be aware that pediatric patients are at risk for airway obstruction should the head fall forward while the child is secured in a car seat.
2. Vital signs should be stable and within acceptable limits.
3. Use of scoring systems may assist in the documentation of fitness for discharge.
4. Sufficient time (up to 2 hours) should have elapsed after the last administration of reversal agents (naloxone, flumazenil) to ensure that patients do not become re-sedated after the reversal agents have worn off.
5. Outpatients should be discharged in the presence of a responsible adult who will accompany them home and be able to report any post-procedure complications.
6. Outpatients and their escorts should be provided with written instructions regarding post-procedure diet, medications, activities, and a phone number to be called in the case of emergency.

[1]Each patient care facility in which sedation-analgesia is administered should develop recovery and discharge criteria that are suitable for its specific patients and procedures. This table outlines some of the basic principles that might be incorporated in these criteria.

Source: American Society of Anesthesiologists Task Force on Sedation and Analgesia by Non-Anesthesiologists. Practice guidelines for sedation and analgesia by non-anesthesiologists. *Anesthesiology.* 2002 Apr;96(4):1004–17.

and severity; alternatives to the procedure being considered and their benefits, risks, and consequences; and the anticipated outcome. In order to thoroughly and efficiently inform patients, videos as well as preoperative and postoperative literature should be standardized. After a patient has had adequate time to review the literature and video presentations, qualified personnel should be available to discuss the procedure with the patient and his or her family.

C. Documentation

Medical records need be decipherable, correct, inclusive, available, and current. It is critical that adverse events are reported. A lack of reporting is an obstacle to peer review and the improvement of patient safety. The American Society of Plastic Surgeons (ASPS) has developed the Tracking Operations and Outcomes for Plastic Surgery (TOPS) database for member use. TOPS is a HIPAA-compliant web-based collection of data compiling plastic surgery procedures and outcomes.

D. Equipment

Another crucial aspect of ensuring patient well-being during office-based surgery is the safety of the equipment. At a minimum, all facilities should have a reliable source of oxygen, suction, resuscitation equipment, and emergency medications (Table 2–4). There should be sufficient space to accommodate all necessary equipment and personnel and to allow for expeditious access to the patient, anesthesia devices (when present), and all monitoring equipment. All equipment should be maintained, tested, and inspected according to the manufacturer's specifications by a certified biomedical technician. Back-up power sufficient to ensure patient protection in the event of an electrical emergency should be available and certified as well.

PATIENT PREPARATION

A. Preoperative Testing and Medical Evaluation

Routine preoperative screening of healthy patients undergoing elective surgery is not recommended. Instead, a selective strategy, as described further, is safe and cost-effective as long as a complete history and physical examination are obtained.

A complete history and physical examination helps the practitioner decide the most appropriate facility in which the surgery will take place. It also provides the necessary baseline information to assist the medical team in their intraoperative and postoperative monitoring of the patient. A thorough preoperative history should include the history of present issues; past medical/surgical history; social history; family history (including bleeding diatheses and adverse reactions to anesthetics); history of medications and supplements (prescribed and over the counter) use as well as allergies; and review of systems. The patient should be prepared to have an adult relative or friend take them home and assist in postoperative care Contact information for the responsible individual should be obtained when possible (see Figure 2–1).

Important aspects of the physical examination include an assessment of the patient's overall condition, height and weight measurements, vital signs, cardiopulmonary auscultation, and a detailed examination of the area undergoing surgery. Patients who are known to have cardiac disease, respiratory disease, diabetes mellitus, or bleeding disorders should be referred to a specialist for evaluation and management recommendations.

A hematocrit should be performed when underlying anemia is suspected and when significant blood loss is expected during surgery. A mild abnormality is not associated with an increase of perioperative morbidity or mortality. A serum creatinine level should be checked for patients older than 40 years and those who take diuretics, especially if large variation in blood pressure or use of nephrotoxic medications are anticipated. Patients with mild-to-moderate renal insufficiency are usually asymptomatic but have an increased risk of perioperative morbidity and mortality. An electrocardiogram (ECG) should be obtained in patients older than 40 years to identify high-risk patients with prior myocardial infarction or arrhythmia. Any rhythm other than sinus, including frequent premature ventricular contraction, is associated with an increase in surgical risk. A higher incidence of cardiovascular death is observed in patients with an

TABLE 2-4. EMERGENCY EQUIPMENT FOR SEDATION AND ANALGESIA[1]

Intravenous equipment
Gloves
Tourniquets
Alcohol wipes
Sterile gauze pads
Intravenous catheters (22 and 24 gauge)
Intravenous tubing (pediatric microdrip)
Intravenous fluid
Assorted needles for drug aspiration, intramuscular injection (intraosseous bone marrow needle)
Appropriately sized syringes
Tape
Basic airway management equipment
Source of compressed oxygen (tank with regular or pipeline supply with flowmeter)
Source of suction
Suction catheters (pediatric suction catheters)
Yankauer-type suction
Facemasks (infant/child)
Self-inflating breathing bag-valve set (pediatric)
Oral and nasal airways (infant and child-sized)
Lubricant
Advanced airway management equipment (for practitioners with intubation skills)
Laryngeal mask airways (pediatric)
Laryngoscope handles (tested)
Laryngoscope blades (pediatric)
Endotracheal tubes 6.0, 7.0, 8.0 mm ID (uncuffed 2.5, 3.0, 3.5, 4.0, 4.5, 5.0, 5.5, 6.0 mm ID)
Stylet (appropriately sized for endotracheal tubes)
Pharmacologic antagonists
Naloxone
Flumazenil
Emergency medications
Epinephrine
Ephedrine
Vasopressin
Atropine
Nitroglycerin (tablets or spray)
Amiodarone
Lidocaine
Glucose 50% (10% or 25%)
Diphenhydramine
Hydrocortisone, methylprednisolone or dexamethasone
Diazepam or midazolam

[1]Appropriate emergency equipment should be available whenever sedative or analgesic drugs capable of causing cardiorespiratory depression are administered. These lists should be used as a guide, which should be modified depending on the individual practice circumstances. Items in brackets are recommended when infants or children are sedated.

Source: American Society of Anesthesiologists Task Force on Sedation and Analgesia by Non-Anesthesiologists. Practice guidelines for sedation and analgesia by non-anesthesiologists. *Anesthesiology.* 2002 Apr;96(4):1004–17.

abnormal ECG than in those with normal ECG results. However, there is no significant difference in the incidence of cardiovascular death in patients, with or without ECG abnormality, who underwent low-risk or low- to intermediate-risk surgery. Any patient over the age of 60 or with underlying cardiac pulmonary disease should receive a preoperative chest radiograph.

B. Patient Positioning

Once the preoperative assessment and work-up have been completed and the procedure and facility have been determined to be appropriate and safe, the patient preparation proceeds to the actual surgical suite. The surgeon must be familiar with correct methods of patient positioning in order to avoid injury. Patient positioning is critical to the maintenance of intraoperative patient safety. Nerve damage was responsible for 16% of the cases in the ASA Closed Claims Database, making it, after death, the second most frequent category of claims for injury. Three risk factors associated with neuropathies after surgery in the lithotomy position are prolonged surgery, very thin body habitus, and recent cigarette smoking.

The **supine position** is the most commonly used position for surgical procedures. Because it is probably also the most commonly used position for natural sleep, it might be considered to be risk free. However, ulnar neuropathies are the most common perioperative nerve injury, and most are associated with surgical procedures done in this position. Pressure on the ulnar groove and the spiral groove of the humerus where the radial nerve passes must be avoided. The ASA Practice Advisory recommends that arm abduction should be limited to 90 degrees and that the forearm and hand be supinated or kept in neutral position (not pronated) when an armboard is used.

The **prone position** is commonly used to provide surgical access to the lower extremities, gluteal region, and back. Before induction of anesthesia, the cervical range of motion the patient can achieve comfortably (laterally and in flexion and extension) should be assessed along with the range of motion of the shoulders. Older patients and those with shoulder problems often cannot move their arms up to 90 degrees, and it is impossible to put their arms out on armboards after the patients are prone; the arms are then tucked at their sides intraoperatively, preventing access to intravenous and arterial lines. Turning the head to the side is safe for most patients as long as pressure on the down eye is avoided; this offers fair access to the airway and endotracheal tube. Turning the neck can be difficult or impossible in the older patient with an arthritic neck. For them, foam pillows are available that support the forehead, cheeks, and chin but have cutouts for the eyes, mouth, and nose.

The **semirecumbent position** may be used for procedures on the head and face as well as for abdominoplasty. Strict attention to detail should be paid to the flexion of the neck in order to prevent excessive flexion and spinal cord ischemia, obstruction of carotid and vertebral arteries, and embolic or thrombotic stroke. The decision about what constitutes excessive neck flexion is difficult; clinical experience and preanesthetic evaluation of range of motion may be most helpful. In general, the surgeon should be able to place two fingers between the chin and the sternum when positioning is complete. In this position, the arms are secured to the armboards with a gauze wrap to prevent them from hanging by the side. When muscle relaxants are used, the downward force caused by the weight of the arms may be sufficient to stretch the brachial plexus. Blankets or foam padding should be placed under the elbow and forearm to support the weight of the arm relieving any downward stretch, and the arm is pushed up slightly, giving the appearance of a slight shoulder shrug. The hips are often flexed because position tends to place the buttocks at an angle to support the weight of the body and because it is thought to aid venous return. The legs must not be outstretched because this places considerable tension on the sciatic nerve. Bending the legs at the knees removes this tension, and placing an artificial fat pad under the buttocks and the sciatic notch of the pelvis may reduce the chances of pressure ischemia of the sciatic nerve.

Occasionally, the **lateral position** is used for liposuction of the flank region. As the patient is rolled onto her side, the superior arm is placed perpendicular to the torso on a pillow or overarm rest to support it. This arm is then secured in position. It is crucial to protect the ulnar nerve at the elbow and the radial nerve as it wraps around the radial groove in the upper third of the humerus. The side of the chest resting on the operating table is generally supported with an axillary roll, which can be fashioned from a 1-liter bag of intravenous fluid wrapped in a blue towel. This intervention displaces the weight of the chest on the rib cage, preventing the shoulder and axilla from being compressed and a brachial plexus injury from developing. In this position, the leg lying against the operating table should be bent, while the upper leg remains straight. A pillow in between the legs and foam cushioning under both ankles completes the set-up.

In any position, pooling of the preparation liquids under the buttocks and lower back can result in a chemical burn; thus, it is wise to remove all drapes in this area after preparation so that puddles of residual solution can be removed. All contact points of the body on the table must be padded for pressure protection.

C. Deep Venous Thrombosis Prophylaxis

Venous thromboembolism (VTE) is a common complication among surgery patients. It affects approximately 25% of hospitalized patients. This results in nearly 450,000 cases of VTE in the United States each year. VTE is the primary cause of preventable deaths in hospitalized patients.

The patient history may be the most important tool in identifying risk factors for deep venous thrombosis (DVT). The presence of inheritable hypercoagulable states, including factor V Leiden mutation, hyperhomocysteinemia, prothrombin gene mutation, protein C and S deficiency, antiphospholipid antibody, antithrombin III deficiency, dysfibrinogenemia, polycythemia vera, and heparin-induced thrombocytopenia, may sometimes be disclosed or suspected based on patient history. Other risk factors for thrombosis include surgery, increased age, malignancy, previous miscarriage, pregnancy, oral contraceptives, smoking, hormone replacement therapy, previous thromboembolism, heart failure, obesity, and paralysis. Entries for bleeding tendencies and clotting disorders should appear on the patient history form.

When surveying plastic surgery procedures, abdominoplasty, especially when combined with other procedures, has the highest reported VTE risk. The most commonly used prophylactic agents are sequential compression devices (SCD), which lowers the incidence of DVT by ~44%; low-dose unfractionated heparin (LDUH); and low-molecular-weight heparin (LMWH) (eg, enoxaparin).

Numerous randomized, prospective trials have proven there is no increase in major bleeding risk with the use of LDUH or LMWH. The risk of minor bleeding is slightly increased with the use of LDUH (approximately 5.9% vs 3.8%).

As a practical matter, all surgical patients should be risk stratified for VTE preoperatively (Figure 2–2). The physician may assign patient risk for venous thromboembolic events using the risk assessment model developed by the American College of Chest Physicians (ACCP). Measures for prophylaxis based on the patient risk profile may then be implemented. The group of patients at highest risk include those with cancer, hypercoagulable states, inflammatory bowel disease, previous DVT or pulmonary embolism, stroke, orthopedic trauma, and acute spinal cord injury with paralysis.

Step I. **Total =**___________

Exposing Risk Factors			
Check the box corresponding to each condition			
1 Factor	**2 Factors**	**3 Factors**	**5 Factors**
Minor surgery ❑	*Major surgery ❑	Previous myocardial infarction ❑	Hip. pelvis, or leg fracture ❑
	Immobilizing plaster cast ❑	Congestive heart failure ❑	Stroke ❑
	Central confined to bed for > 72 hrs ❑	Severe sepsis ❑	Multiple trauma ❑
	Central venous access ❑	Free flap ❑	Acute spinal cord injury ❑

*Major surgery is defined by the use of a general anesthesia or any procedure lasting longer than 1 hour.

Step II. **Total =**___________

Predisposing Risk Factors		
Check the box corresponding to each condition		
Clinical Setting	**Inherited**	**Acquired**
Age 40 to 60 (1 Factor) ❑	Any genetic hypercoaguable disorder (3 Factors) ❑	Lupus anticoagulant (3 Factors) ❑
Age > 60 (2 Factors) ❑		Antiphospholipid disorders (3 Factors) ❑
History of DVT/PE (3 Factors) ❑		Myeloproliferative disorders (3 Factors) ❑
Pregnancy or < 1 month postpartum (1 Factor) ❑		Heparin-induced thrombocytopenia (3 Factors) ❑
Malignancy (2 Factors) ❑		Hyperviscosity (3 Factors) ❑
Obesity > 20% IBW (1 Factor) ❑		Homocystinemia (3 Factors) ❑
Oral contraceptive/hormone replacement therapy (1 Factor) ❑		

Step III. **Total Step I and Step II =** ________________ **Factors**

Step IV. Orders

1 Factor	Low risk	Ambulate patient TID ❑
2 Factors	Moderate risk	Intermittent pneumatic compression stockings with elastic compression stockings on at all times when not ambulating ❑
3–4 Factors	High risk	Intermittent pneumatic compression stockings with elastic compression stockings on at all times when not ambulating ❑
> 4 Factors	Highest risk	Intermittent pneumatic compression stockings with elastic compression stockings on at all times when not ambulating ❑ + 1. Enoxaparin (Lovenox) 40 mg SQ once daily post op ❑ *For 1: Give first dose 12 hours post Op*

Signature ______________________________ Date/Time ____________________
Print Name Pager #

Figure 2–2. Venous thromboembolism risk and prevention. IBW, ideal body weight; DVT, deep venous thrombosis; PE, pulmonary embolism. (Reproduced, with permission, from Davison SP et al. Prevention of venous thromboembolism in the plastic surgery patient. *Plast Reconstr Surg.* 2004 Sep 1;114(3):43E–51e.)

Moderate risk factors include age older than 40 years, cardiac dysfunction (including myocardial infarction and congestive heart failure), estrogen use, nephrotic syndrome, obesity, recent pregnancy, more than 3 days of bed rest, surgery lasting longer than 45 minutes and the presence of varicose veins.

According to the ACCP 2005 guidelines, SCD and LDUH are not considered sufficient prophylaxis for patients at highest risk for VTE. Low-dose LMWH may be used instead of LDUH for moderate- and high-risk patients. Antiembolic stockings are ineffective unless properly fitted; however, SCD are considered more effective. LMWH dose must be lowered in patients with poor kidney function.

VTE chemoprophylaxis timing recommendations for most plastic surgery procedures are similar to general surgery. In patients at highest risk for VTE, the initial dose of LMWH or LDUH should be given 2 hours before surgery. For all procedures performed under intravenous sedation or general anesthesia lasting longer than 45 minutes, intraoperative recommendations for VTE prophylaxis suggest SCD (unless contraindicated) and pillow under knees (5 degree knee flexion) if possible.

According to the ACCP guidelines, in low-risk general surgery patients who are undergoing minor procedures, are younger than 40 years, and have no additional risk factors, no specific prophylaxis other than early ambulation is recommended (grade 1C). For moderate-risk general surgery patients undergoing minor procedures who have additional thrombosis risk factors as well as those having non-major surgery between the ages of 40 and 60 years with no additional risk factors and those undergoing major operations who are younger than 40 years with no additional clinical risk factors, prophylaxis with LDUH, LMWH, elastic stocking (ES), or intermittent pneumatic compression (IPC) is recommended (all grade 1A in comparison to no prophylaxis). Higher-risk general surgery patients—including those having non-major surgery over the age of 60 years or with additional risk factors, or patients undergoing major surgery over the age of 40 years or with additional risk factors—should receive thrombosis prophylaxis with LDUH, LMWH, or IPC (all grade 1A in comparison to no prophylaxis). In higher-risk general surgery patients with a greater than usual risk of bleeding, the ACCP recommends the use of mechanical prophylaxis with ES or IPC, at least initially (grade 1C).

In very-high-risk general surgery patients with multiple risk factors, the ACCP recommends that effective pharmacologic methods (LDUH or LMWH) be combined with ES or IPC (grade 1C based on small studies and on extrapolation of data from other patient groups). Lastly, in selected very-high-risk general surgery patients, it is recommended that clinicians consider postdischarge LMWH or perioperative warfarin (international normalized ratio [INR] 2.0 to 3.0) (grade 2C).

VTE prophylaxis is highly effective in reducing VTE incidence; however, it is underutilized. At present, up to 60% of plastic surgeons do not use any form of thromboprophylaxis, despite DVT and pulmonary embolism being among the most common postoperative surgical complications. Only one-third of patients with clearly identifiable VTE risk factors receive appropriate prophylaxis.

D. Antibiotic Prophylaxis

Today, there is increasing concern about the inappropriate use of prophylactic antibiotics in surgery. Surgical site infections are a significant source of increased morbidity and mortality, prolonged hospital stays, and increased hospital care costs. Every day, approximately 85,000 Americans undergo surgical procedures. Surgical site infections are estimated to occur in ≈3% of cases, with estimated costs varying widely but approaching $5000/case. The appropriate use of prophylactic antibiotics has been demonstrated to decrease surgical site infections in a number of procedures (eg, breast, hernia).

Antibiotics should be appropriate for the procedure, and administered prior to the skin incision (ideally within 1 hour for cefazolin and clindamycin and within 2 hours for vancomycin). Antibiotics need not be continued after incision closure. Interestingly, prophylactic antibiotics are not indicated for most procedures (specifically cosmetic). Cefazolin, a first-generation cephalosporin with wide gram-positive skin flora coverage, is an appropriate choice for virtually all plastic surgery procedures. In patients who are allergic to β-lactams, clindamycin is recommended.

Prolonged and inappropriate use of antibiotics increases adverse drug reaction risk, increases resistant bacteria, increases associated infectious morbidity (ie, yeast infections, bacterial enterocolitis), and increases unnecessary health care costs. The appropriate use of prophylactic antibiotics lowers the incidence of surgical site infections.

E. Herbal Supplements

Natural herbal supplements are purported to boost the immune system, provide more energy, and make patients healthier. However, many of these "harmless" supplements can cause dangerous side effects during plastic surgery by interacting with anesthetic agents, promoting bleeding, or interfering with wound healing. While 24% of the general public take supplements without informing their physician, the ASPS has shown that 55% of plastic surgery patients take supplements and often do not tell their surgeons. Patients often assume herbal agents are safe and only think to mention prescription medicines when asked about pharmaceutical use. Of the plastic surgery patients taking herbal medicine, all took at least two different types of pills and at least one on a daily basis.

The most popular common supplements were chondroitin (18%), ephedra (18%), echinacea (14%), and glucosamine (10%). Chondroitin is often used to treat osteoarthritis. Chondroitin is advertised as a remedy for aching joints by maintaining the structure and function of cartilage by acting as an anti-inflammatory. Patients using chondroitin may suffer from bleeding complications during surgery, particularly when used in combination with prescribed anticoagulants or antiplatelet medications. Ephedra is taken to promote weight loss; increase energy; and treat respiratory tract conditions, such as asthma and bronchitis. This agent has been banned by the US Food and Drug Administration (FDA) because it can raise blood pressure, heart rate, and metabolic rate, ultimately causing heart attacks, heart arrhythmia, stroke, and even death. This can be a lethal combination with anesthetic agents. Echinacea is often used for the prevention and treatment of viral, bacterial, and fungal infections, as well as, chronic wounds, ulcers, and arthritis. On the other hand, it can trigger immunosuppression, causing poor wound healing and infection. Glucosamine, often taken in conjunction with chondroitin, contains chemical elements that mimic human insulin and may artificially cause hypoglycemia during surgery. Other common supplements taken by patients in the study that may cause dangerous side effects included *Gingko biloba,* goldenseal, milk thistle, ginseng, kava, and garlic (Table 2–5).

F. Cosmeceuticals

Cosmeceuticals are a hybrid category created by merging cosmetics and pharmaceuticals. The desire for the improvement of aging skin has resulted in a plethora of products designed to improve the appearance beyond the simple camouflage of cosmetics. These products claim to diminish fine lines and wrinkles, decrease redness, smooth texture, and fade discoloration. They are topically applied and purport to alter dermal biology. It is important to remember, however, that for benefit to be realized, the final product must be stable in formula, absorbed into the skin, and biologically active at the target for clinical benefit. Cosmeceuticals

▶ **TABLE 2-5. USES AND POSSIBLE SIDE EFFECTS OF COMMON HERBAL SUPPLEMENTS**

Common Name	Uses	Surgical Concern	Recommendation
Chondroitin	Osteoarthritis	Perioperative hemorrhage	Stop 2–3 weeks preoperatively
Ephedra	Energy, weight loss, asthma	Hypertension, cardiac instability mixed with anesthetics	Stop at least 1 day preoperatively
Echinacea	Infection, ulcers, arthritis, prevention of bruising	Potentiates barbiturate and halothane toxicity, allergic reaction and immunosuppression	Stop 2–3 weeks preoperatively
Glucosamine	Osteoarthritis	Hypoglycemia	Stop 2–3 weeks preoperatively
Gingko biloba	Dementia, vascular disease, tinnitus, asthma, colds, anti-inflammatory	Postoperative sedation, perioperative bleeding	Stop 1.5 days preoperatively
Goldenseal	Laxative, anti-inflammatory, infection	Volume depletion, postoperative sedation, photosensitization	Stop 2–3 weeks preoperatively
Milk thistle	Hepatoprotective, anti-inflammatory	Volume depletion	Stop 2–3 weeks preoperatively
Ginseng	Antioxidant, energy, lowers blood glucose	Perioperative bleeding	Stop 1 week preoperatively
Kava	Anxiolytic, muscle relaxant	Postoperative sedation	Stop at least 1 day preoperatively
Garlic	Infection, hypertension, hypercholesterolemia, cancer prevention	Perioperative bleeding	Stop 1 week preoperatively
Saw palmetto	Sedative, anti-inflammatory, benign prostatic hypertrophy, aphrodisiac	Perioperative bleeding	Stop 2–3 weeks preoperatively
St. John's wort	Depression, anxiety, pain, insomnia, infection	Postoperative sedation, cardiovascular collapse, photosensitization, swelling	Stop 5 days preoperatively Do not combine with monoamine oxidase inhibitors
Valerian	Insomnia, anxiolytic	Postoperative sedation	Stop 1 week preoperatively
Ginger	Antiemetic, sore throat, anti-inflammatory	Perioperative bleeding	Stop 2–3 weeks preoperatively
Eicosapentaenoic acid	Cardioprotective, skin disorders, asthma	Perioperative bleeding	Stop 2–3 weeks preoperatively
Vitamin E	Cardioprotective, antioxidant	Perioperative bleeding, prolonged wound healing	Stop 2–3 weeks preoperatively

Adapted, with permission, from Heller J et al. Top-10 List of Herbal and Supplemental Medicines Used by Cosmetic Patients: What the Plastic Surgeon Needs to Know. *Plast Reconstr Surg.* 2006;117(2):436–445.

are not subject to review by the FDA nor is the term recognized by the Federal Food, Drug, and Cosmetic Act. Cosmeceuticals are tested for safety by the manufacturer; however, there are no requirements for proof that the formulation satisfies its advertising claims. The most frequently used botanicals marketed as cosmeceuticals include teas, soy, pomegranate, date, grape seed, pycnogenol, horse chestnut, German chamomile, curcumin, comfrey, allantoin, and aloe. Out of this group, only green and black tea, soy, pomegranate, and date have been studied in published clinical trials. Many ingredients have been added to these products based on theoretical benefits discovered from in vitro studies on wound healing and other metabolic processes. Few botanical-based cosmeceuticals have uses that are supported by evidence-based science (Table 2–6).

OUTCOMES ASSESSMENT

In the publication "To Err is Human," the Institute of Medicine (IOM) declared that preventable medical errors were the eighth leading cause of death in the United States. When preventive medicine and the focus of research dollars are considered, cancer, heart disease, and vehicular trauma are often the first to come to mind. This landmark publication on public safety showed that up to 98,000 Americans die each year as a result of preventable medical errors. In the United States, the annual cost was estimated to be between $55 and $89 billion dollars. The IOM has called for a national effort to make health care safe. Progress has been slow; however, that study helped shift the focus onto changing systems, stimulating a broad array of medical personnel

TABLE 2–6. COSMECEUTICALS AND THEIR PURPORTED EFFECTS

Common Name	Uses
Retinoids	Antioxidant, reducing wrinkles, decreasing skin laxity, bleaching hyperpigmented spots
Hydroxy acids	Decrease the signs of aging
Vitamin C	Decrease the signs of aging
Vitamin E	Reduce erythema, edema, sunburn cells, immunosuppression caused by sunlight
Panthenol	Humectant
Lipoic acid	Antioxidant
Niacinamide	Increased epidermal turnover and exfoliation
Dimethylaminoethanol	Improved skin firmness, lift sagging skin
Melatonin	Free radical scavenger, suppresses UV radiation-induced erythema
Superoxide dismutase	Decreases UV radiation-induced erythema, antioxidant
Allantoin	Cell proliferant, epithelialization stimulant, and a chemical debrider
Chamomile	Anti-inflammatory, inhibits histamine release
Curcumin	Anti-inflammatory
Aloe vera	Accelerate wound healing, protect and soothe skin
Hyaluronic acid	Accelerate wound healing, epidermal regeneration
Papain	Exfoliate keratotic skin and treat hypertrophic scars
Epidermal growth factor	Accelerates re-epithelialization in burn and excision wounds
Transforming growth factor	Promote wound healing
Estrogen	Improves skin elasticity, firmness, wrinkle depth, and pore size
Clostridium botulinum	Temporary chemical denervation

to engage in patient safety, and motivating hospitals to adopt new safe practices and a culture of patient safety.

One of the most critical aspects of the practice of plastic surgery is the maintenance of patient safety. Cosmetic surgery presents the unique scenario of a strictly elective surgical procedure being performed to enhance an individual's aesthetic appearance. This scenario magnifies the importance of adhering to the oath chosen by plastic surgeons—"primum non nocere." Technologic advances in plastic surgery techniques and anesthesia have transported the cosmetic surgical procedure largely from the hospital setting to the office-based operative facility. Consumer driven demand for privacy, convenience, efficiency, and cost containment has perpetuated this transition. The social acceptance and accessibility of plastic surgery has steadily increased such that the number of cosmetic surgery procedures being performed over the past decade in the office-based setting has burgeoned. Today, over 80% of procedures performed by plastic surgeons are done in the outpatient setting.

Concurrent transfer of regulatory oversight has lagged behind the advancement of science and technology. In 2003, the *US News and World Report* publicized a 10-fold increase in the risk of serious injury from procedures performed in a private office as opposed to an ambulatory surgery facility. In response to this information and the IOM report citing preventable deaths caused by physician and system error, plastic surgeons have taken a proactive role in creating a safe operating environment for patients. The ASPS task force, created in 2002 after publicized plastic surgery deaths in Florida, developed office-based surgery practice advisories emphasizing patient safety as a foremost concern. For plastic surgeons, liposuction, which can result in large fluid shifts, is of particular concern in the outpatient setting. The ASPS and The American Society for Aesthetic Plastic Surgery have set precedence in maintaining focus on patient safety through a tripartite initiative to support the Patient Safety and Quality Improvement Act of 2005. This legislation encourages voluntary reporting of errors without fear of retribution. Data, stripped of identifiers, will be maintained by public or private entities. The analysis of the information collected will be used to improve medical systems and practice.

The safety of office-based surgical procedures has more recently been confirmed by studies revealing low morbidity comparable to other operative settings. This may be in part due to the adoption of a culture of safety posture by plastic surgery as a discipline. Plastic surgeons must continue to foster this culture to protect and safely provide care to the cosmetic surgery population.

REFERENCES

American Society of Anesthesiologists Task Force on Sedation and Analgesia by Non-Anesthesiologists. Practice guidelines for sedation and analgesia by non-anesthesiologists. *Anesthesiology.* 2002 Apr;96(4):1004–17. [PMID: 11964611]

Bitar G et al. Safety and efficacy of office-based surgery with monitored anesthesia care/sedation in 4778 consecutive plastic surgery procedures. *Plast Reconstr Surg.* 2003 Jan;111(1):150–6. [PMID: 12496575]

Byrd HS et al. Safety and efficacy in an accredited outpatient plastic surgery facility: a review of 5316 consecutive cases. *Plast Reconstr Surg.* 2003 Aug;112(2):636–41. [PMID: 12900627]

Hasen KV et al. An outcome study comparing intravenous sedation with midazolam/fentanyl (conscious sedation) versus propofol infusion (deep sedation) for aesthetic surgery. *Plast Reconstr Surg.* 2003 Nov;112(6):1683–9. [PMID: 14578803]

Heller J et al. Top-10 list of herbal and supplemental medicines used by cosmetic patients: what the plastic surgeon needs to know. *Plast Reconstr Surg.* 2006 Feb;117(2):436–45. [PMID: 16462323]

Horton JB et al. Patient safety in the office-based setting. *Plast Reconstr Surg.* 2006 Apr;117(4): 61e–80e. [PMID: 16582768]

Iverson RE; ASPS Task Force on Patient Safety in Office-Based Surgery Facilities. Patient safety in office-based surgery facilities: I. Procedures in the office-based surgery setting. *Plast Reconstr Surg*. 2002 Oct;110(5):1337–42. [PMID: 12360080]

Iverson RE et al; ASPS Task Force on Patient Safety in Office-Based Surgery Facilities. Patient safety in office-based surgery facilities: II. Patient selection. *Plast Reconstr Surg*. 2002 Dec;110(7):1785–90. [PMID: 12447066]

Kohn L, Corrigan JM, Donaldson M, eds. *To Err is Human: Building a Safer Health System*. Washington, DC: National Academy Press, 2000.

Platt R et al. Perioperative antibiotic prophylaxis for herniorrhaphy and breast surgery. *N Engl J Med*. 1990 Jan 18;322(3):153-60. [PMID: 2403655]

Rohrich RJ. Patient Safety and Quality Improvement Act of 2005: what you need to know. *Plast Reconstr Surg*. 2006 Feb;117(2):671–2. [PMID: 16462357]

CHAPTER 3

Nonsurgical Skin Care

Lawrence S. Reed, MD & Vikisha Fripp, MD

Nonsurgical skin care is a feasible alternative for patients who are looking to delay or avoid surgical interventions and treat unwanted hair. The wide array of options available and minimal recovery time make these procedures very attractive.

The growing trend toward nonsurgical skin care has been confirmed in the latest data from the American Society of Plastic Surgeons, which shows that from 2007 to 2008 minimally invasive cosmetic procedures jumped 5% to 10.4 million procedures. The top five procedures performed in 2008 were Botox therapy, hyaluronic acid fillers (Restylane, Hylaform, and Hylaform plus), chemical peel, laser hair removal, and microdermabrasion.

Fortunately, several skin conditions, including acne and acne scarring, age spots (senile keratosis), hyperpigmentation, rosacea, actinic keratosis, sun damage, wrinkles, and hair removal, can all be treated without surgery. The addition of a medical grade skin care regimen can act to complement these procedures and often reverse sun damage. Several medical grade regimens exist, including the Obagi line of products, LaRoche-Pasay by Biomedics, Method Physioderme, SkinMedica, and Jurlique.

Most nonsurgical procedures are performed in the doctor's office with minimal recovery time. The procedure begins with a complete analysis of the patient's skin, including a complete history of sun exposure, prior procedures and surgery, and the determination of the patient's skin type. The most commonly used classification is the Fitzpatrick typing, which divides patients into six types based on color and response to sunlight. This classification helps determine a patient's risk for post-procedural hyperpigmentation.

A new tool in the plastic surgeon's armamentarium is Visia, which evaluates the skin for porphyrins, sun damage, pore size, and the texture of the skin, brown spots, and wrinkles. This painless analysis is done in the doctor's office and provides a comparison of the patient to their age-matched group. The information gathered from this analysis helps determine the appropriate treatment plan for the patient.

▶ CHEMICAL PEELS

PATIENT EVALUATION & SELECTION

Patient desiring chemical peels are evaluated with a thorough history and clinical examination of the skin. Chemical peels are used to treat patients with photoaging- actinic keratosis, solar elastosis, solar lentigo, superficial rhytids, pigmentary disturbances (eg, melasma, postinflammatory pigmentation), acne, acne scarring, and rosacea. The type of chemical peel selected depends on the patient's *desires* (rejuvenation of the skin or treatment of a specific condition), *skin type* (as determined by the Fitzpatrick classification), *condition* of the skin, (thin vs thick, oily vs dry), and the amount of *recovery time* available.

Patient desiring superficial epidermal peels are best treated with low concentrations of trichloroacetic acid (TCA) (20%), glycolic acid, lactic acids, or combination peels (Vitalize peels). Patients desiring complete epidermal resurfacing are treated with higher concentration TCA, up to 50%. Phenol, the strongest chemical peel, was used in the past to treat coarse facial wrinkles, areas of sun-damaged skin, and a precancerous growth. However, because of its cardiotoxicity, its use has fallen out of favor.

Glycolic acid and lactic acid are used to treat patients with acne-prone skin and pigmentation issues and deliver a more gradual peel. The strength of glycolic and lactic acid peels are titrated to achieve these goals with lower concentrations used on patients who have not had prior chemical peels. Using the Vitalize peels (combination of lactic acid, salicylic acid, and resorcinol with an added layer of liquid retinoic acid) or alternating peels is also an option for patients with acne-prone skin. Rosacea has been found to respond best to lactic acid peels.

Typically, Fitzpatrick skin types I–IV can be treated with any of the chemical peels available, while skin types IV–VI are treated with milder, superficial glycolic, lactic acid, or Vitalize peels. Thin-skinned individuals are better suited for lactic acid peels, which are ideal for sensitive skin or skin unable to tolerate glycolic acid, while thicker skinned individuals can tolerate TCA peels. The recovery time associated with TCA peels varies depending on the depth of the peel used, while the recovery time associated with lactic acid, glycolic acid, and Revitalize peels is so short that they are referred to as the "lunch time" peels.

PATIENT PREPARATION

Pretreatment may consist of placing a patient on Retin-A, to thin out the skin's surface layer allowing for better penetration. Hydroquinone is prescribed for a week preceding chemical peels for patients with hyperpigmentation or blotchy skin. Patients are instructed to avoid direct sunlight and sun tanning procedures prior to the treatment. Before the procedure, the skin is cleansed with an oil-free cleanser to remove makeup and debris and Acetone is applied to allow better penetration. No anesthetic is used for the procedure.

TECHNIQUE

A. TCA

The face is washed with an oil-free cleanser or foaming gel cleanser and patted dry. The TCA is then placed over the area, avoiding the eyes, lips, and mucous membranes. The solution should not be rubbed into the face. The product is then observed for the presence of precipative/frost. Subsequent layers are applied until the desired epidermal/dermal layer is visualized. Ice soak gauze is then applied to the face and heavy emollients, moisturizers, and sunscreen is applied. Three days after the peel, an eschar is established. After 3 to 5 days, the eschar begins to separate and desquamation begins, usually in the perioral and periorbital areas. The majority of peeling has finished at 1 week, with flaking persisting for several additional days.

B. Lactic Acid, Glycolic Acid, and Vitalize Peel

The face is washed with an oil-free cleanser or foaming gel cleanser and pat dry. The chemical solution is then placed over the area, avoiding the eyes, lips, and mucous membranes. The solution should not be rubbed into the face. The product is left on the face for 2 to 6 minutes depending on the skin sensitivity.

Glycolic acid is the only product that requires neutralization of the acid to prevent further penetration of the product. The others are rinsed from the skin with lukewarm water. Post peel, moisturizer-containing sunscreen is applied. The process is repeated weekly for lactic acid. Vitalize peels require fewer treatments with a series of three to six peels, 3 to 4 weeks apart. For best results, glycolic acid peels are done at monthly intervals. Post-treatment, heavy emollient, moisturizers, and sunscreen are applied.

COMPLICATIONS

Treatment with TCA typically requires significant recovery time and several weeks between treatments. Complications include erythema, sensitivity to sunlight and temperature, herpes simplex virus reactivation, ulcerations, and hyperpigmentation. Glycolic acid, lactic acid, and Revitalize peels are less irritating and patients return to daily activities after treatment. All patients, especially those treated with TCA, are advised to wear sunscreen and avoid direct sunlight.

OUTCOMES ASSESSMENT

No clinical studies have been done to evaluate the efficacy of TCA, glycolic acid, and Vitalize peels. Lactic acid has been proven to be effective in treating melasma. Pure lactic acid, full strength (92%; pH 3.5), was used by Sharquie et al in 12 patients with melasma, all skin type IV. The chemical peeling sessions were done every 3 weeks until the desired response was achieved, but not more than six sessions. Follow-up was done for 6 months after the last session. All 12 patients in the study showed marked improvement, as calculated by the Melasma Area and Severity Index (MASI) score before and after treatment, and the response was highly statistically significant. No side effect was recorded in all treated patients.

REFERENCES

Collawn SS et al. Ultrastructural study of the skin after facial chemical peels and the effect of moisturization on wound healing. *Plast Reconstr Surg.* 1998 Apr;101(5):1374–79. [PMID: 9529229]

Sharquie KE et al. Lactic acid as a new therapeutic peeling agent in melasma. *Dermatol Surg.* 2005 Feb;31(2):149–54. [PMID: 15762205]

▶ HAIR REMOVAL

PATIENT EVALUATION & SELECTION

Hair removal is a growing area of plastic surgery with more and more patients opting for this procedure versus electrolysis and waxing. Unwanted hair on the face, neck, axilla, groin, and back are the most common areas patients request to be treated. Patients with darker skin may need more sessions as their skin may require lower energy levels for safe treatment since the target of the energy is melanin. Laser hair treatments are less effective on light blond or gray hair.

The patient's skin type is the major determinant in the type of treatment used for hair removal. The Q switched Nd:YAG laser is ideal for dark-skinned (Fitzpatrick IV–VI) individuals while the long-pulsed alexandrite is better suited for lighter skinned patients (Fitzpatrick I–III). The diode is another laser that can be used for hair removal in light-skinned patients. Intense pulse light (IPL) is a nonlaser option for hair removal and has the benefit of use on darker-skinned individuals.

PATIENT PREPARATION

Patients are asked to refrain from plucking the hair in the treatment areas after the procedure. Most patients have a topical anesthetic agent applied prior to the procedure to avoid discomfort. The only other pretreatment required is trimming of the hair. Patients wear protective goggles for all hair removal techniques.

TECHNIQUE

After each session, most of the treated hairs are stunned and fall out. After approximately 6 weeks, the surviving hair follicles gradually start growing hair. As the follicle must be in the anagen phase, only a third of the hairs treated never return and are permanently removed. The remaining hairs tend to be lighter in color and smaller in size. Multiple treatments maximize the opportunity to treat hair follicles in more susceptible parts of their growth cycle with intervals of 2 to 3 months between treatments. Most patients require four to six sessions to achieve their hair loss goals.

The diode laser uses an 810-nm wavelength for selective photothermolysis. Through a sapphire chilled tip, which protects the skin, a highly concentrated light energy is directed at the melanin pigment located in the hair follicles. The laser pulses for a fraction of a second, just long enough to vaporize the pigment, disabling several follicles at a time to eliminate or significantly impede hair growth. Only one pass is done per treatment area.

Before treatment with the Nd:YAG laser, mineral oil or hydrogel dressing containing carbon particles are placed over the area. A low-fluence first pass is done, followed by a high-fluence second pass. This method has been demonstrated by Goldberg to provide permanent hair follicle destruction. The alexandrite laser works similar to the other lasers in that the target of the laser is the melanin in the hair follicle. Larger areas can be treated in a shorter period of time with the Ruby laser. A single pass is done per treatment session using fluences of 25 to 40 J/cm^2 and pulse durations of 2 msec. Most patients are treated with three to five sessions.

Another option for hair removal is the nonlaser IPL. This modality has the advantage of being effective on all skin types. The settings are adjusted based on the patient's skin type (Fitzpatrick), density of hair (thick vs sparse) and type of hair (fine vs coarse). A single pass is done per session.

COMPLICATIONS

The patients may experience mild redness following treatment, which will disappear in the first day or two. Hyperpigmentation or hypopigmentation of the skin can occur; however, it is usually transient.

OUTCOMES ASSESSMENT

There are no data comparing the efficacy of laser hair treatment with nonlaser hair treatment. However, Sadick et al report a mean hair removal efficiency of 76% after a mean of 3.7 treatments with IPL photoepilation. Side effects were reported as mild and reversible and occurred in a small number of patients. The adverse effects were hyperpigmentation in 3 of 34 patients and superficial crusting in 2 of 34 patients.

REFERENCES

Goldberg DJ et al. Topical suspension assisted Q-switched Nd:YAG laser hair removal. *Dermatol Surg.* 1997 Sep;23(9):741–5. [PMID: 9311366]

Lawrence WT. Hair removal laser and nonlaser light systems. Plastic Surgery Educational Foundation DATA Committee. *Plast Reconstr Surg.* 2000 Jan;105(1):459–61. [PMID: 10627017]

Sadick NS et al. Long-term photoepilation using a broad-spectrum intense pulsed light source. *Arch Dermatol.* 2000 Nov;136(11):1336–40. [PMID: 11074695]

▶ MICRODERMABRASION

PATIENT EVALUATION & SELECTION

Patients with senile keratosis, fine rhytids, and acne scarring are the best candidates for microdermabrasion. Microdermabrasion removes the top layer of the skin resulting in a firmer, more even skin tone.

PATIENT PREPARATION

No anesthetics or pain medication is required, and the therapy is most effective when done on a weekly basis.

TECHNIQUE

The procedure is performed in the office and takes approximately 45 minutes. The excess, dead skin present on the top layer of skin is removed with the use of fine crystals. With the aid of a vacuum, the crystals and the skin's cellular debris are removed from the skin surface. The size of the hand piece is determined based on the condition of the skin and level of tolerance. Typically, a less abrasive hand piece is chosen for the first treatment. The initial passes of the hand piece are done over the treatment area in a criss-cross pattern and additional passes are performed over problem areas (ie, hyperpigmented areas, depressed scars). It is strongly recommended that sunscreen be applied for the duration of the treatment.

COMPLICATIONS

Mild redness can be expected for a couple of hours following the treatment; however, makeup can be used immediately after the procedure.

OUTCOMES ASSESSMENT

No clinical trials are currently available.

▶ IPL PHOTOFACIAL

PATIENT EVALUATION & SELECTION

Patients requiring improvement in brown or red discoloration (poikiloderma) secondary to sun damage, vascular lesions, redness, pore size, skin surface irregularities, rosacea, and fine rhytids with minimal recovery time are ideal for this procedure. This procedure is also used by patients desiring a preventive and maintenance plan for general signs of aging. In addition to treating conditions on the face, it can be used to treat the skin on the neck, chest, hands, and arms. The patient undergoes a clinical examination of the skin to identify areas of concern as well as a Visia analysis, if available. Patients with Fitzpatrick skin types V and VI may not use the IPL for facial rejuvenation; however, they can be treated for hair removal. Patients with skin type IV require pretreatment with hydroquinone.

PATIENT PREPARATION

The treatment area is cleansed of makeup and cellular debris. Protective goggles are worn by the patient and the skin care professional during the procedure. Topical anesthetics are not required but can be used for patient comfort.

TECHNIQUE

The IPL delivers a precise amount of light energy through the skin's surface that works to reorganize the dermal collagen. Topical anesthetics and cool gel help minimize discomfort during the treatment. The IPL hand piece is not directly applied to the skin but rather aimed at the area of treatment. The settings are adjusted according to the condition being treated, the skin type, and level of patient comfort. Some patients describe the feeling as a rubber band snap. More often than not, only one pass is done. Treatment consists of five to six sessions done in 3-week intervals.

COMPLICATIONS

After the procedure, the skin may appear pink/red and feel warm and have increased visibility of small capillaries. These symptoms usually begin to disappear within a few hours of treatment. Blistering and bleeding has been reported in very rare cases, and hyperpigmentation and hypopigmentation (darkening and lightening of the skin) have been reported as well. Scarring has been reported, but this too is very rare. However, within a few hours makeup can be applied and most patients return to work immediately after treatment. It is important to wear sunscreen after all laser treatments.

OUTCOMES ASSESSMENT

No clinical trials are available.

► ALUMA

PATIENT EVALUATION & SELECTION

This treatment works best for patients desiring improvement in fine rhytids and laxity of the skin in the jowl area, neck, and areas of the trunk. It is effective for all Fitzpatrick skin types; however, patients with autoimmune disease should not have Aluma done. Patients are clinically evaluated for skin tone, texture, and amount of adipose tissue.

PATIENT PREPARATION

When Aluma therapy is performed on the face, the skin is cleansed to remove makeup and cellular debris. No spot testing is required prior to therapy.

TECHNIQUE

Aluma uses radiofrequency to deliver heat to the deep dermal layer of the skin stimulating collagen formation. The design of the Aluma tip along with the vacuum apparatus enables deeper skin layers to be reached as the radiofrequency flows in a straight path to the dermal tissue. This also allows only the tissue located between the two electrodes to be treated, increasing safety and efficacy and decreasing pain.

The settings are made depending on the amount of adipose tissue, level of patient comfort, and area of the body. Darker skin types may require higher settings as the skin may be thicker in some anatomic areas. A gel is applied over the area and a series of passes (up to three) are made over the treatment area in different directions. The goal of the Aluma therapy is to tone and tighten the overlying epidermis resulting in healing in the lower layers of the skin with little or no discomfort.

The procedure is done at weekly intervals for 6 weeks for optimal outcome.

COMPLICATIONS

Complications of Aluma are few and are limited to minor bruising in the treatment area.

OUTCOMES ASSESSMENT

Gold and Goldman performed a prospective, self-controlled trial of 46 patients who underwent full-face treatments at 1- to 2-week intervals for a total of eight treatments. They used the Fitzpatrick-Goldman Classification of Wrinkles for Degree of Elastosis (ES) to measure the results and found 85% showed improvement of at least one ES unit.

In addition, 90% of participants in the study expressed satisfaction with the treatment and its outcome.

REFERENCE

Gold MH, Goldman MP. Treatment of Wrinkles and Skin Tightening Using Aluma Skin Renewal System with FACES (Functional Aspiration Controlled Electrothermal Stimulation) Technology. Whitepapers/Lumenis. 2005:1–4.

▶ LASER SKIN RESURFACING: Ablative (CO_2 Laser Therapy)

PATIENT EVALUATION & SELECTION

The type of laser used for epidermal and dermal resurfacing is highly dependent on the patient's desires. The amount of recovery time available is the main factor considered. CO_2 laser therapy is an ablative laser that requires significant recovery time but is effective for treating deeper rhytids around the mouth and eyes, resurfacing of photodamaged skin, and removal of epidermal skin lesions without surgical scars. It is not appropriate for Fitzpatrick skin types V and VI.

PATIENT PREPARATION

Intravenous sedation with or without nerve blocks or general anesthesia is required. It is therefore not amenable to office settings. If general anesthesia is being used, attention is paid to wrapping the endotracheal tube with wet sponges/gauzes and decreasing the exposure to oxygen, which can precipitate a fire during laser use. The eyes are lubricated with Lacrilube and metal corneal eye protectors are placed. All personnel in the operating room should wear protective eyewear with side shields.

TECHNIQUE

The laser settings should be pretested on a dry tongue depressor to confirm the spot size, pattern, and energy to be delivered and to verify coincidence between the CO_2 and indicating beams. Once this is confirmed, the laser is directed toward the treatment area and fired. If there is no indwelling evacuator, an assistant holds the plume evacuator close enough to the surgical field to capture the smoke. Typically two or three passes are made over the treatment area and Aquafor or Vaseline is applied.

▶ LASER SKIN RESURFACING: Nonablative (ActiveFX, MaxFX, Fraxel)

PATIENT EVALUATION & SELECTION

Those patients unable to tolerate long recovery times are better suited for the nonablative laser resurfacing via ActiveFX, MaxFX. The

ActiveFX is best used for dyschromias, comedones, clogged pores, fine lines, fine wrinkles, and skin tightening with minimal recovery time. MaxFX is best suited for damaged and scarred skin and treats heavier lines, wrinkles, acne scars, and deeper dyschromias and significant skin tightening. They can both be used for incisional, excisional, and ablative purposes.

Fraxel laser therapy is also used for patients who desire no recovery time because it can be done in the office setting. Fraxel laser therapy is used to treat acne scars, senile keratosis, melasma, and fine lines and wrinkles around the eyes.

PATIENT PREPARATION

The patient's face is cleansed of makeup and debris. For nonablative treatments, a topical anesthetic cream is applied to the area of treatment. The anesthetic is kept on the area for 30 minutes to 1 hour. The face is then wiped clean of the cream and the hair is swept away from the face. The eyes are irrigated with saline and plastic corneal protectors are placed.

TECHNIQUE

The settings and grinds are determined based on the skin type, areas of treatment, and level of patient discomfort. Typically, only one pass is made over the treatment area. As the heat is deposited in the skin, it stimulates collagen formation with continued improvement in the tone and texture of the skin for 3 to 6 months. After the procedure, Aquafor or Vaseline is applied to the treatment area as well as ice.

For both ablative and nonablative techniques, the patient is instructed to avoid direct sunlight, keep the area moisturized and use pain medication as needed. Follow-up is scheduled 3 to 4 days postoperatively. The procedure can be repeated after 6 months when reepithelization is completed.

COMPLICATIONS

Severe edema and excessive weeping of the skin secondary to desquamation is more commonly seen with CO_2 and MaxFX, as the entire epidermis is removed. Oral corticosteroids are prescribed for the edema, and the weeping usually subsides as reepithelization beings. Severe pain, herpes virus reactivation, and conjunctivitis can also occur after treatment. These adverse effects are treated with opioids, acyclovir, and Tobradex eye drops. Patients with active suntans or darker pigments may experience color variations post-procedure.

OUTCOMES ASSESSMENT

No clinical trials are available for ActiveFX, MaxFX, Fraxel.

REFERENCE

Rohrich RJ et al. CO_2 laser safety considerations in skin resurfacing. *Plast Reconstr Surg.* 1997 Oct;100(5):1285–90. [PMID: 9326794]

▶ BLU-U PHOTOFACIAL LIGHT THERAPY

PATIENT EVALUATION & SELECTION

Blu-U photofacial light therapy is a new treatment for patients with acne, rosacea, and actinic keratosis. Patients with recalcitrant acne vulgaris are particularly good candidates for the procedure. Prior to the therapy, all potential candidates are clinically examined and a Visia is performed to determine the cellular condition of the skin. The Visia is also performed after the treatment to chart the improvement of the skin. This procedure is good for all skin types and also patients with active suntans.

PATIENT PREPARATION

The patient's face is cleansed with acetone and the makeup and debris are removed. No pretreatment is required.

TECHNIQUE

This technique combines the topical agent aminolevulinic acid hydrochloride (Levulan) with blue light in a procedure termed "Levulan photodynamic therapy" (PDT). This topical medication is placed on the skin for an hour after which the Levulan is then activated by a painless, blue light for 16 minutes. This light therapy kills acne-causing bacteria, overactive oil glands, and premalignant skin cells. This procedure is repeated in 2- to 3-week intervals for a total of four treatments. The procedure requires that the patient avoid direct sunlight for 3 days after the procedure and wear sunscreen at all times.

COMPLICATIONS

Post-procedural redness, peeling, burning, and the appearance of sunburn are expected.

OUTCOMES ASSESSMENT

No clinical trials are available.

▶ SKIN CARE REGIMEN

PATIENT EVALUATION & SELECTION

Before a skin care regimen is chosen, the patient's goals as well as level of compliance are ascertained. Some product lines have multiple steps and require patients to use the products at least twice daily; therefore, patients with poor compliance are not candidates for those regimens. A history of sun exposure, tanning bed use, laser therapy, and medications are obtained. This is followed by a clinical examination to determine the skin type, presence of any dermatologic conditions as well as fine lines and wrinkles. Patients who request improvement in the texture of the skin, appearance of senile keratosis, hyperpigmentation, acne vulgaris, and sun damage are candidates for being on a skin care regimen.

Several regimens are on the market with each having a target area and catchment group but sharing many similarities. The Obagi skin care system works well in sun-damage skin, hyperpigmented areas, melasma, and fine rhytids (Figure 3–1). The Biomedic line of products of LaRoche-Pasay are used to treat acne and works well on sensitive skin, especially rosacea. Glytone distributed by Genesis pharmaceuticals is another product in the armamentarium for skin care specialists used for hyperpigmentation and anti-aging. The Jurlique line of products is a holistic, natural skin care line available for sensitive skin and can be used to treat acne, burns, and rosacea. SkinMedica provides a system that allows comprehensive treatment of the skin, and the skin care professional can add products as the patient's skin dictates.

PATIENT PREPARATION

Patients are advised to use only one skin care regimen and refrain from mixing different programs without consulting with their skin care professional.

TECHNIQUE

Each line has different morning and evening regimens, which are outlined by the skin care professional. These regimens work at the epidermal and dermal layers as well as the cellular level.

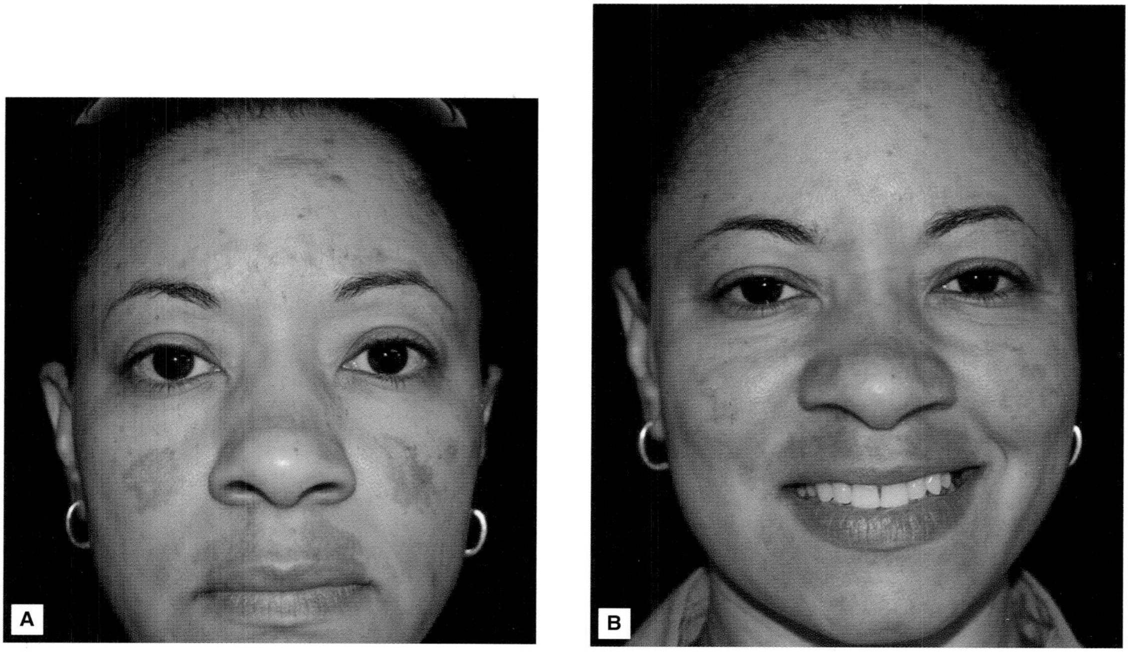

Figure 3–1. Obagi skin care system works well in treating sun damaged skin, hyperpigmented areas, melasma, and fine rhytids. **A:** Hyperpigmented areas on the forehead, bridge of nose, cheeks, and upper lip. **B:** Marked improvement in the skin tone with resolution of hyperpigmentation.

COMPLICATIONS

Most regimens produce mild redness and burning with the initiation of therapy. These symptoms subside as the skin adjusts to the therapy and rarely, the regimen has to be diluted or discontinued.

OUTCOMES ASSESSMENT

No clinical trials are currently available.

CHAPTER 4

Injectable Fillers

Lawrence S. Reed, MD & Vikisha Fripp, MD

The role of injectable fillers in soft tissue augmentation continues to expand. Ideally, an injectable implant should not cause a significant inflammatory response, be easily introduced into the recipient site, and produce an acceptably long period of volume retention. There are a plethora of agents being used for soft-tissue augmentation (Table 4–1). There are four types of semipermanent and permanent injectable fillers currently in use: polymer gels (silicone), nondegradable polymer microspheres (ArteFill), slowly degradable polymer microspheres (Sculptra and Radiesse), and autologous fat. The nonpermanent fillers are the hyaluronic acids and collagen derivatives, which are enzymatically degraded and offer short-term results. Determining the ideal filler depends on the patient's areas of concern and the condition of the skin.

From 2007 to 2008, the number of minimally invasive cosmetic procedures jumped 5% to 10.4 million procedures. The top five procedures were Botox (5 million), hyaluronic acid fillers (1.1 million), chemical peel (1 million), laser hair removal (892,000), and microdermabrasion (842,000). Hyaluronic acid fillers debuted in the top five, bumping out sclerotherapy, which had been among the top five minimally invasive procedures for the previous 3 years.

As the skin ages, hyaluronic acid, collagen, and elastin are gradually lost from the dermis. The end result is volume loss, skin laxity, and wrinkles. Although superficial perioral and periorbital wrinkles can be treated effectively with laser and chemical peel and those around the mouth can be treated with dermabrasion, deeper wrinkles and folds may require soft-tissue fillers for dermal replacement. Most injectable fillers require no pretreatment, and basic guidelines of nontreatment during active skin infection and inflammation are followed. In addition, patients with prolonged bleeding, such as those taking aspirin and ibuprofen, are cautioned.

Placement of injectable fillers requires knowledge of the anatomy of the facial muscles and the blood supply to the face in order to achieve the desired results and avoid untoward effects (Figure 4–1). Physicians may reduce the risk of complications by selecting the appropriate patients and by using proper injection technique. In general, thin skin (0.4 mm thick, as in the lids) is a contraindication

▶ TABLE 4–1. COMPARISON OF PERMANENT AND SEMIPERMANENT FILLERS

Filler Manufacturer	Composition	Particle Size	Injection Technique	Depth	Permanency	Skin Testing	Anatomical Sites	Adverse Effects
ArteFill Artes Medical, Inc., San Diego, Calif.	20% homogenous polymethylmethacrylate microspheres evenly suspended in a solution of partly denatured 3.5% bovine collagen (derived from calf skin of a closed herd in the United States) and 0.3% lidocaine	30- to 50-μm-diameter microspheres	26-gauge needle; layered, tunneling technique	Reticular dermis	Permanent	Collagen skin test	Glabellar frown lines, nasolabial folds, upper lip lines, and mouth corners	Allergy to collagen, hypertrophic scarring, and granuloma formation
Aquamid Ferrosan A/S, Copenhagen, Denmark; marketed and distributed by Contura International S.A., Soeberg, Denmark	Gel composed of 97.5% apyrogenic water bound to 2.5% crosslinked polyacrylamide	30- to 40-μm-diameter microdroplets	27-gauge needle, injected into subcutaneous tissue using fine multiline retrograde technique	Subcutaneous	Permanent	None	Lip augmentation, nasolabial folds, mouth corners, perioral wrinkles, glabella; cheek, chin, nose, and vermillion horder contouring	Hematoma, edema, skin pigment changes, granuloma
Silicone Bausch & Lomb Pharmaceuticals, Inc., Rochester, N.Y. (Adatosil 5000): Alcon Laboratories, Inc., Fort Worth. Texas (Silikon 1000)	Highly purified injectable long-chain polydimethylsiloxane silicone oil of 5000- or 1000-S viscosity	20- to 100-μm-diameter microdroplets (after injection)	28- to 30-gauge needle; microdroplet technique with a tuberculin syringe through either a linear or fanning subdermal or a multiple-stab technique	Intradermal	Permanent	None	Facial rhytides and scars, augmentation of facial eminences, correction of facial asymmetries, lip augmentation	Hardness, nodules, granuloma

Radiesse BioForm Medical, Inc., San Matteo, Calif.	Suspension of 30% calcium hydroxylapatite microspheres in a 70% gel consisting of 1.3% sodium carboxymethyl cellulose, 6.4% glycerin, and 36.6% sterile water for injection	25- to 45-μm-diameter microspheres	26-gauge needle; without overcorrection	Deep dermis	9–18 mo	None	Soft-tissue filling of nasolabial folds, lipodystrophy of cheeks, acne scars, wrinkles and hand, and liposuction contour defects	Ecchymosis, hematoma, nodules (lip augmentation), granuloma
Sculptra Dermik Laboratories, Berwyn, Pa.	Powder of poly-L-lactic acid microspheres, sodium carboxymethylcellulose, nonpyrogenic mannitol, and sterile water for injection	40- to 63-μm-diameter microspheres	26-gauge needle; tunneling or threading, depot injection (zygoma, temples), massage	Deep dermis or 1-2 yr subcutaneous	1–2 yr	None	Cheeks and temples of HIV patients on HAART	Ecchymosis, edema, subcutaneous papules, granulomas
Fat Autologous	Autologous liposuctioned fat	0.1-cc aliquots	17- to 18-gauge needle or blunt cannulae; withdrawing technique	Subcutaneous on intramuscular	Months to years	None	Lips, nasolabial folds, postliposuction deformities, hands	Resorption, fat cysts, edema

HAART, highly active antiretroviral therapy; N/A, not applicable
Reproduced with permission from *Plast Reconstr Surg.* 2006;118:974.

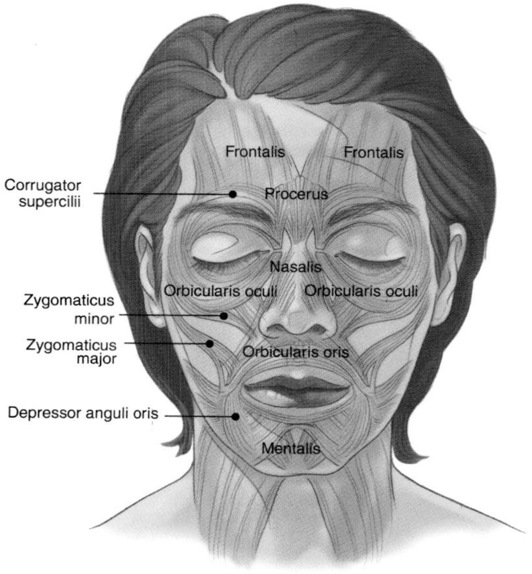

Figure 4–1. Knowledge of facial anatomy is essential for proper placement of both Botox and injectable fillers.

for all fillers, especially around the eyes and in cheeks that have many tiny wrinkles. Also, lighter skinned patients are more prone to allergic reactions. The level of injection into the skin depends on the filler being used; however, most fillers are placed within or below the dermis. The indications for more superficial placement include treatment of acne or surgical/traumatic scars.

Touch-up injections are required in most patients to maintain the desired results. Different injectable fillers may be used within the same setting without adverse effects, and because fillers are placed at the level of the dermis, laser treatments can also be done in the same setting. There are few medical contraindications to injectable fillers, including diabetes, HIV infection, immunosuppression, autoimmune and rheumatoid disease, and lupus.

REFERENCES

Broder KW et al. An overview of permanent and semipermanent fillers. *Plast Reconstr Surg.* 2006 Sep;118(3 Suppl)7S–14S. [PMID: 16936539]

Eppley BL et al. Injectable soft-tissue fillers: clinical overview. *Plast Reconstr Surg.* 2006 Sep 15; 118(4):98e–106e. [PMID: 16980841]

► NONPERMANENT FILLERS

HYALURONIC ACIDS (RESTYLANE, CAPTIQUE, JUVÉDERM, HYLAFORM)

A. Patient Evaluation and Selection

Before any hyaluronic acid filler is selected for use, a complete history is required because severe effects can be seen in patients with certain conditions. Restylane, Captique, and Juvéderm are all derived from *Streptococcus equi,* and patients with allergies to bacterial proteins should avoid its use. Patients with certain neuromuscular disorders such as amyotrophic lateral sclerosis (ALS), myasthenia gravis, or Lambert-Eaton syndrome may be at increased risk for serious side effects as well. Hylaform is a chemically modified hyaluronic acid derived from a bird (avian) source and patients with avian allergies should refrain from using this product (Table 4–2).

Restylane was approved by the FDA in 2003 for mid-dermal applications such as deeper wrinkle reduction, especially around the mouth and nose and for lip augmentation; nasolabial folds; and glabellar creases. It has even been successfully used in the treatment of tear trough deformities (Figures 4–2A and 4–2B). Restylane Fine Lines is indicated for thin superficial wrinkles. Perlane is intended for shaping facial contours and correcting deep folds and for lip augmentation. Restylane typically lasts up to 6 months or longer.

▶ TABLE 4-2. **HYALURONIC ACID DERMAL FILLER OPTIONS**

	Restylane	Captique	Hylaform	Hylaform Plus
Source	Bacterial fermentation	Bacterial fermentation	Nongender chicken combs	Nongender chicken combs
Cross-linking agent	1,4-Butandiol diglycidylether	Divinyl sulfone	Divinyl sulfone	Divinyl sulfone
Degree of concentration	1%	20%	20%	20%
Hyaluronic acid concentration	20 mg/mL	4.5-6.0 mg/mL	4.5-6.0 mg/mL	4.5-6.0 mg/mL
Gel particle size	400 pm	500 pm	500 pm	750 pm

Captique is derived from the same nonanimal source as Restylane but through a different manufacturing process. Patients requiring improvement in facial wrinkles have Captique as another option. It is indicated for fine lines and wrinkles with longevity of 3 to 6 months. Patients concerned about bruising and swelling may benefit from this self-purported advantage.

Juvéderm Ultra and Juvéderm Ultra Plus are indicated for injection into the mid to deep dermis for contouring and volumizing of moderate to severe facial wrinkles and folds. It is the first FDA-approved hyaluronic acid dermal filler with demonstrated safety and efficacy in persons of color. It is not to be used in patients with presence of multiple severe allergies and history of allergies to gram-positive bacterial proteins. Patients with certain neuromuscular disorders such as ALS, myasthenia gravis, or Lambert-Eaton syndrome may be at increased risk for serious side effects. It is purported to last 6 to 9 months.

Like other hyaluronic acids, Hylaform is used to replenish the dermal volume loss that allows wrinkles to form. It is also used to enhance lips and fill in acne scars. Hylaform's effects are immediate and last for about 12 weeks.

B. Patient Preparation

The patient's skin is examined for the presence of active infection, inflammation, or bruising. The skin is cleansed with alcohol gauze and topical anesthetic is applied. The areas of concern are then identified and marked with an eyebrow pencil or marking pen.

C. Technique

All hyaluronic acid fillers are placed into the dermis. They are injected beneath the wrinkle or fold at the dermal layer in a linear fashion, using a 27- or 30-gauge needle. Overcorrection is not required because the product draws water to the area. Results are seen immediately and are fully evident within 1 week. As degradation occurs over time, water is attracted to the material at the site of implantation. This feature is what probably accounts for its longer volume retention effects than bovine collagen; however, follow-up treatments are needed. The amount of hyaluronic acid used per session depends on the depth of the wrinkle or fold and the number of areas being treated.

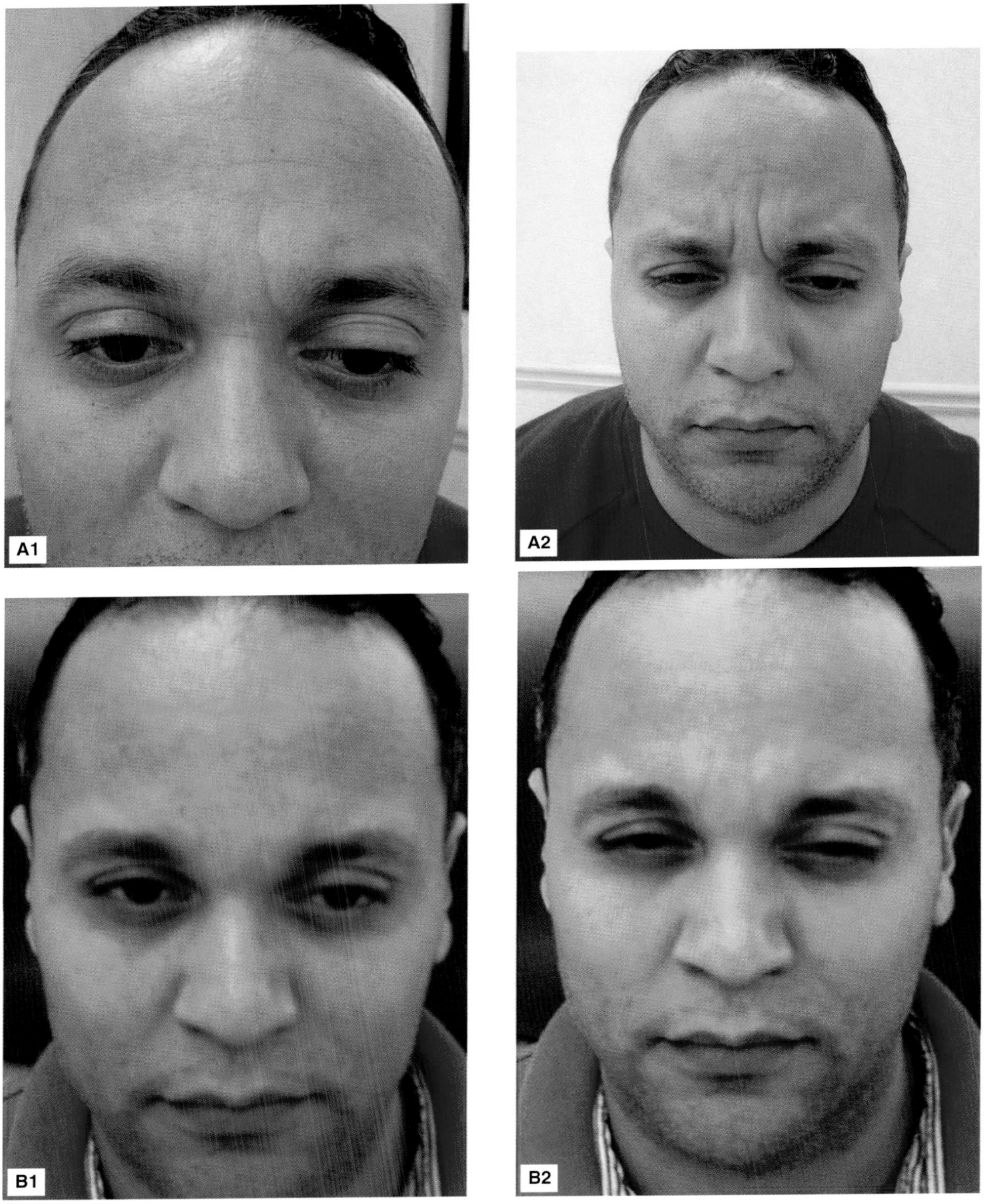

Figure 4–2. **A:** *Before* treatment with Botox and Restylane, the glabellar crease is pronounced. **B:** *After* treatment with Botox and Restylane, notice the softening of the glabellar crease.

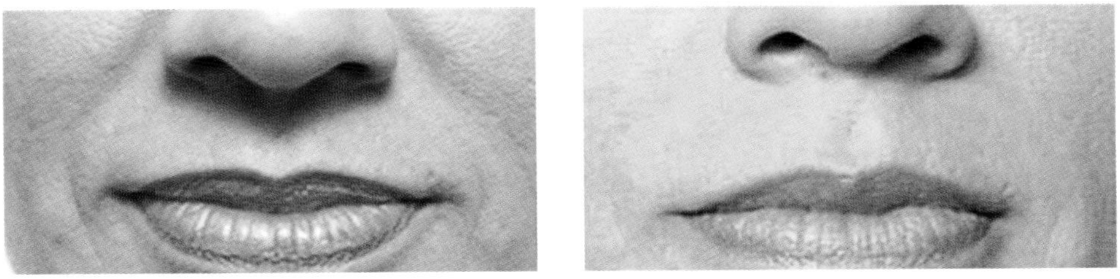

Figure 4–3. The nasolabial folds have been treated with Juvéderm (left, before; right, after) (Used with permission from Allergan.)

D. Complications

The most common side effects of Restylane include headache, nausea, flu-like symptoms, redness, and pain at the injection points. Infrequently, patients experience muscle weakness, which resolves itself within days or, in some cases, months after the procedure. There may also be pronounced swelling lasting 2 or 3 days. Severe contour irregularities and pronounced pain may necessitate removal of the product, which is accomplished by injecting hyaluronidase to dissolve the product. Captique, Juvéderm, and Hylaform share temporary injection site reactions, such as redness, pain, firmness, swelling, and bumps. Hylaform has also been reported to cause temporary eyelid droop and nausea.

E. Outcome Assessment

In 2006, Matarasso et al and the Restylane Consensus group compared Restylane, Captique, Hylaform, and HylaformPlus. The factor that distinguished the products was the four-fold increase concentration of hyaluronic acid in Restylane and small particle size. These properties allowed Restylane to maintain its volume through isovolumetric degradation, increasing its longevity. An independent three-arm clinical trial done by Juvéderm enrolled 349 patients and compared their product with control and Zyplast. At 6 months post-treatment, 78% to 88% of patients preferred Juvéderm. Figure 4–3 shows the results of Juvéderm 6 months after the injection.

REFERENCES

Kane MA. Treatment of tear trough deformity and lower lid bowing with injectable hyaluronic acid. *Aesthetic Plast Surg.* 2005 Sep–Oct;29(5):363–7. [PMID: 16151656]

Matarasso SL et al; Restylane Consensus Group. Consensus recommendations for soft-tissue augmentation with nonanimal stabilized hyaluronic acid (Restylane). *Plast Reconstr Surg.* 2006 Mar; 117(3 Suppl):3S–34S. [PMID: 16531934]

Product inserts for Juvéderm.

COLLAGEN

A. Patient Evaluation and Selection

Collagen's use has markedly declined with the emergence of hyaluronic acid dermal fillers. Patients generally request treatment on the day of evaluation, and the pretesting required for collagen does not allow this option. Collagen remains an option for soft-tissue augmentation in areas such as the lips and treatment of superficial to moderate facial wrinkles and scars on the face, neck, back, and chest.

B. Patient Preparation

Pretesting is required for collagen products. Bovine-derived products require a series of testing, which delays treatment for at least 1 month. However, human-derived collagen products can be tested on the day of initial consultation and evaluated in 72 hours, after which treatment can begin. Skin testing is most commonly done on the volar forearm.

The skin over the treatment area is cleansed of makeup and debris; a topical anesthetic agent is applied, or a nerve block is performed. The areas to be treated are then marked with an eyebrow pencil or a marking pen.

C. Technique

With the skin held slightly taut, the collagen product is delivered into the superficial/mid dermis layer through a 30-gauge needle. Multiple passes are used to layer the product under the area of the wrinkle. The skin is watched for blanching, which indicates that the product has been delivered into the appropriate depth. Approximately, 20% to 30% overcorrection is recommended.

D. Complications

Chronic granulomatous reactions have been seen with lip augmentation. When the placement is too superficial, irregularities, which appear as lightly pigmented globules, may result. Allergies to the bovine component of bovine-derived collagen is a known adverse reaction.

E. Outcomes Assessment

There are no clinical trials comparing collagen products with other available dermal fillers.

REFERENCE

Fagien S. Facial soft-tissue augmentation with injectable autologous and allogeneic human tissue collagen matrix (autologen and dermalogen). *Plast Reconstr Surg.* 2000 Jan;105(1):362–74. [PMID: 10627006]

► SEMIPERMANENT FILLERS

RADIESSE

A. Patient Evaluation and Selection

Radiesse is approved by the US Food and Drug Administration (FDA) for use in oromaxillofacial defects. Off-label uses include reduction of the appearance of wrinkles and skin folds around the mouth and nose; lip augmentation; and soft-tissue filling of the nasolabial folds, acne scars, post liposuction defects, and facial lipodystrophy. There has been some concern regarding the use of Radiesse in the lips after Zide cited white, hard calcium nodules in approximately 50% of patients after the methylcellulose component dissipated. Jansen et al explained that the highly mobile environment of the lip combined with overly aggressive volume injection led to nodule formation; to lessen this complication, precise placement of the product in the potential space between the orbicularis oris muscle and the mucosa is recommended.

B. Patient Preparation

The patient's skin is examined for the presence of active infection, inflammation, or bruising. The skin is cleansed with alcohol gauze to remove makeup and debris and topical anesthetic is applied. The areas of concern are then identified and marked with an eyebrow pencil or marking pen (Figure 4–4A).

C. Technique

Radiesse injections are performed in the clinician's office with the use of topical anesthesia. The product is injected into the deep dermis using a 25-gauge needle and no overcorrection

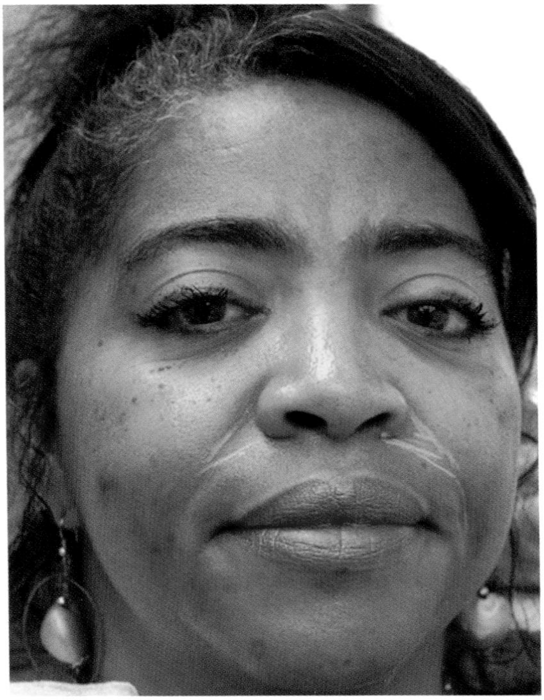

Figure 4–4A. White soft pencil is used to mark the area of depression.

is required (Figure 4–4B). Patients may experience minimal discomfort from the needle injection. Depending on the extent of the treatment, the procedure can take a few minutes to 20 minutes. Radiesse is fully evident within a week and can last 2 years or more, though touchups may be necessary throughout this time period. Results are expected to be evident from 9 to 18 months (Figure 4–4C–E).

D. Complications

The adverse affects of Radiesse injection are ecchymosis, erythema, edema, pain, and pruritus, which are usually minimal and subside within 24 to 36 hours. A rare complication is the appearance of nodules, which may require corticosteroid treatment (Figure 4–4F) or surgical intervention. Patients return to normal activity after the treatment with the advice to stay out of the sun.

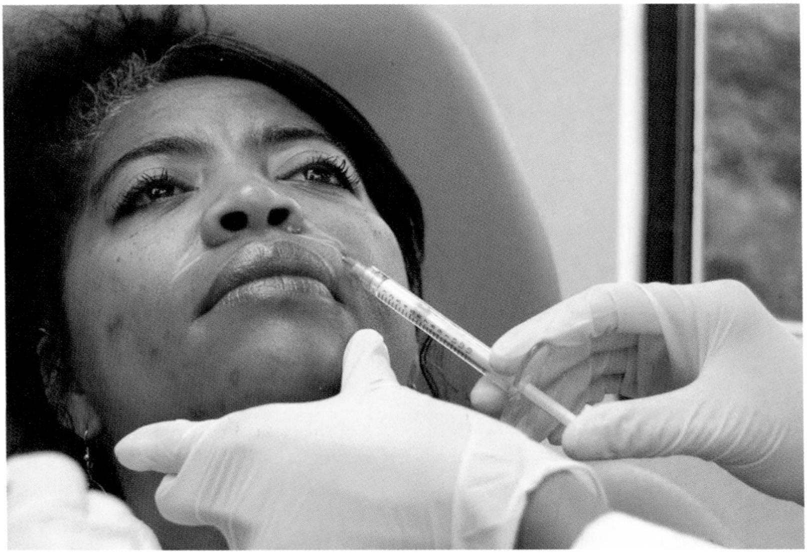

Figure 4–4B. The needle is inserted in the dermis/subcutaneous interface.

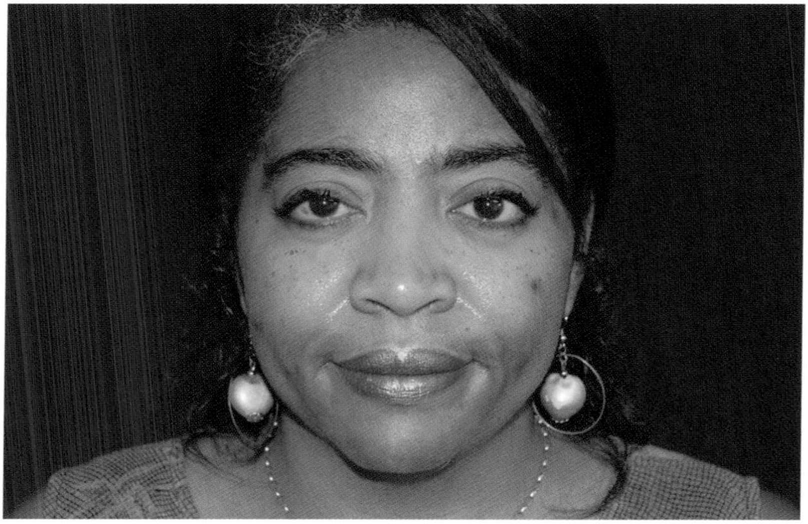

Figure 4–4C. *Before* treatment, the nasolabial folds are moderately deep.

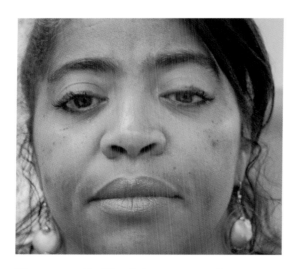

Figure 4–4D. The *left* nasolabial fold has been treated; notice the difference in the volume between the treated and untreated side.

E. Outcomes Assessment

Silvers et al report that of the 100 HIV-infected patients participating in their study, 99% of the patients would "recommend Radiesse treatment" and 98% felt that the treatment had been "beneficial," at 12 months. The safety of the product was assessed by the same group. They recorded the incidence, severity, and duration of all adverse events from baseline through 18 months. Their clinical trial established Radiesse as being a safe medical device for soft-tissue augmentation for the treatment of facial lipoatrophy.

In a larger study done by Jansen et al, 155 participants reported an overall treatment satisfaction at 6 months of 3.94 (on a scale of 1 to 5, with 5 being the highest). In addition, 89% of participants said they would chose to receive the same treatment again. At 12- to

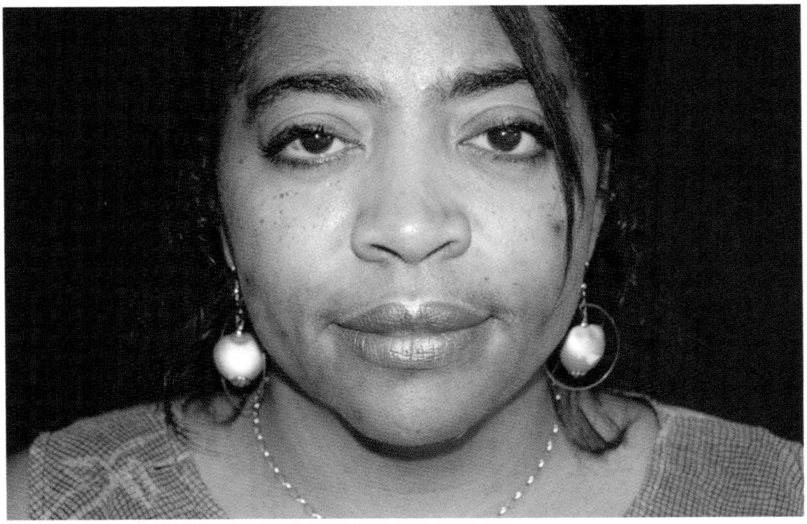

Figure 4–4E. Both nasolabial folds have been treated; notice the softening of the nasolabial folds and lack of alar depression.

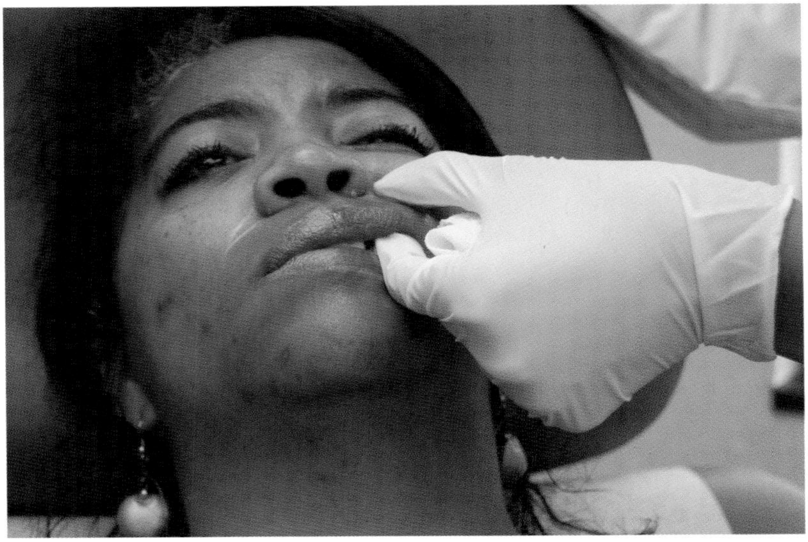

Figure 4–4F. To avoid the rare complication of nodules, it is important to massage the treatment area after injection.

24-month follow-up, 69% reported continued satisfaction and 74% stated they would have repeat application, if desired.

REFERENCES

Jansen DA et al. Evaluation of calcium hydroxlyapatite-based implant (Radiesse) for facial soft-tissue augmentation. *Plast Reconstr Surg.* 2006 Sep;118(3 Suppl):22S–30S. [PMID: 16936541]

Silvers SL et al. Prospective, open-label, 18-month trial of calcium hydroxylapatite (Radiesse) for facial soft-tissue augmentation in patients with human immunodeficiency virus-associated lipoatrophy: one-year durability. *Plast Reconstr Surg.* 2006 Sep;118(3 Suppl):34S–45S. [PMID: 16936543]

Zide BM. Radiance Short-term experience. *Aesthet Surg J.* 2003 Nov–Dec;23(6):495–9. [PMID: 19336126]

SCULPTRA

A. Patient Evaluation and Selection

This product is FDA approved for restoration and correction of the signs of facial fat loss (lipoatrophy) in people with HIV infection. Its off-label use in patients without HIV infection mirrors its approval indications.

B. Patient Preparation

The patient's skin is examined for the presence of active infection, inflammation, or bruising. The skin is cleansed with alcohol gauze to remove makeup and debris, and topical anesthetic is applied. The areas of concern are then identified and marked with an eyebrow pencil or marking pen.

C. Technique

The product is packaged as two vials of sterile freeze-dried preparation, which have to be hydrated by the addition of 5 mL of sterile water prior to use. Most users add 1 mL of lidocaine with 4 mL of sterile water to aid in anesthesia. The reconstitution is recommended a minimum of 2 hours before the procedure with the best product obtained with 24 hours or more of reconstitution. It is shaken vigorously before drawing up into a tuberculin syringe and is usable for 72 hours. It is stored at room temperature before and after hydration.

Sculptra is injected between the deep dermis and subcutaneous layer with a 25- to 26-gauge, 1-inch needle. The product is administered in 0.1 to 0.2 mL aliquots in a depot technique in the temporal region or zygoma areas or via tunneling techniques. Overcorrection of the area is not needed as collagen formation cannot be precisely predicted. The area is massaged after the procedure to avoid clumping and to evenly distribute the product. Self-massage is then done three to four times daily for the first few post-procedure days. Ice is applied to the areas immediately after the injections.

The quantity of Sculptra and the number of injection sessions will vary by patient. A typical treatment course for severe facial fat loss involves three to six injection sessions, with sessions separated from 2 to 3 weeks to 3 months. The original skin depressions may initially reappear, but the depressions should gradually improve within several weeks as the treatment effect of Sculptra occurs. Full effects of the treatment course are evident within weeks to months. The patients should be reevaluated no sooner than 2 weeks after each injection session to determine whether additional correction is needed. Patients should be advised that supplemental injection sessions may be required to maintain an optimal treatment effect.

D. Complications

Immediately following an injection session with Sculptra, redness, swelling, and bruising may be noted in the treatment area. The most common adverse effect is the delayed occurrence of subcutaneous papules, which are confined to the injection site typically palpable, asymptomatic, and nonvisible. The patient should minimize exposure of the treatment area to excessive sun and UV lamp exposure until any initial swelling and redness has resolved.

E. Outcomes Assessment

Valantin et al and Moyle et al report improved quality of life and anxiety and depression in HIV-positive patients.

REFERENCES

Moyle GJ et al. A randomized open-label study of immediate versus delayed polylactic acid injections for the cosmetic management of facial lipoatrophy in person with HIV infection. *HIV Med.* 2004 Mar;5(2):82–7. [PMID: 15012646]

Valantin MA et al. Polylactic acid implants (New-Fill) to correct facial lipoatrophy in HIV-infected patients: results of the open-label study VEGA. *AIDS.* 2003 Nov;17(17):2471–7. [PMID: 14600518]

▶ AUTOLOGOUS FAT

PATIENT EVALUATION & SELECTION

Fat is used to restore volume to the nasolabial, tear trough areas, Marionette lines, submental grooves, lips, hands, and postliposuction deformities. Most patients are candidates for autologous fat injection because it can be taken from multiple donor sites and is easy to harvest. The site chosen for harvest depends on the ease of accessibility and the area of most favorable site for contour improvement.

PATIENT PREPARATION

Patients are either under sedation during this process or a local anesthetic is used. The patient is then positioned in the optimal position to aid in harvesting of the fat graft.

TECHNIQUE

Autologous fat is usually harvested using a Coleman cannula and a Luer-Lok syringe setup. The cannula is guided into the harvest site with multiple passes done until the syringe is filled. Once filled, the syringe alone is then placed in the centrifuge. The oil, blood, water, and debris are separated from the fat in this process and the pure, filtered fat is injected subcutaneously or intramuscularly using an 18-gauge blunt tip needle. Blunt tip needles allow for more precise, less traumatic placement of the fat grafts. The autologous fat is injected at an interval of 0.1 mL per site during withdrawal to minimize resorption and act as scaffolding for further treatment.

COMPLICATIONS

The major complications of autologous fat are placement of inappropriate quantities as well as irregularities and overgrowth of fat grafts with or without weight gain. Post-procedural swelling is an expected occurrence and can be minimized by elevation, cold therapy, and external pressure on the area.

OUTCOMES ASSESSMENT

No objective data have been published on the satisfaction level of patients receiving autologous fat grafts or on the true longevity of the injected product. Ersek et al reported promising results from the lipo-layering technique they discovered, with clinically acceptable results with up to an 8-year postoperative follow-up. Thirty to fifty percent of implants do not survive; however, it is quite simple to repeat this procedure under local anesthesia as an outpatient procedure in a few minutes. Therefore, several repeated episodes can accumulate enough viable fat cells to maintain the desired augmentation. Long-term storage of fat in liquid nitrogen is being studied so that harvested and processed material may be available for injection months or years later.

REFERENCES

Coleman SR. Structural fat grafting: more than a permanent filler. *Plast Reconstr Surg.* 2006 Sep;118(3 Suppl):108S–120S. [PMID: 16936550]

Ersek RA et al. Lipo layering of autologous fat: an improved technique with promising results. *Plast Reconstr Surg.* 1998 Mar;101(3):820–6. [PMID: 9500405]

▶ PERMANENT FILLERS

Although semipermanent injectable fillers offer immediate correction of varying superficial rhytids, they are biologic agents that are metabolized and degraded. The typical half-life of these agents ranges from 6 to 9 months. The desire for longer lasting agents prompted the search for permanent injectable fillers. ArteFill and silicone are discussed below. Other dermal fillers being used in Europe and Asia include the polymethylmethacrylate microspheres (eg, Aphrodite Gold of the Netherlands, Metacrill of Brazil, Bioplasty of Brazil, and Precise of Mexico), which remain unchanged throughout the patient's life and provide a scaffold for continuously renewed connective tissue formation and vascularity. These permanent agents provide the prospect for an ideal agent for use in facial rejuvenation; their existence should be noted and watched for their emergence into the U.S. market.

ARTEFILL

A. Patient Evaluation and Selection

ArteFill is best used to treat wrinkles of the glabella, nasolabial folds, radial upper lip lines, and corners of the mouth. Patients seeking long-term dermal fillers are candidates for treatment with this product.

B. Patient Preparation

Patients must be skin tested for allergy to the bovine collagen component. Before injection of the product, topical anesthetic cream/ointment is applied and, for the upper lip, local anesthesia is used when indicated.

C. Technique

ArteFill is implanted into the dermal/subcutaneous fat interface with a 26-gauge needle using a higher constant pressure because of its high viscosity. The product is delivered using the tunneling technique and is deposited in a layered fashion. ArteFill then settles into the deep dermis and, if necessary, is reinjected deep into the deep dermis to "fill" in the wrinkle. In patients with thin skin, the implant may appear erythematous for several weeks, and the implant may be visualized as small white granules. The material is then massaged with the fingertip, and slight pressure is applied to detect any lumps.

D. Complications

One study reported a less than 0.02% incidence of complication with the use of ArteFill. The most common adverse effects were inaccurate depth of injection, allergy to the collagen component, hypertrophic scarring, and granuloma formation.

E. Outcomes Assessment

After deep dermal injection of ArteFill, the collagen carrier is degraded by the body within 1 to 3 months and completely replaced by the body's own collagen at a similar rate, ensuring a steady augmentation result. Because the polymethyl microspheres are nonbiodegradable and too large to migrate or to be phagocytosed by macrophages, the tissue augmentation is expected to be permanent, consisting of

80% of autologous connective tissue volume. The results of a 4- to 5-year study from Broder et al showed that the quantity of ArteFill used was nearly half that of collagen. Patients' satisfaction rating and investigator success rating for the ArteFill group were also higher than for collagen in each of the injection sites (glabellar folds, nasolabial folds, upper lip lines, and mouth corners) at 6 months after implantation. Human histologic examination reported by Lemperle reveals that at 9 months, the ArteFill injection is unchanged in size, which suggests a lack of microsphere dissipation, phagocytosis, or migration to lymph nodes.

REFERENCES

Broder KW et al. An overview of permanent and semipermanent fillers. *Plast Reconstr Surg*. 2006 Sep;118(3 Suppl):7S–14S. [PMID: 16936539]

Lemperle G et al. Human histology and persistence of various injectable filler substances for soft tissue augmentation. *Aesthetic Plast Surg*. 2003 Sep–Oct;27(5):354–66. [PMID: 14648064]

SILICONE

A. Patient Evaluation and Selection

Another option for patients requesting longer lasting dermal fillers are the silicone oils. Silicone oil (eg, AdatoSil 5000 and Silikon 1000) is only FDA approved for use in the treatment of severe retinal detachment and use during eye surgery to prevent or treat detached retina. Its off-label uses include acne scars; glabella, nasolabial, and marionette folds; cheek hollows; tear troughs; chin and cheek augmentation; and post-rhinoplasty defects.

B. Patient Preparation

The patient's skin is examined for the presence of active infection, inflammation, or bruising. The skin is cleansed with alcohol gauze to remove makeup and debris, and topical anesthetic is applied. The areas of concern are then identified and marked with an eyebrow pencil or marking pen.

C. Technique

The microdroplet technique is used, delivering miniscule amounts of product at very precise depths in the subdermal plane. Benedetto et al describe the microdroplet technique as 0.01 to 0.02 mL of silicone injected subdermally with a tuberculin syringe through a 28- to 30-gauge needle. Either the linear fanning or multiple stab technique is used. Multiple injections sessions are needed at monthly intervals.

D. Complications

The complications of silicone use are bruising, edema, and erythema, although their incidence is reported by Orentreich to be less than the other available fillers. Other complications are beading, which occurs when it is placed too superficially; granuloma formation; cellulitis; ulcerations; migration; and nodule formation. The most severe complications are pneumonitis from large-volume injections, severe edema, and localized discoloration of the area injected.

E. Outcomes Assessment

Clinical trials are underway in the United States for the use of silicone oil as a facial soft-tissue filler; however, no current study is available.

REFERENCES

Benedetto AV et al. Injecting 1000 centistoke liquid silicone with ease and precision. *Dermatol Surg*. 2003 Mar;29(3):211–4. [PMID: 12614410]

Orentreich DS. Liquid injectable silicone: techniques for soft tissue augmentation. *Clin Plast Surg*. 2000 Oct;27(4):595-612. [PMID: 11039892]

CHAPTER 5

Cosmetic Uses of Botox

Nicholas Clavin, MD, Vikisha Fripp, MD, Brooke Burkey, MD, Lawrence S. Reed, MD, & Mia Talmor, MD

In the past decade, there has been an enormous rise in the number of cosmetic procedures performed in the United States. As public exposure to the field of cosmetic surgery grows, more and more people are considering facial enhancement procedures than ever before. Aesthetic plastic surgery is no longer restricted to the very wealthy. A large part of this expanding accessibility is due to advances in technology and the boom of both nonsurgical and minimally invasive techniques of facial enhancement. These techniques are typically less expensive and require less recovery time than open surgical procedures. Leading the way since its reinvention as a cosmetic injectable in the early 1990s, botulinum toxin type A (Botox, Allergan, Inc., Irvine, Calif.) injection has remained the most common cosmetic procedure performed in the United States. The American Society for Aesthetic Plastic Surgery maintains a Cosmetic Surgery National Data Bank that is the authoritative source for statistics on cosmetic surgery in the United States. In 2005, almost 11.5 million total cosmetic procedures, both surgical and non-surgical, were performed by the plastic surgeons, dermatologists, and otolaryngologists surveyed. Of these procedures, 9.5 million (83%) were nonsurgical. Botox injections rank at the top of the nonsurgical list, with 3.2 million procedures performed in 2005. Compare these figures to those from 1997 when 65,000 Botox injection procedures were performed comprising only 3.1% of the total 2.1 million procedures. With these trends in mind, it is obvious that Botox procedures are a crucial element in the current armamentarium of the plastic surgeon.

PATIENT SELECTION

Although Botox is not an injectable filler, it is used in combination with dermal fillers to provide comprehensive treatment of facial laxity and rhytids. The ideal patient has wrinkles in the periocular and glabella region, which can be softened with Botox. Although some dermal regeneration occurs once the dermal fat is lost, a filler is generally needed to diminish the wrinkle depth. Patients with perioral wrinkles, platysmal banding, and mentalis overactivity can also be treated with Botox therapy.

A crucial component of the evaluation is the anatomy and interaction of the facial musculature (Figure 5–1). The Consensus group points out that eyebrow shape is altered with injections into the procerus, corrugators, and orbicularis oculi muscles; therefore, the patient's desires have to be known before the procedure. This is important because the positions of the brows mold the aesthetics of the face and have different positions between the genders. The same holds true when Botox is injected around the mouth; the position of the mouth shapes the lower portion of the face.

PATIENT PREPARATION

Botox injections are performed in the doctor's office, usually without anesthesia. However, a numbing cream may be applied to the treatment area. No pretreatment is required; however, patients with active skin infection or inflammation, and those currently taking aspirin are not treated. Prior to the start of the procedure, the skin is cleansed with alcohol and the injection sites are marked with a marking pencil.

TECHNIQUE

The product is reconstituted with 2 to 4 mL of preserved saline and the increments are units per 0.1 mL. The Botox Consensus group recommended refraining from agitation and foam to avoid issues with potency. It is drawn into a tuberculin needle and injected at points where the muscle contracts not within the wrinkle itself.

A. Glabellar and Periocular Rhytids (Crow's Feet)

Some experts advocate touching the periosteum and then pulling back to ensure the product is administered into the muscle, while others advocate piercing the skin and delivering the product directly below the level of the skin. The glabella is typically treated with 20 to 25 units of Botox, while the periocular rhytids are injected with 5 to 10 units per side (Figures 5–2 and 5–3).

B. Perioral

With the lips pursed the orbicularis oris muscle is easily identified. The Botox, 2 units, is typically injected at each corner of the lip, adjacent to the vermillion border (Figures 5–4 and 5–5).

C. Platysmal Banding

To decrease the appearance of these bands, 25 to 50 units of Botox is injected into the muscle. The injection sites are 1.5 cm apart, and the product is placed directly into the muscle.

D. Mentalis Overactivity

The mentalis muscle is identified coursing from the inferior edge of the symphysis to the skin of the lower lip. The patient is asked to tense the muscle by pressing the lips together. Three to five units of Botox is injected directly into the muscle belly.

The treatment typically takes less than 15 minutes. The effects of Botox are typically seen 7 to 10 days after treatment and can be expected to last from 3 to 6 months.

COMPLICATIONS

When properly administered to the appropriately selected patient population, Botox injection can be considered safe and with minimal risk of complication. The most common side effects of Botox include headache, nausea, flu-like symptoms, redness, and pain at the injection points. Most problems that occur after injection are unwanted side effects that can be avoided with careful and meticulous technique. In order to minimize complication risk, there are several crucial points that exist

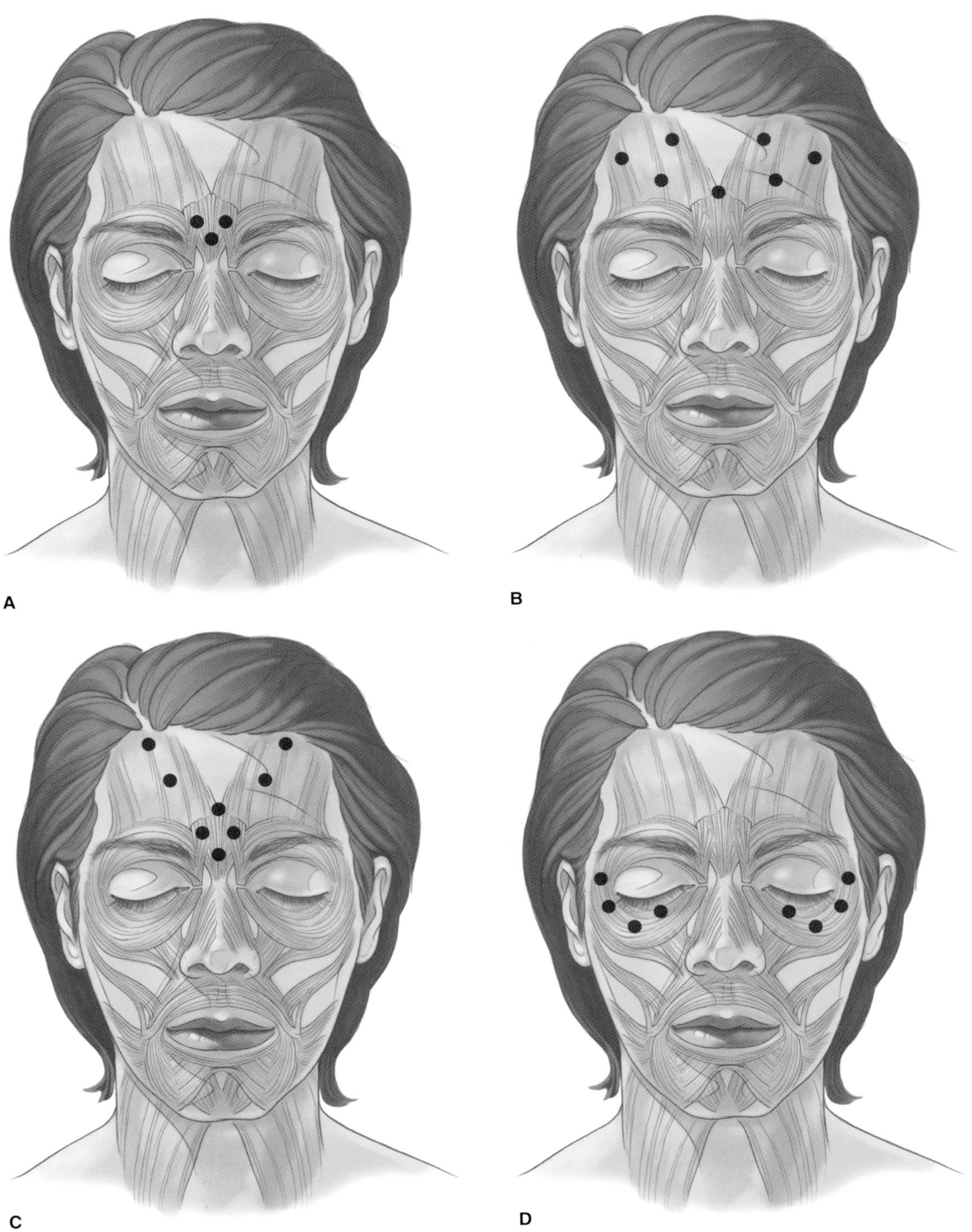

Figure 5–1. Approximate areas of injection of Botox for the following areas of concern. **A:** Glabellar creases. **B:** Transverse forehead furrows. **C:** Technique for brow elevation in patients with brow ptosis. **D:** Lateral canthal rhytids (subcutaneous injection).

Before

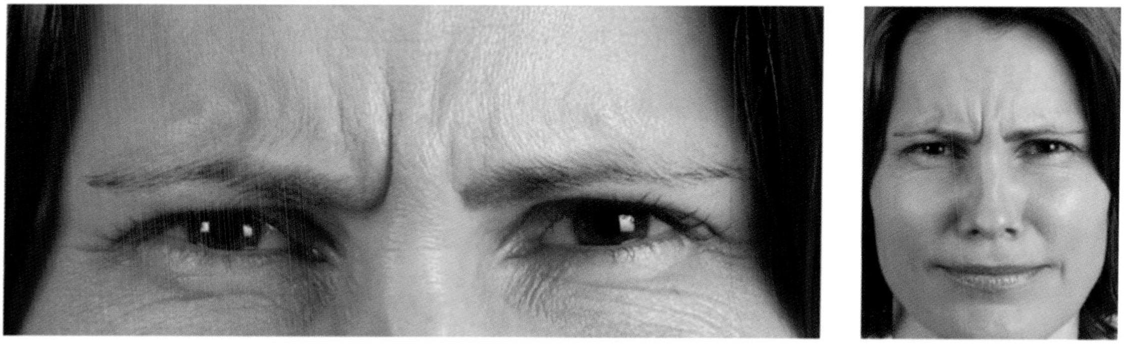

After

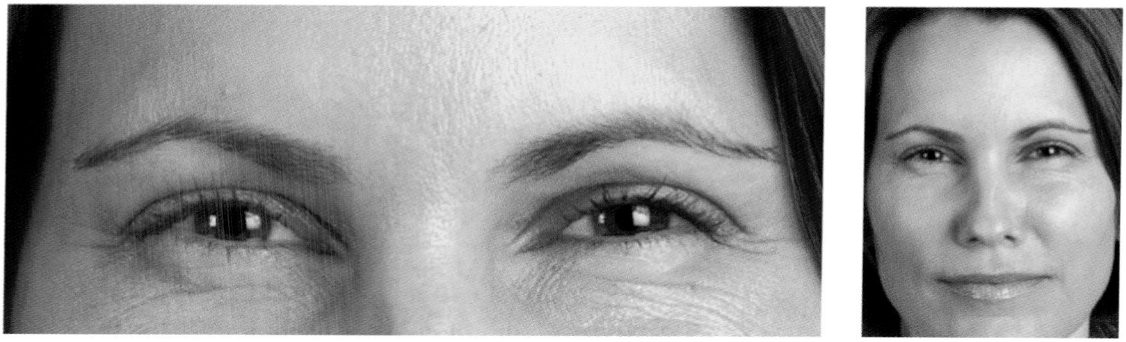

Figures 5–2 and 5–3. Before and after Botox injection for glabellar and periocular rhytids. (Used with permission from Allergan.)

that must be addressed *prior* to the procedure. The first is patient selection. The emphasis here should be on both identifying contraindications as well as patients with unrealistic expectations. The second point is preparation and storage of the solution. Errors in this process can cause a myriad of problems. The third point is the procedure itself, in which meticulous technique can prevent problems that range from minor ecchymoses to dysphagia. Finally, postoperative counseling with care instructions and "what to expect" information should be completed before and after the procedure. Serious or permanent complications are extremely rare.

There are many potential unwanted effects of Botox injections that relate specifically to imprecise targeting of the facial muscles (Table 5–1). The first is a general "overparalysis," which results in a masklike facies and loss of facial expression. Avoiding this complication mandates the appropriate dose be delivered to the desired muscle group. It has been observed that large volumes of dilute toxin are more likely to diffuse to unwanted muscles. For example, in an attempt to minimize the complication of brow ptosis, many surgeons avoid treating multiple areas of the upper third of the face at once. Injection should also be administered at least 1 cm above the eyebrow.

Before

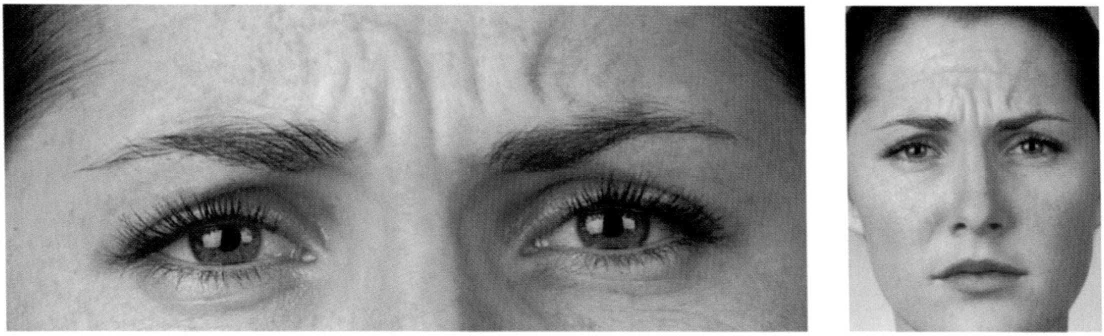

After

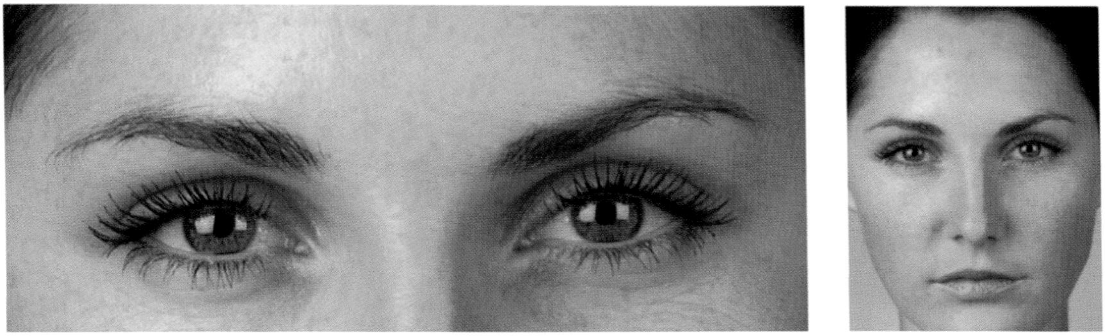

Figures 5-2 and 5-3. (Continued)

This preserves both brow position and movement for expression.

The second complication that relates to imprecise targeting of the facial muscles is insufficient paralysis, resulting in residual rhytids. Causes include insufficient dosing of the toxin and failure to accurately target the involved muscles. When determining the dose of Botox, the clinician must take into account the bulk of the muscle mass to be injected. This varies among individual muscles as well as between men and women, with men typically having more muscle bulk than women. In some cases, skin thickness must also be taken into account. On occasion, weakening of the muscle is preferred to complete paralysis. The forehead region is an example where some patients and clinicians may prefer to retain some function to avoid the masklike facies, at the expense of some residual rhytids.

A corollary problem to insufficient paralysis of a given muscle is insufficient treatment of a muscle complex. This problem is well-demonstrated in the forehead area where treatment of the central portion of the frontalis muscle without adequate treatment of the lateral frontalis will result in a perplexed expression, where the peak of the eyebrow is farther from the midline than would appear naturally. This complication can be avoided by cautiously and conservatively injecting the lateral frontalis, with the knowledge that

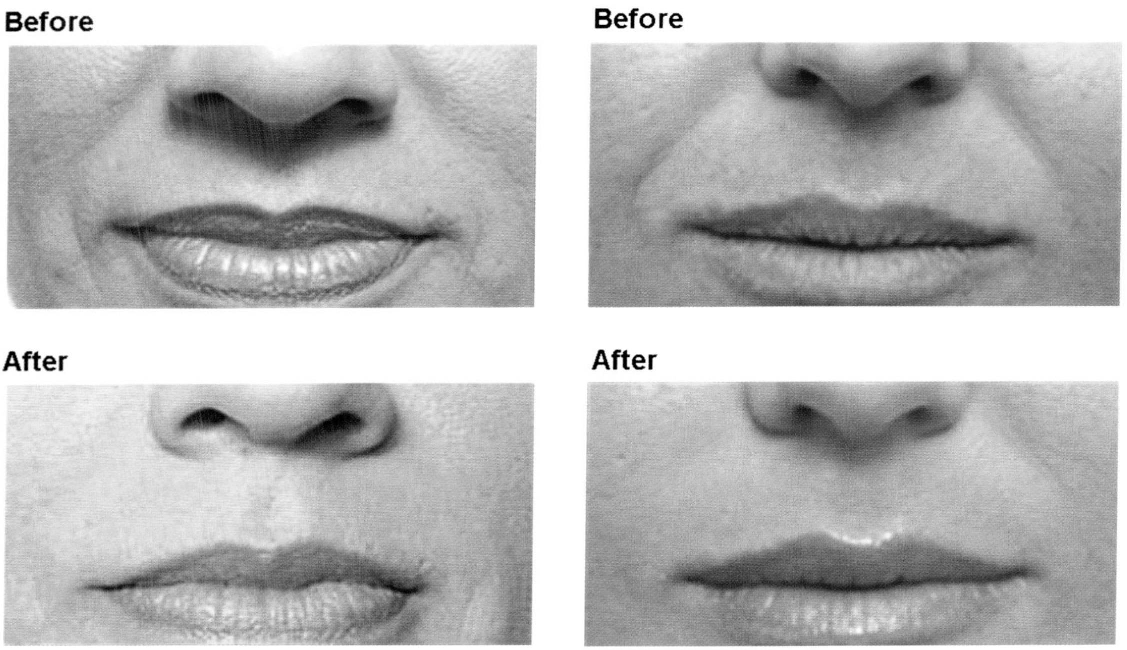

Figures 5–4 and 5–5. Before and after Botox injection for perioral rhytids. (Used with permission from Allergan.)

▶ **TABLE 5–1. RATES OF ADVERSE EVENTS REPORTED IN THE LITERATURE ARE EXTREMELY LOW, DESPITE THE WIDE RANGE OF POSSIBLE COMPLICATIONS**

Anatomic Area	Unwanted Effect	Etiology	Prevention/Treatment
Glabella	Ptosis	Diffusion to levator muscle	Accurate, low-volume injections, α-adrenergic agonists
Forehead	Mask-like facies Heavy brow Brow ptosis	Complete paralysis of frontalis muscle	Restrict injections to 1 cm above eyebrow
	Perplexed/quizzical appearance	Incomplete treatment of lateral frontalis muscle	Judicious supplemental injections
Crow's feet	Lower lid droop Ectropion Exposure keratitis	Weakening of Orbicularis muscle support	Injections at least 1 cm from lateral canthus and above zygoma
	Diplopia	Lateral rectus muscle paralysis	
Perioral	Lateral lip droop	Levator labii superioris, zygomaticus, or orbicularis oris paralysis	Accurate technique
Neck	Dysphagia Neck weakness	Diffusion or direct injection into SCM, diffusion into muscles of deglutition	Accurate technique Reassurance Diet modification

SCM, sternocleidomastoid.

CHAPTER 6

Aesthetic Laser Surgery

Kenneth O. Rothaus, MD

Lasers have been used clinically by physicians and surgeons for decades. The use of lasers in the operating rooms and offices of aesthetic plastic surgeons, however, surged in the mid-1990s. This coincided with the introduction of carbon dioxide (CO_2) lasers as an alternative to chemical peels and microdermabrasion. Since that time, plastic surgeons have seen the numbers of lasers and intense pulse light (IPL) devices introduced into the aesthetic market place expand exponentially as the field has advanced both clinically as well as technically. Lasers and IPL devices are used today not only to resurface or smooth skin but also to tighten and rejuvenate the texture and pigmentation of the skin of the face and neck as well as the other parts of the body.

▶ APPROPRIATE LASER SELECTION

Selecting a laser requires choosing the proper wavelength of light as well as paying attention to multiple other parameters such as energy and pulse duration, to achieve the desired clinical effect with minimal complications. This selection is based in part on the basic tenets of the theory of selective photothermolysis.

The first tenet explains that the wavelength of light must be selectively absorbed by the target tissue. For example, the target of the laser surgeon who wishes to treat hirsutism is melanin. Lasers that emit light in the range selectively absorbed by melanin, which include the alexandrite (755 nm), the ruby (694 nm), and the diode (810 nm) wavelength lasers, would be appropriate choices.

The second tenet explains that the energy of the laser light must be of a high enough energy to destroy the target tissue.

Finally, the laser must produce sufficient energy to destroy the target without damaging the surrounding structures. In other words, if the laser generated so much heat in destroying the hair follicle that the surrounding skin blistered and scarred, the clinical result would obviously be unsatisfactory.

In order to achieve destruction of the target tissue, the target must be heated faster than the rate that the heat dissipates. This rate is defined as **the thermal relaxation time of tissue** (TRT). The TRT is a measurement of how long it takes for any tissue or structure to lose half the heat put into it by a laser or other heat source.

► LASER–TISSUE INTERACTION

When light is directed onto the surface of the skin, the light is transmitted, reflected, scattered, or absorbed. Achieving the desired clinical or therapeutic effect requires an understanding of the laser-tissue interaction as well as the spectral absorption properties of the tissue being targeted. The three types of laser tissue interactions include photothermal, photoacoustic, and photochemical.

Photothermal effects represent the most common type of laser-tissue interaction clinically encountered in aesthetic treatments. The laser light is selectively absorbed by the chromophore, or target. The energy in the laser light is converted to thermal energy, which alters or destroys the target tissue. An example of a clinical situation in which the target is altered includes targeting the melanin around hair shafts for laser hair removal. Similarly, an example of a clinical situation in which the tissue is destroyed is targeting water in skin when using the CO_2 or erbium lasers. In this situation, the temperature of the tissue is elevated until protein denatures and eventually is expressed as a plume of particulate organic matter and steam.

Photoacoustic effects are another common type of laser-tissue interactions. Very high fluences of laser are delivered in a very short time, usually in nanoseconds. The elevation of temperature in the target tissue occurs so rapidly that the tissue literally disrupts or explodes apart. Q-switched lasers rely on this type of laser-tissue interaction to achieve their desired result. This type of interaction is commonly used for the removal of tattoos.

Photochemical laser-tissue interactions are commonly used by dermatologic surgeons. One such example is photodynamic therapy for the treatment of hyperpigmentation or acne. Tanning is another example of a photochemical effect.

► LASER HAZARDS & PREVENTION

Beam-related hazards can involve the eye, the skin, and the respiratory tract. The most devastating injuries involve the lens, cornea, and retina. Each of these structures absorbs the various wavelengths of the spectrum differently. Severe visual disruption can occur with even a brief unprotected exposure of the eye to the laser light. Burns of the skin can occur due to accidental exposure to laser light. Finally, inhalation of laser plume can expose the patient, clinician, and staff to aerosolized biologic material including tissue, bacteria, and viruses.

Non-beam hazards include mechanical hazards, electrical hazards, and fire hazards. Mechanical hazards can be caused by laser devices because of their size, weight, or shape. Injuries can occur during the movement of the laser or its delivery device.

Due to the high energies often required to achieve production of the laser light, electrical hazards can occur. For this reason, lasers that are not functioning properly should only be opened by trained laser technicians.

Finally, fires can be related to equipment failure or electrical malfunction. They can also be started by the interaction between the laser and surgical drapes or between the laser and oxygen and anesthetic gases.

Methods to prevent laser injury include the following:

- Installing door interlocks and warning sounds.
- Posting signs about laser use.
- Educating and training staff.

- Creating up-to-date policy and procedure manuals.
- Using nonreflective instruments as well as wet towels around treatment sites.
- Wrapping anesthesia tube.
- Providing protective equipment to patients and staff (eg, eye shields and goggles, smoke evacuators). All glasses and goggles should be checked before the operation of the laser to make sure that they offer adequate protection against the wavelength in use.

► CATEGORIES OF TREATMENT METHODS

Current aesthetic laser treatments can be divided into two categories: nonablative and ablative.

Nonablative laser treatment spares the overlying epidermis, leaving it intact after the treatment. An example of a nonablative laser treatment would be using 532 nm and 1064 nm lasers for photorejuvenation (reduction in brown pigment and superficial vessels in the skin as well as stimulation of collagen production).

Ablative laser treatment removes the overlying epidermis, exposing the underlying dermis. Ablative laser treatments are often used for skin resurfacing, for improvement and reductions of wrinkles, and for skin tightening. The classic example and gold standard for ablative skin resurfacing is the CO_2 laser.

Both ablative and nonablative laser treatments can each be divided into fractional and nonfractional treatments. The classic laser treatments for facial resurfacing were all fully ablative (ie, the entire anatomic area was evenly treated). Recently, more laser procedures have been applied as fractional treatments. In fractional treatments, islands of tissue are treated but the intervening tissue is left intact. The concept is that the treated tissue can recover or heal faster if the zone of treatment is small and surrounded by uninjured tissue. These treated areas have been referred to as microscopic treatment zones.

Thus, treatments can be referred to as nonfractional, nonablative; fractionally nonablative; nonfractional, ablative; and fractionally ablative.

An example of a **nonfractional, nonablative treatment** would be the use of the KTP laser or an IPL device for treatment of a patient with extensive facial rosacea. The entire area is evenly treated using a scanning or stamping technique. The epidermis is intact after the treatment and there are no areas left untreated.

An example of a **fractionally nonablative treatment** would be resurfacing using devices operating at the 1540 nm or 1550 nm to reduce wrinkles, improve skin texture, and reduce hyperpigmentation (Figure 6–1). The epidermis is left intact at the end of the procedure, but there are islands of injury within the dermis surrounded by normal tissue. Multiple treatments are usually necessary in order to attain complete coverage and maximal results.

The nonfractional ablative treatment is probably the first type of laser treatment performed by most aesthetic surgeons. Laser resurfacing with the CO_2 and erbium lasers are classic examples of this type of treatment. The epidermis is ablated entirely. When a CO_2 laser is used, the dermal wound is deep; when the erbium laser is used, the dermal wound is more superficial.

Fractionally ablative treatments are the newest type of aesthetic laser treatments. Wavelengths such as 10,600 nm (CO_2 laser) or 2940 nm (erbium laser) are used to resurface the skin and, perhaps, tighten it as well without creating the wounds and healing time associated with nonfractionally ablative treatments that use the same wavelengths (Figure 6–2).

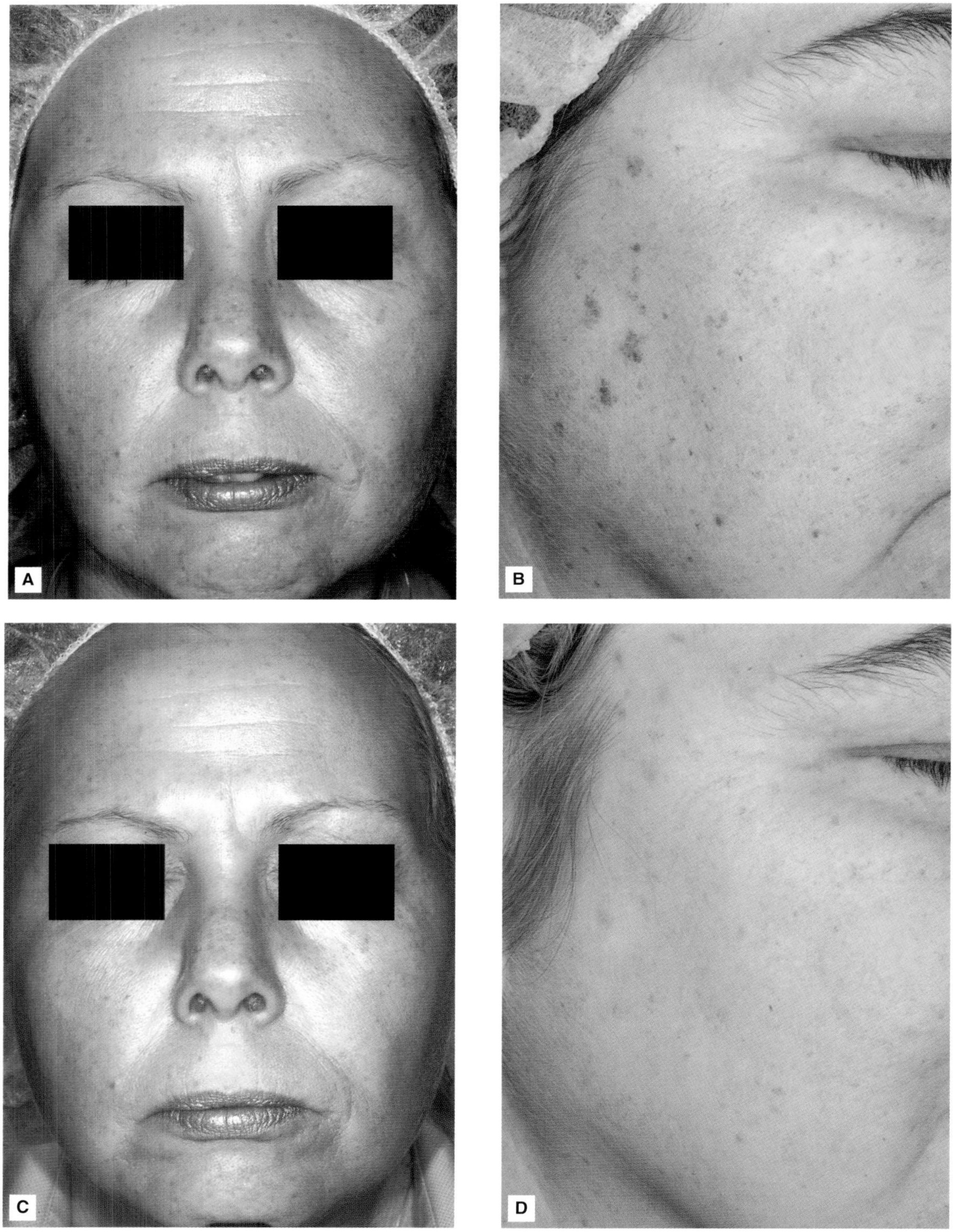

Figure 6–1. Pretreatment (**A, B**) and posttreatment (**C, D**) with 1540 nm laser.

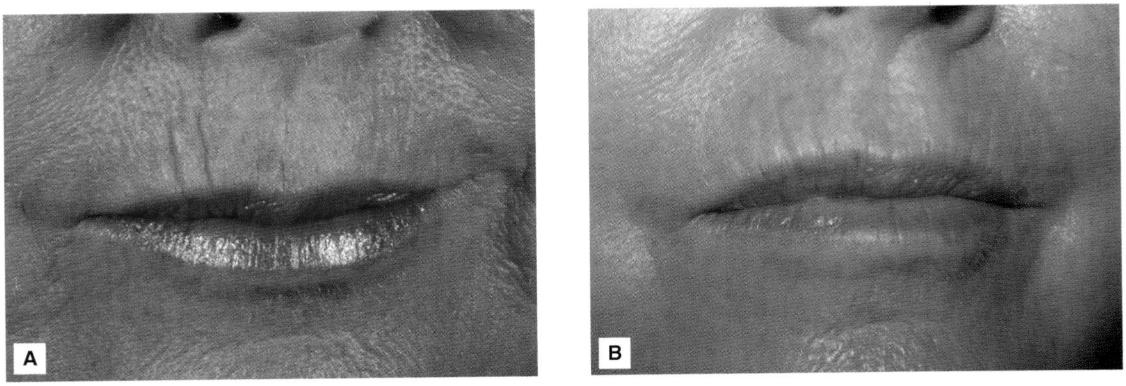

Figure 6–2. **A:** Pretreatment with erbium laser. **B:** Posttreatment with erbium laser.

▶ CLINICAL APPLICATIONS

Aesthetic laser surgery includes the treatment of patients for the following clinical conditions:

- Vascular abnormalities.
- Hyperpigmentation.
- Wrinkles and scarring.
- Skin laxity.
- Tattoos.
- Hirsutism.

1. Vascular Abnormalities

FACIAL VASCULAR LESIONS

Patients seek treatment of superficial and visible facial vessels and rosacea not only because they consider these lesions unattractive but also because they associate them with aging (Figure 6–3).

A. Patient Selection

Proper patient selection is crucial. The physician must take a detailed history and perform an appropriate examination. Recent sun exposure and accurate Fitzpatrick skin classification must be documented. With rare exceptions, patients who have a recent tan or a history of unprotected sun exposure in the last 30 days should not undergo laser or IPL treatments. Table 6–1 outlines the six categories of the Fitzpatrick skin type classification.

B. Technique

In the past, nonselective conservative topical therapies or electrosurgical devices were often

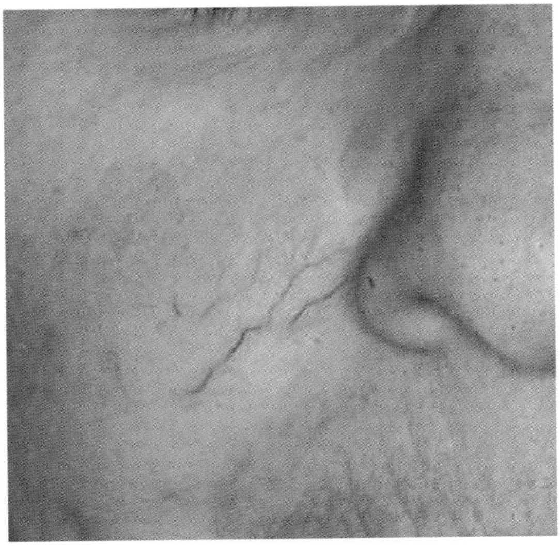

Figure 6–3. Pretreatment of facial vessels.

▶ **TABLE 6–1. FITZPATRICK CLASSIFICATION OF SKIN TYPES**

Type	Description
I	Patients have extremely fair skin; they will always burn and never tan.
II	Patients have fair or white skin; they will usually burn, and if they tan, they will lose it very quickly.
III	Patients have more olive color in their skin; they sometimes burn and retain their tan for longer periods of time.
IV	Patients have dark or olive in skin color; they rarely burn, tan easily, and stay tan for very long periods of time.
V	Patients have darker brown skin color, tan very easily, and very rarely burn.
VI	Patients have black skin and never burn.

used to treat such lesions. The latter were, at times, successful but often left the patients with scarring, pitting, and pigmentary changes in the skin. Approximately a quarter of a century ago, laser surgeons began to selectively target the chromophores oxyhemoglobin and deoxyhemoglobin with the goal of ablating vascular lesions. These chromophores had absorption peaks at 538 and 578 nm, respectively. Initially, argon, copper vapor, and krypton lasers were all used in an effort to treat these lesions with mixed success. The development of the pulse dye laser soon replaced the argon, copper vapor, and krypton lasers in most surgeons' armamentariums. Although the pulse dye laser is very effective for the treatment of vascular lesions (especially larger lesions such as hemangiomas and port wine stains), it is often problematic in cases of small visible blood vessels or rosacea because of the associated purpura. Q-switched lasers at 532 nm were also effective for treatment but similarly associated with purpura.

The development of longer pulse (non–Q-switched) 532 nm wavelength lasers (KTP) and IPL devices enable aesthetic laser surgeons to treat patients with these facial vascular lesions satisfactorily without purpura.

Treatment of benign facial epidermal vascular lesions (such as capillaries, spider veins, rosacea, and hemangiomas) is relatively fast, simple, and pain-free. No anesthesia is required.

C. Outcomes Assessment

Patients usually have some erythema that may last from several hours up to the next morning following treatment. No post-treatment care is required by the patient. Make-up may be applied almost immediately afterward. A series of treatments (especially for rosacea) is often necessary for clearance of these vascular lesions.

LEG VEINS

A. Patient Selection

Although more women than men seek treatment for spider veins, telangiectasia, and reticular and varicose veins of the lower extremities, these conditions are seen in both sexes.

B. Technique

Laser treatment of these veins without purpura is most commonly achieved with 532 nm and long-pulse 1064 nm lasers (Figure 6–4). The KTP (532nm) laser can be used successfully for the more superficial and smaller red vessels. Because the KTP laser is highly absorbed by oxyhemoglobin as well as melanin, its

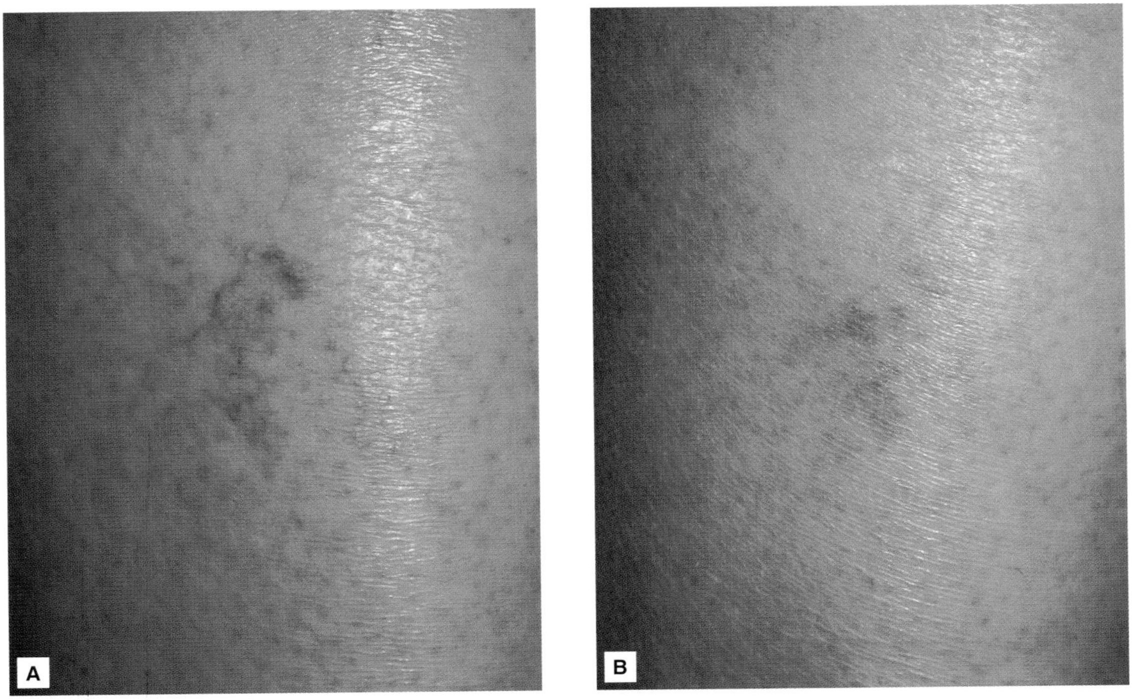

Figure 6–4. **A:** Pretreatment of leg vessels. **B:** Posttreatment of leg vessels.

use for the treatment of deeper vessels or in patients with darker skin is limited. Long-pulse Nd:YAG (1054 nm) lasers can be used to treat the larger and deeper vessels, which are bluer in appearance. These lasers can achieve deep penetration, have lesser absorption by melanin, and can seal vessels up to 4 mm in diameters due to their longer wavelengths.

Lasers of other wavelengths, such as 1320 nm, are being used to treat larger veins and even ablate the greater saphenous vein, thus, obviating the need for surgical stripping. The laser energy is delivered through a fiber that is percutaneously passed into the vein and up the leg using ultrasonic guidance. The activated laser fiber is mechanically withdrawn under ultrasonic guidance resulting in ablation of the vein in an outpatient setting under a local or tumescent anesthesia.

2. Hyperpigmentation

PATIENT SELECTION

Patients selected for treatment must meet the following criteria: absence of histologically suspicious lesion in the area to be treated and no sun exposure for 30 days prior to treatment. In addition, the surgeon must choose the appropriate device for the patient's skin type (using the Fitzpatrick classification system).

The clinician must be 100% confident that any pigmented lesion being treated is benign. If there is any question of a malignancy being present, such as a melanoma or pigmented basal cell carcinoma, then further evaluation (including obtaining tissue for the dermatopathologist) must be performed prior to any laser treatment.

TECHNIQUE

Benign epidermal lesions and areas of hyperpigmentation, such as solar keratosis and melasma, are easy to treat. The thermal relaxation time of the melanosome and melanin in the skin is such that very short pulse durations must be used in order to effectively treat the targeted pigmented lesions. Classically, Q-switched lasers, such as the Q-switched Alexandrite (755 nm), Q-switched Ruby (694 nm), and the Q-Switch Nd:YAG (1064 nm and 532 nm) lasers, were used. Higher levels of energy may be required for lesions that are lighter in color. The Q-switched Nd:YAG lasers do cause some purpura. The Q-switched Ruby and the Alexandrite lasers can also be used for treatment of many tattoos as well as for hair removal. In addition, the Q-switch Nd:YAG can be used for treatment of hyperpigmentation, vascular lesions (with purpura resulting), facial rejuvenation, and as a temporary solution for hair removal as well as removal of tattoos.

Devices such as the KTP laser (532 nm) and IPL devices can achieve excellent clearance of these benign pigmented lesions and probably at this time represent the devices of choice (Figures 6–5 and 6–6). Treatment is relatively simple and rapid. Patients do not require any anesthesia. The lesions are treated at fluences recommended by the manufacturer until there is a darkening or crusting of the lesion. These areas of superficial darkening will slowly flake off over the next 10 days and require only topical moisturizers. The result will be a total removal or lightening of the lesion. Several treatments a month apart may be necessary.

3. Wrinkles & Scarring

RESURFACING: ABLATIVE

A. Patient Preparation

Patients treated for ablative resurfacing are usually treated with an antiviral agent as a

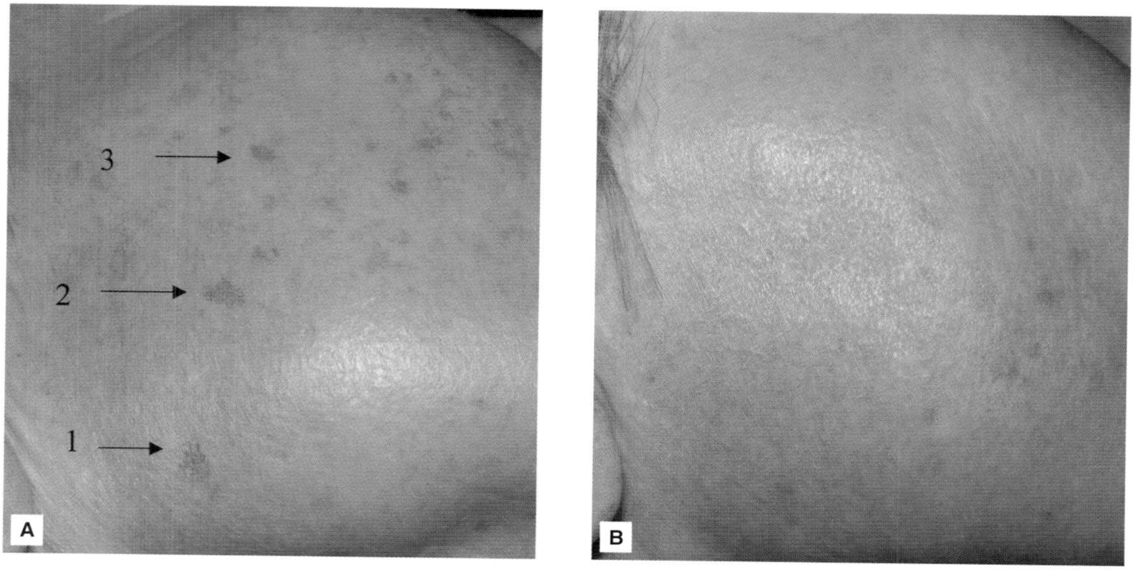

Figure 6–5. A: Pretreatment of pigmented cheek. **B:** Posttreatment of pigmented cheek.

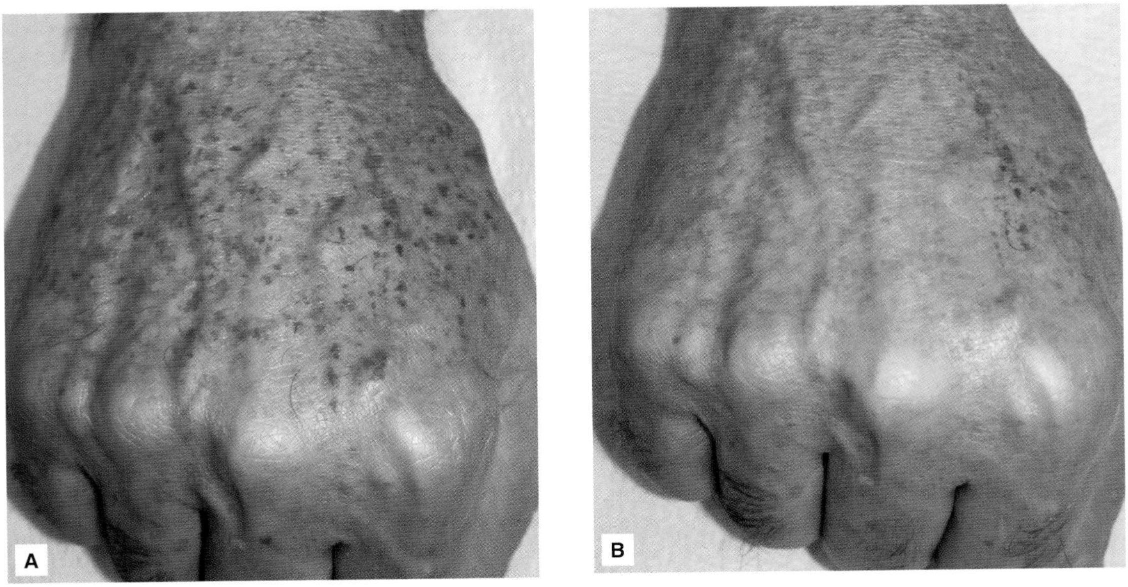

Figure 6–6. **A:** Pretreatment of pigmented hand. **B:** Posttreatment of pigmented hand.

prophylactic measure against a herpetic outbreak and with an antibiotic as prophylaxis against infection. Although there is no clear data to support the following, many clinicians give hydroquinone as pretreatment to patients undergoing CO_2 laser therapy in an attempt to reduce the incidence of postinflammatory hyperpigmentation (PIH).

B. Technique

The CO_2 and erbium lasers still represent the mainstays in the armamentarium of those aesthetic laser surgeons who perform fully ablative skin resurfacing. The CO_2 laser, which is modestly absorbed by water at 10,600 nm, is a powerful ablative device that achieves deep ablation as well as heating of tissue. Treatment with the CO_2 laser results in depth of ablation of the epidermis and dermis of 150–200 μm or greater and even deeper zones of thermal heating or modification of the deeper dermis. This deep ablation and heating is a consequence of the incomplete absorption of light by water at this wavelength and the large amount of heat that is released.

Although this treatment is considered the gold standard because of the improvement in skin texture, reduction of wrinkles, and tightening that can be achieved, it is not without its downsides. Patients treated with the CO_2 laser require a period of 10 to 20 days to heal, are left with a period of erythema that lasts 3 to 6 months, and the treatment is associated with a high incidence of both PIH and delayed hypopigmentation.

Ablation with the erbium laser (2940 nm), however, achieves much thinner zones of ablation (approximately 20–50 μm) and heating (approximately 15–20 μm) than the CO_2 laser. Patients heal faster and have shorter periods of erythema, a lower incidence of PIH, and minimal delayed hypopigmentation. The downside is that the degree of improvement is reduced compared with the CO_2 laser. In addition, the treatment is non-hemostatic so that pinpoint bleeding occurs as one ablates deeper, it requires many more passes than the CO_2 laser, and there is no associated skin tightening.

RESURFACING: FRACTIONAL

In fractional resurfacing, the laser or IPL device is used to create microscopic zones of thermally modified, damaged or ablated tissue that are surrounded by normal untreated tissue. This treatment is used to achieve stimulation of collagen production, wrinkle improvement, pigmentation reduction and, in some instances, skin tightening. There is little or reduced healing time compared with CO_2 and erbium resurfacings; each microscopic thermal zone heals quickly because it is surrounded by normal, untreated tissue.

A. Technique

Fractionally nonablative resurfacing can be applied to the face, neck, chest, and extremities. The most common wavelengths for this treatment are 1540 nm and 1550 nm. The overlying epidermis is left intact or minimally changed by the treatment. Although there is no skin tightening with this procedure, the patients see a significant improvement in their skin texture, pigmentation, and reduction in wrinkles.

Fractionally *ablative* resurfacing differs from fractionally nonablative resurfacing in that a core of tissue consisting of epidermis as well as a varying portion of the dermis is ablated by the laser. These microscopic columns of ablation are surrounded by intact tissue. Depending on the fluence and wavelength used, the "intact" tissue may exhibit significant thermal modification. The goal of these treatments is to see greater improvement in wrinkle reduction, acne scarring, and skin tone and texture as well as tightening.

The main wavelengths used in these treatments are 10,600 nm (CO_2) and 2940 nm (erbium). For most laser surgeons, ablative resurfacing laser treatments are best limited to the face when CO_2 lasers are used and to the face and neck when the erbium laser is used.

B. Outcomes Assessment

Fractionally nonablative resurfacing is repeated several times on a monthly schedule and may require topical anesthetic at higher fluences but has minimal to no healing time. Complications are also minimal.

Patients undergoing a **fractionally ablative treatment** may only require a single treatment but may require up to a week or more to heal.

4. Skin Laxity

The concept of nonablative fractional resurfacing has been applied to the deeper dermis and adjacent subcutaneous tissues in order to achieve skin tightening. IPL devices using infrared wavelengths in the range of 850 to 1350 nm have been used to achieve islands of thermal injury to these tissues, sparing the overlying tissues and tightening the skin. These IPL devices are currently used clinically in attempts to achieve tightening of the face, neck, abdomen, and upper arms.

5. Tattoos

Traditional treatment for removal of tattoos before the application of lasers included surgical excision, skin grafting, and dermabrasion. None of these treatments were satisfactory because of the resultant scarring or incomplete results.

A. Technique

Laser surgeons are able to treat tattoos by selectively targeting each pigment in the tattoo with an appropriate wavelength of light. Tattoos with multiple colors require treatment with multiple wavelengths. The laser treatment results in the destruction and breakdown of the pigment so that it can be removed by phagocytes. Fortunately, the most common pigments in tattoos—black, blue-black, and red—are the colors most easily removed with the available lasers. The most commonly used lasers are the Q-switched Ruby (694 nm), Q-switched Alexandrite (755 nm), and Q-switched Nd:YAG lasers (1064 nm/532 nm). Other colors, such as light greens, sky blues, and yellow, require different wavelengths and can be more problematic.

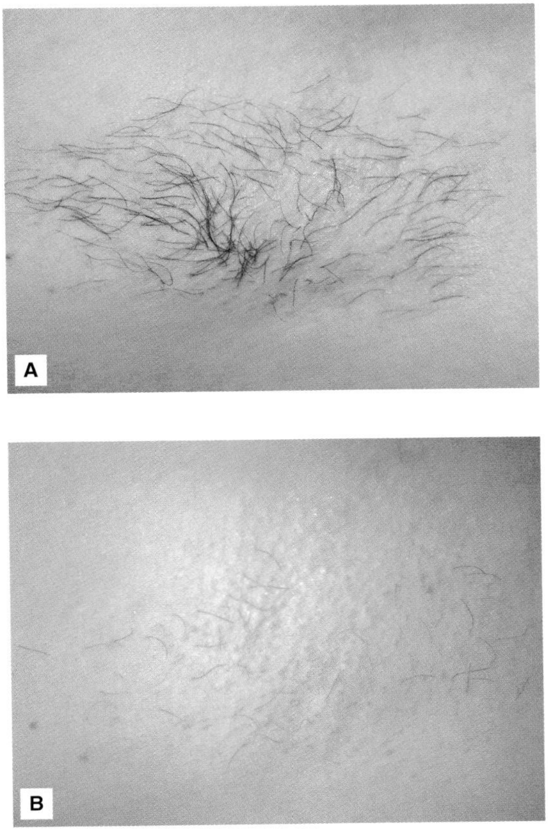

Figure 6–7. Pretreatment (**A**) and post-treatment (**B**) of hirsutism of axilla.

B. Outcomes Assessment

Laser treatments for tattoo removal are best performed at least 6 or more weeks apart; can require as few as 4 to 6 treatments and as many as 12 treatments; and can result in scarring, skin textural changes, and hypopigmentation.

6. Hirsutism

PATIENT EVALUATION & SELECTION

Patients with darker hair are better candidates for this procedure. Photoepilation is at best difficult, if not impossible, in patients with blonde, red, gray, and white hair. Patients with darker skin types represent greater challenges for the clinician practicing photoepilation and can only be treated with a narrow range of laser and IPL devices.

TECHNIQUE

Probably one of the most common applications of laser and IPL technology is for laser hair removal or photoepilation (Figures 6–7 through 6–10). The concept is that the pigment in the hair shaft and, perhaps, the hemoglobin in the vessels surrounding the hair follicle absorb the laser light, the light energy is converted to heat, and the follicle is modified so that no further hair is produced. This must be accomplished without damaging the skin around the hair shaft and follicle.

OUTCOMES ASSESSMENT

Excellent results can be achieved in patients in a series of 4 to 6 treatments. Many patients, however, undergoing photoepilation will see

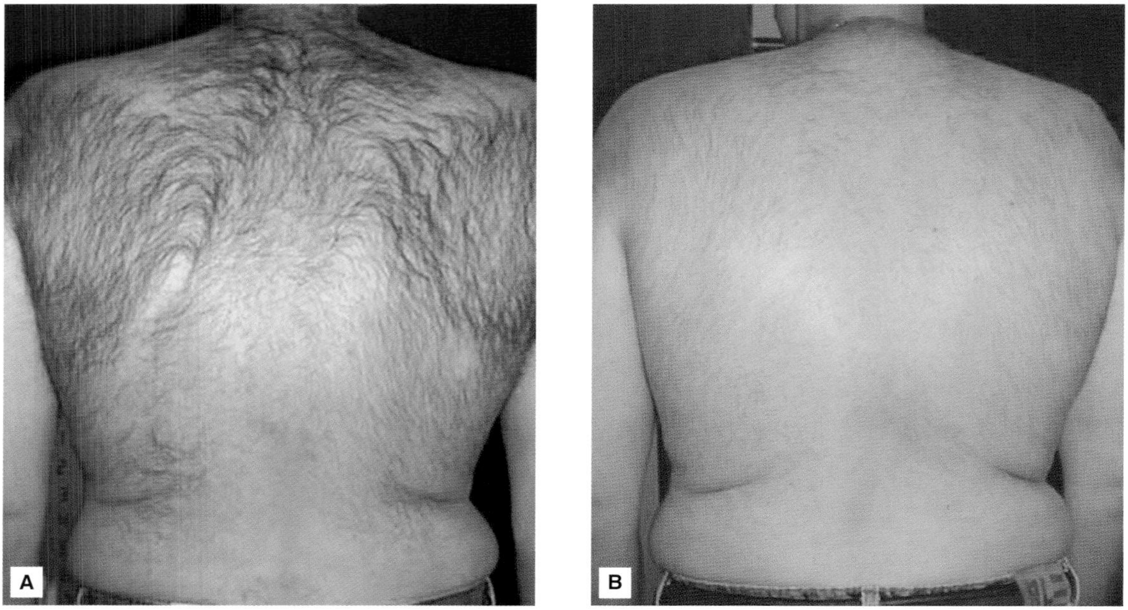

Figure 6–8. Pretreatment (**A**) and posttreatment (**B**) of hirsutism of back.

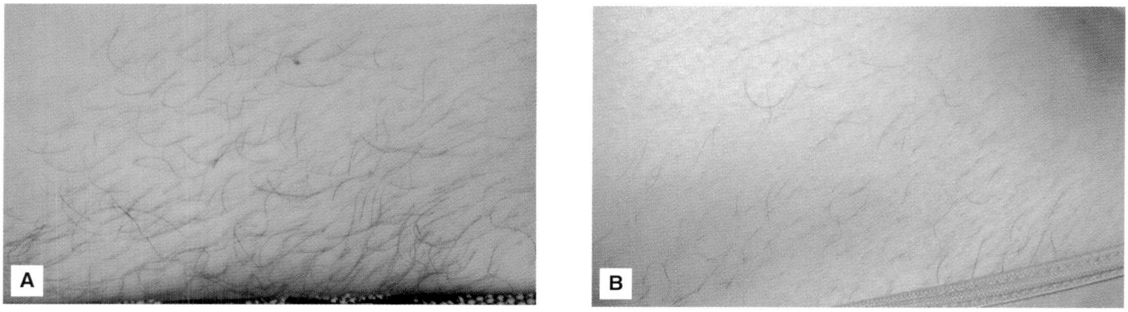

Figure 6–9. Pretreatment (**A**) and posttreatment (**B**) of hirsutism of bikini.

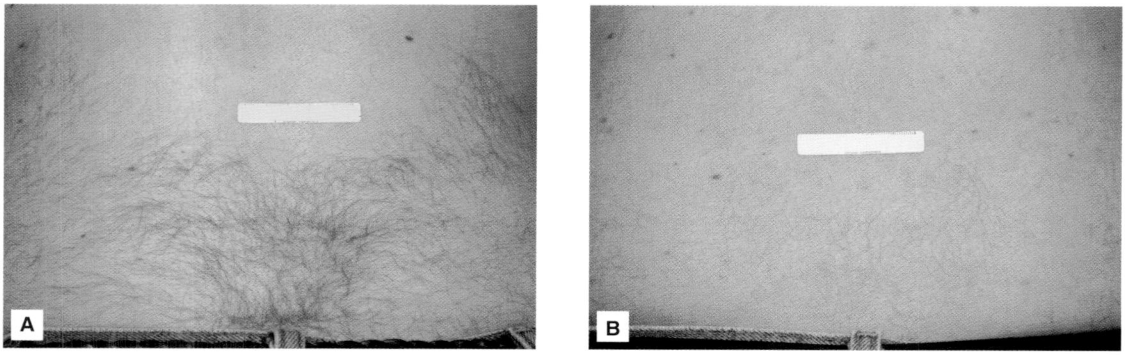

Figure 6–10. Pretreatment (**A**) and posttreatment (**B**) of hirsutism of lower back.

different results depending on the anatomic site treated, can require 12 or more treatments in some sites, and can expect to require a life-long maintenance program.

▶ COMPLICATIONS

Hospitals and clinicians should have policies and procedures in place to ensure the safe and proper use of lasers. In addition to blindness and inhalation injuries, the most common complications of laser therapy include blistering, scarring, PIH, and hypopigmentation.

PIH is best treated using a combination of three topical therapeutic agents: a corticosteroid (reduce inflammation), a hydroquinone (blocks melanin production), and a retinol (mild peeling). Resolution of PIH usually occurs in a matter of months in almost 100% of the cases.

▶ OTHER RELATED TECHNOLOGIES

1. Light Emitting Diodes

Light emitting diodes (LED) represent low level lights that are being used to achieve photomodulation of the skin. The yellow LED at 585 nm has been clinically shown to treat hyperpigmentation, eliminate small vascular lesions, deposit collagen for wrinkle reduction, and reduce inflammation.

These LED treatments are painless, rapid (35 seconds), and can be used in conjunction with laser treatments to decrease inflammation and improve results.

Investigations are currently underway using low level light and LED treatments for further manipulation of the skin including fat modulation, cellulite treatment, treatment of acne, and stimulation of hair growth for treatment of alopecia.

2. Laser Lipolysis

One of the newest areas for the application of laser technology is in the area of liposuction. There are multiple devices currently in use which operated at 924, 975, 980, 1064, 1320, and 1440 nm. The concept of this procedure is that the laser energy is used to render the fat suitable for aspiration in a less traumatic fashion than traditional liposuction. The energies mentioned interact with the fat in a variety of ways: the fat is either melted, disrupted by photoacoustic mechanisms, or thermally injured by heating of the soft tissues which results from the absorption of laser energy by water. The interaction of these wavelengths of laser light with the water in the dermis is felt to have the added benefit of resulting in tightening of the skin as well.

Energies other than those already discussed in this chapter that are currently being used and/or investigated to modulate the soft tissues and achieve skin tightening, wrinkle reduction, correction of cellulite, or fat reduction. These other energies include RF (radiofrequency), IR (infrared), low level energy lasers, focused ultrasound, nitrogen plasma, and even cold.

Although innovative energy-based technology has put exciting new tools in the surgeons' hands, the clinician must be judicious in their use of such new devices until their clinical efficacy and safety has been clearly demonstrated.

CHAPTER 7

Brow Lift

P. Pravin Reddy, MD, Gregory S. LaTrenta, MD, FACS, Robert C. Silich, MD, FACS, Gerald Imber, MD, & Robert T. Grant MD, MSc, FACS

Since the introduction of the endoscopic brow lift in 1994, open brow lifts have seen a decline in popularity. However, the open coronal technique remains effective and is the gold standard against which all other forehead rejuvenation procedures are compared. In selected patients, it remains the best approach to achieving forehead rejuvenation.

The open approach affords the advantage of superior exposure, release of adhesions, muscle excision, brow mobilization, and excess scalp excision. Disadvantages include a significant scar, numbness, dysesthesia, and alopecia. Compared with the endoscopic brow lift, the open procedure is a better alternative for patients with a high receding hairline and a convex frontalis bone. These morphologic features present insurmountable problems to instrumentation during an endoscopic brow lift.

Endoscopic brow lifting has achieved wide physician and patient acceptance as a means for achieving rejuvenation of the upper face. The procedure is associated with durable results and can be effectively combined with other procedures. The advantages of endoscopic brow lifting include short camouflaged scars, resection of glabellar muscles under direct and magnified vision, preservation of scalp sensation by avoidance of nerve transection, and decreased alopecia.

▶ ANATOMY

When performing a brow lift, the surgeon should appreciate the following anatomic features:

- The temporalis muscle.
- Relationship of deep temporalis fascia and parietotemporal fascia.
- The course of the frontal branch of the facial nerve.
- The temporal crest.
- Supraorbital ligaments.
- Arcus marginalis.
- The lateral and medial (sentinel) temporoparietal veins.
- The course and branching of the supratrochlear and supraorbital nerves.
- The origin and insertions of the corrugator, supercilii; and procerus muscles as well as their relationship to the supratrochlear and supraorbital nerves.

▸ PATIENT EVALUATION & SELECTION

The ideal candidate for brow lifting has brow ptosis with caudad migration of the brow line, deep static forehead rhytides, dynamic glabellar rhytides, or asymmetry of brows. Patients usually describe these findings as "constantly appearing to be tired." Descent of the brows may be the result of senescence, trauma, or hereditary factors. Asymmetry of the brows may exist as a congenital condition.

The aforementioned criteria are excellent indications for brow elevation; however, in addition, patients with a low thick hairline combined with a short flat, as opposed to tall convex, forehead are suited for endoscopic brow lifting. A tall convex shaped forehead may pose technical challenges as the convexity and length may not admit endoscopic instruments as easily as a flat short forehead. The open brow lift is a better approach for these patients.

As with most elective cosmetic procedures, the patient's general health status should be carefully reviewed before the patient undergoes surgery. Clear contraindications are preexisting cardiac conditions, presence of bleeding diathesis, previous frontal craniotomy, and frontal sinus fracture.

Advanced age does not disqualify a patient from undergoing brow lifting, providing a review of their general health does not reveal acceptable anesthetic risks.

A history of dry eyes should be noted and if necessary, a Schirmer test used to confirm that adequate tearing is present. Brow lifting may potentially exacerbate tearing problems.

The presence of soft tissue connective disorder is an uncertain risk.

▸ PATIENT PREPARATION

Routine preoperative evaluation is performed and age appropriate diagnostic testing is performed in accordance with American Society of Anesthesiology guidelines.

Patients are instructed to halt all routine medications carrying a risk of bleeding. Care is taken to review all herbal supplemental medications preoperatively.

The patient is brought to the operating room where they are placed in a comfortable supine position. Routine measures, such as sequential compression stockings, to minimize venous thromboembolic disease, are applied. Preoperative markings are made with the patient seated upright. The sentinel vein, temporal crest, supraorbital, and supratrochlear nerves are all marked. Furthermore, the direction and position of the desired vectors are marked.

Hair may be braided or shaved in order to provide optimum exposure; however, a simple separation of hair with petrolatum or bacitracin gel serves just as well in most cases and is far less time-consuming.

The patient is positioned supine with slight head elevation. Once under general anesthesia, the patient is repositioned on the table so that the vertex extends slightly beyond the table, ensuring that the surgeon has excellent access to the frontal region.

The endoscopic brow lifting procedure relies on appropriate and properly functioning equipment. Typically, a 30-degree angled rigid endoscope is preferred with a 3-chip color processing unit. A halogen light source, high definition video monitor and anti-fogging solution are essential for optimal viewing. In addition, a selection of periosteal elevators, curved and square tipped, should be available.

Once the landmarks have been identified, the operative field is prepared and draped. The surgeon stands at the head of the operating room table.

▸ TECHNIQUE

Figure 7–1 shows preoperative and postoperative photographs of a patient who underwent brow lift.

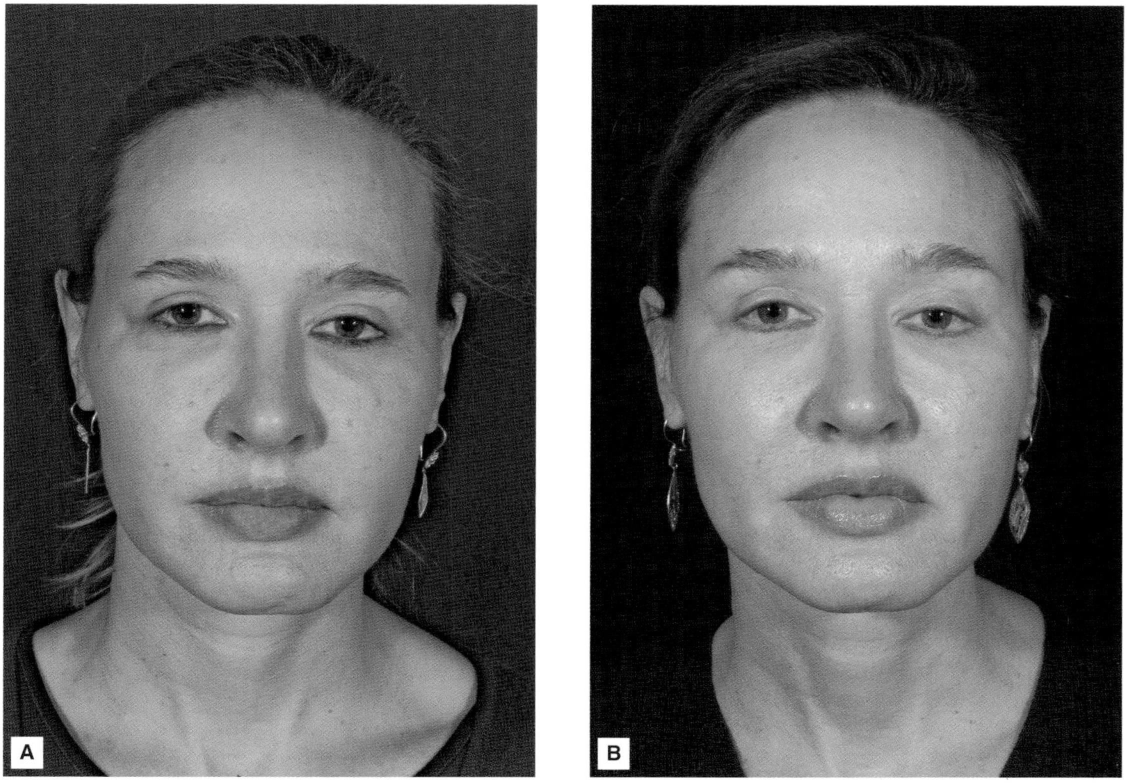

Figure 7–1. Preoperative and postoperative photographs of patient who underwent brow lift. (Used with permission from Robert C. Silich, MD, FACS.)

OPEN BROW LIFT

After satisfactory anesthesia has been achieved, the line of incision is marked and infiltrated with a vasoconstrictive local anesthetic. Full thickness skin incisions are made parallel to the hair follicles in an attempt to preserve them. The following incisions may be used depending on the patient's hairline: standard coronal incision, modified coronal incision, anterior hairline incision.

In those cases where either a standard or modified coronal incision is selected, the plane of dissection is between the temporoparietal fascia and the deep temporal fascia laterally and the periosteum medially. Elevation of the brow proceeds to the level of the supraorbital rims. When the anterior hairline incision is used, dissection proceeds in the subcutaneous plane, thus preserving sensation to the forehead.

The goal of dissection is to visualize the following muscles: procerus, corrugator, and depressor supercilii. Once these muscles have been visualized, muscle modification may proceed with division or avulsion. The frontalis muscle is modified with one of several techniques. The frontalis muscle may be divided horizontally, cross-hatched, or a strip excision may be performed.

Care is taken to avoid injury to the supraorbital neurovascular bundle or its branches.

The forehead flap is then placed under gentle traction and stapled to the scalp along the previously determined vectors of fixation. Excess skin is excised and the brow fixed to its final position with absorbable sutures and staples. Drains are typically not employed during this procedure.

As with any procedure aimed at rejuvenating the forehead, the open brow lift seeks to reposition the brow and correct ptosis, eliminate rhytides, address crow's feet and lateral orbital crowding, and eliminate excess skin in the glabellar and nasal radix.

Repositioning of the brow is achieved by mobilization of the brow, lysis of adhesions, and muscle modification. The procedure is usually performed in conjunction with procedures aimed at rejuvenating the periorbit. In fact, it is considered unusual to perform the brow lift without at least an upper blepharoplasty. Figures 7–2 and 7–3 show preoperative and postoperative photographs of patients who underwent open brow lift.

ENDOSCOPIC BROW LIFT

First, relevant anatomic landmarks including the temporal crest, sentinel vein, and the course of the frontal branch of the facial nerve are identified with the patient in a seated upright position. With the patient in the seated position, the vectors necessary for rejuvenating the brow line are noted.

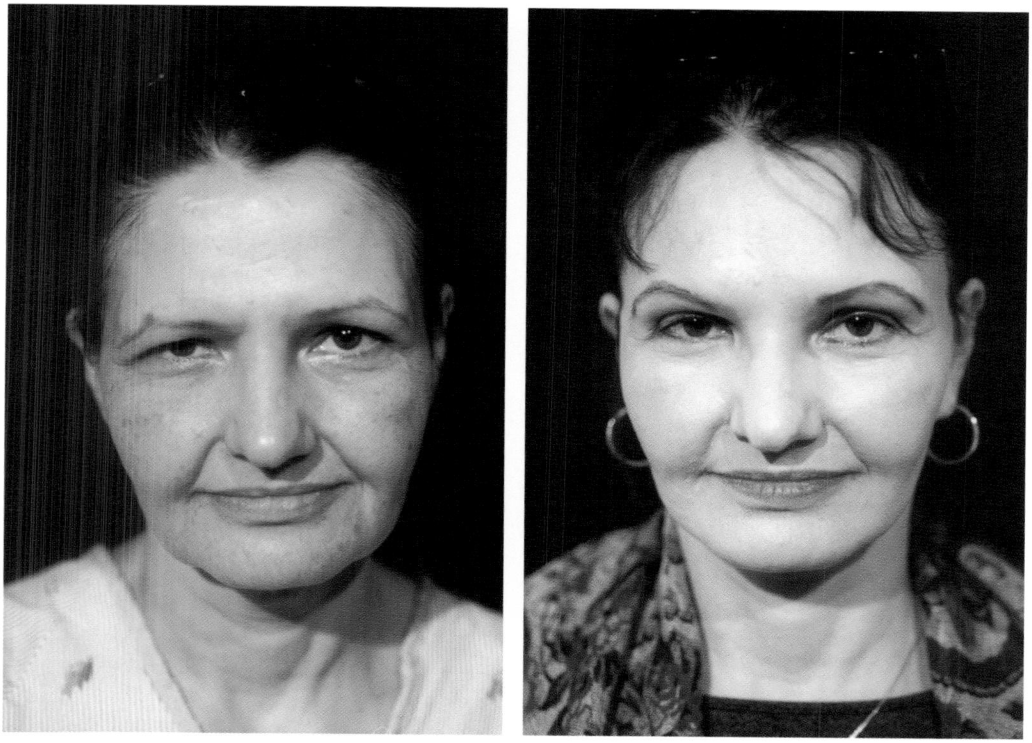

Figure 7–2. Preoperative and postoperative photographs of patient who underwent open brow lift. (Reproduced, with permission, from LaTrenta G. *Aesthetic Face & Neck Surgery*. Philadelphia: W.B. Saunders Company; 2003.)

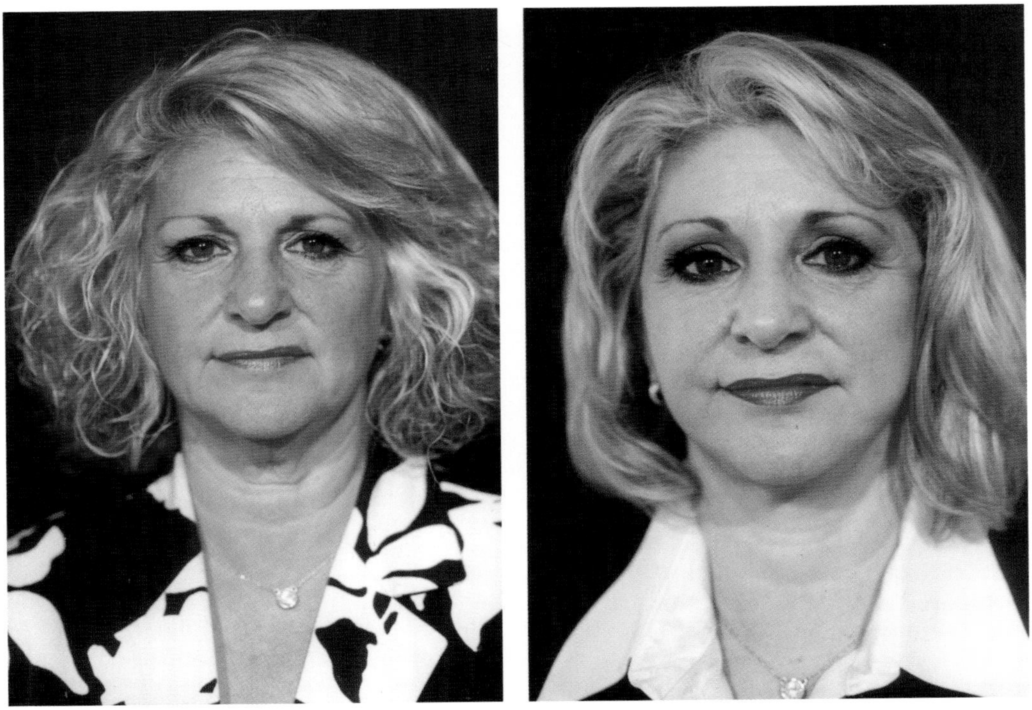

Figure 7–3. Preoperative and postoperative photographs of patient who underwent open brow lift. (Reproduced, with permission, from LaTrenta G. ***Aesthetic Face & Neck Surgery***. Philadelphia: W.B. Saunders Company; 2003.)

The youthful brow has its apex at the lateral canthus. The nadir of the brow arch is located at the medial limit of the brow. In some cases, despite a normal brow position, the effect of rejuvenation may not be apparent. This is usually due to hollowing of the orbit, and a separate procedure is required to achieve the full effect of rejuvenation.

Once the patient has undergone satisfactory anesthesia and appropriate positioning, the surgery begins with the placement of incisions. Transverse-oriented temporal incisions are placed approximately 4 cm behind the hairline. Care is taken to bevel the incisions across the hair shafts. This maneuver allows the hair to grow through the scar, thus camouflaging the incision. Dissection is carried down to the plane between the deep layer of the superficial temporal fascia and the deep temporal fascia. Dissection in this plane may be performed safely because the frontal branch of the facial nerve is elevated with the temporoparietal fascia. A Freer dissection spatula is then gently introduced into this plane and dissection is carried anteriorly to the level of the lateral orbital rims using the temporal crest as a landmark.

Release of the supraorbital ligaments is approached through a radially oriented midline incision strategically placed posterior to the frontal hairline for a distance of 2.5 cm. Sharp dissection is carried down to periosteum, and the frontalis muscle is bluntly elevated to a level approximately 2.5 cm superior to the supraorbital ridges in the subperiosteal plane. Dissection in the subperiosteal plane yields a superior optical window with minimal bleeding.

Since the sentinel vein is identified preoperatively, dissection can proceed rapidly until the vein is approached. Once an adequate optical window has been developed, the endoscope is introduced and the sentinel vein is directly visualized.

An endoscopic grasping instrument is then introduced, and the sentinel vein carefully skeletonized. This process serves the dual purpose of releasing supraorbital periosteal attachments and isolating branches of the supratrochlear and supraorbital nerves.

Subperiosteal dissection is then completed by elevating the periosteum to the level of the supraorbital rims taking care to avoid injury to the supraorbital nerves. Once this optical window has been fully developed, the periosteum is then divided in its entirety extending from lateral orbital rim to the contralateral side. It is only after dividing the periosteum that additional mobility can be realized and the glabellar complex visualized.

A. Supraorbital and Supratrochlear Nerve Preservation with Modification of Glabellar Muscle Complex

Following division of the periosteum, the glabellar complex, which consists of the procerus, corrugator, and depressor supercilii muscles, is visualized.

Using a Takahashi forceps, the glabellar complex muscles are gently grasped and lysed. Injury to the supratrochlear nerves is avoided by directly visualizing the nerves during the process of muscle lysis. The muscles of the glabellar complex will yield readily to forcep lysis relative to the nerves, and this tactile feedback aids in the dissection. The degree to which muscles are lysed varies depending on the thickness of the complex and the extent of glabellar rhytides.

B. Elevation and Fixation of Brow Line

After achieving adequate mobilization of the brow, the brow is elevated in the desired vector and fixed in the new position. The brow is elevated starting laterally and progressing medially. An assistant maintains the new brow position while the surgeon accomplishes fixation.

A variety of fixation techniques are available including tapes, fibrin glue, external screw fixation, internal screws, Mitek anchors, cortical tunnels, and the Endotine device. Whatever the fixation technique selected, whether temporary or permanent, the surgeon should appreciate that the mobilized periosteum does not adhere to the new position for a minimum of 8 days.

The Endotine device, a biodegradable fixation device, has several distinct advantages including permanent fixation with multiple vectors, absorbable material, and reproducible results. The device is associated with low complication rates.

Once the lateral temporal brow is fixed, the central brow is fixed using absorbable sutures anchoring the temporoparietal fascia to the deep temporal fascia. Excess skin is then excised following which 10 Fr drains are inserted. The drain is removed within 24 hours of the procedure. Incisions are then closed routinely. Figures 7–4 and 7–5 show preoperative and postoperative photographs of patients who underwent endoscopic brow lift.

▶ POSTOPERATIVE CARE

After undergoing open or endoscopic brow lift, the patient is instructed to maintain head elevation, and cold compresses are applied to the operative site. Judicious control of blood pressure and postoperative nausea and vomiting

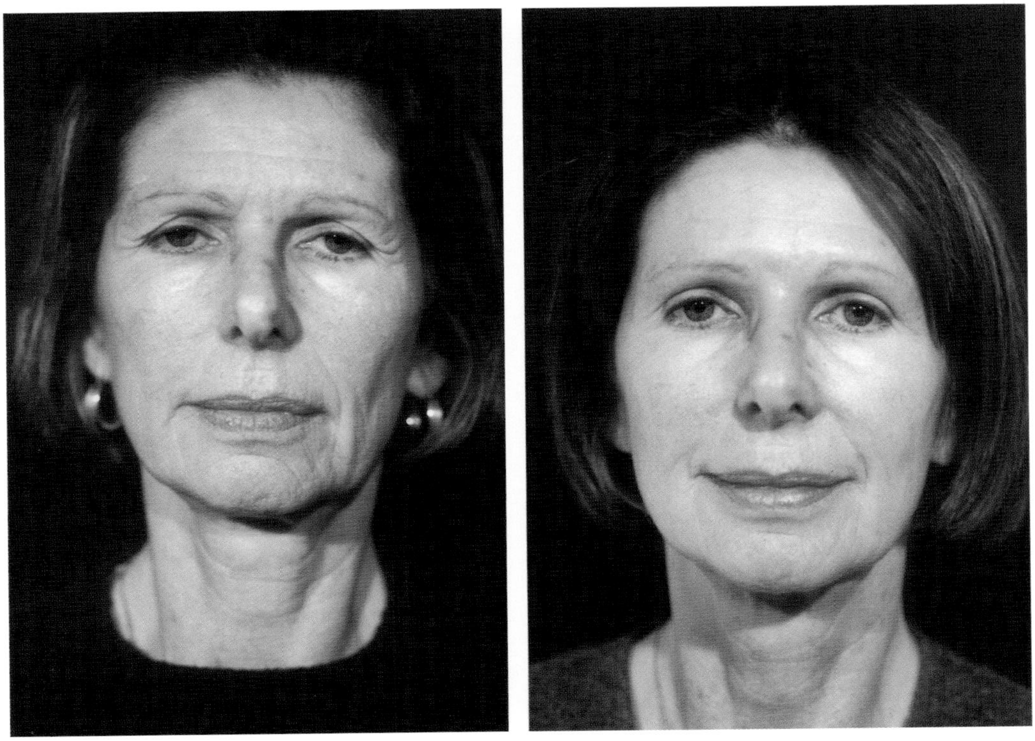

Figure 7–4. Preoperative and postoperative photographs of patient who underwent endoscopic brow lift. (Reproduced, with permission, from LaTrenta G. ***Aesthetic Face & Neck Surgery***. Philadelphia: W.B. Saunders Company; 2003.)

is implemented. The procedure is ambulatory and any skin sutures or staples that were placed are usually removed on postoperative day 5.

▶ COMPLICATIONS

OPEN BROW LIFT

Immediate postoperative complications are bleeding and infection. Delayed complications include numbness, dysesthesia, and alopecia.

ENDOSCOPIC BROW LIFT

Complications associated with endoscopic brow lifting include injury to the frontal branch of the facial nerve, hypoesthesia of the frontal area and scalp as a result of injury to the supratrochlear and supraorbital nerves, hematoma, alopecia associated with scar placement, persistent pruritus, and loss of brow position. Rare cases of meningitis have been reported in cases where cortical tunnels or screw fixation of the brow is applied.

▶ OUTCOMES ASSESSMENT

Patient satisfaction reports from multiple authors describing their experience with both the open and endoscopic techniques exceeds 95%. The rates of nerve injury or permanent areas of sensory loss in the scalp are estimated to be below 3%. The late 1990s saw the transition of popularity of techniques used by

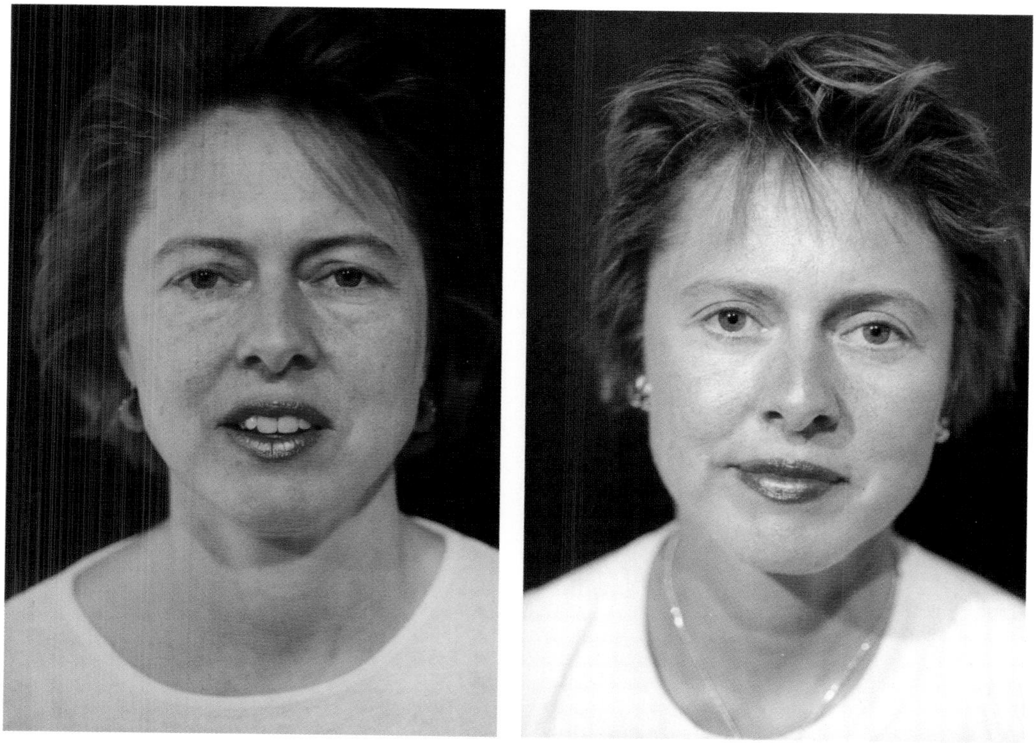

Figure 7–5. Preoperative and postoperative photographs of patient who underwent endoscopic brow lift. (Reproduced, with permission, from LaTrenta G. ***Aesthetic Face & Neck Surgery***. Philadelphia: W.B. Saunders Company; 2003.)

plastic surgeons change from the open technique to the predominantly endoscopic technique because of reduction in scarring. There was therefore a potential theoretical decrease in incidence of postoperative nerve dysfunction, visible scarring, and hair loss associated with scarring. However, some anecdotal reports also indicated that the duration of the result following endoscopic brow lifts was less than that seen with the open technique. More recently, the introduction of neurotoxin administration (Botox) in 2001 was responsible for a paradigm shift in the evaluation and approach toward brow and forehead rejuvenation. Results, albeit temporary and of limited duration, that could only formerly be achieved by surgery could now be obtained through nonsurgical means and without any surgical risks. Skillful administration of Botox has served as a beneficial adjunct to the open and endoscopic brow lift techniques. Multiple literature reports confirm that both surgeons and patients describe extremely high levels of satisfaction with the quality and predictability of the brow and forehead rejuvenation results that are currently achieved.

REFERENCES

Byrne PJ. Efficacy and safety of endotine fixation in endoscopic brow lift. *Arch Facial Plast Surg.* 2007 May–Jun;9(3):212–4. [PMID: 17519210]

De Cordier BC et al. Endoscopic forehead lift: review of technique, cases, and complications. *Plast Reconstr Surg.* 2002 Nov;110(6):1558–68. [PMID: 12409778]

Elkwood A et al. National plastic surgery survey: brow lifting techniques and complications. *Plast Reconstr Surg.* 2001 Dec;108(7):2143–50. [PMID: 11743421]

Friedland JA. Open approach for upper facial rejuvenation. *Plast Reconstr Surg.* 1997 Sep;100(4): 1040–2. [PMID: 9290676]

Maas CS et al. Temporal brow lift using botulinim toxin A: an update. *Plast Reconstr Surg.* 2003 Oct;112(5):109S–112S. [PMID: 14504491]

Puig CM et al. A retrospective comparison of open and endoscopic brow-lifts. *Arch Facial Plast Surg.* 2002 Oct–Dec;4(4):221–5. [PMID: 12437426]

Tabatabai N et al. Limited incision nonendoscopic brow lift. *Plast Reconstr Surg.* 2007 Apr 15; 119(5):1563–70. [PMID: 17415251]

Wise DM. Limited incision foreheadplasty. *Plast Reconstr Surg.* 1999 Dec;104(7):2334–7. [PMID: 11149813]

CHAPTER 8

Face & Neck Lift

Mehul Kamdar, MD, Gerald Imber, MD, & Robert C. Silich, MD, FACS

For the last four decades, the full subcutaneous face lift has been the procedure of choice to treat the facial effects of aging. Superficial musculoaponeurotic system (SMAS) plication, platysma tightening, and deep-plane surgery have improved face lift results. However, to achieve optimal results, it is important for the surgeon to understand and appreciate all available techniques. All face lifts are not the same: all procedures are not necessarily indicated for all patients, and physical findings dictate the choice of specific procedure.

In the last 15 years, less invasive techniques have been proven appropriate for earlier signs of aging. Such techniques have assumed increased importance as a younger group of patients (eg, those in their fourth and fifth decade) seek to counter the effects of aging.

The limited-incision face lift technique (LIFT) offers an effective procedure for meeting the needs of many patients. A principal advantage of this procedure is the elimination of the postauricular, neck, and often temporal scalp incision and the scarring and sequelae that accompany each incision. The LIFT allows full correction of upper, mid, and lower facial aging without the pulled look that often results from traditional subcutaneous procedures (Figure 8–1). It also allows a more rapid recovery and return to activity as well as ease and safety of performance.

ANATOMY

A thorough understanding of the normal facial anatomy and the changes associated with aging is paramount to successful aesthetic surgery. Facial **skin** undergoes atrophy with aging and the most significant effect is seen in the dermis. Fine facial rhytids are caused by the combination of actinic damage, gravitational forces, genetics, and the repeated use of facial muscles. Deep to the skin is a layer of **subcutaneous fat**, which is the dissection plane of the traditional rhytidectomy. In the face, this plane separates the SMAS-muscle layer from the overlying skin. It is convenient to think of the facial planes of the scalp-temporal region-face-neck as continuous units. Superiorly, the **SMAS-muscle layer** of the face continues above the zygomatic arch as the temporoparietal fascia and further on as the galea in the scalp. Inferiorly, the SMAS-muscle layer continues in the neck as the **superficial cervical fascia** investing the **platysma**. The SMAS,

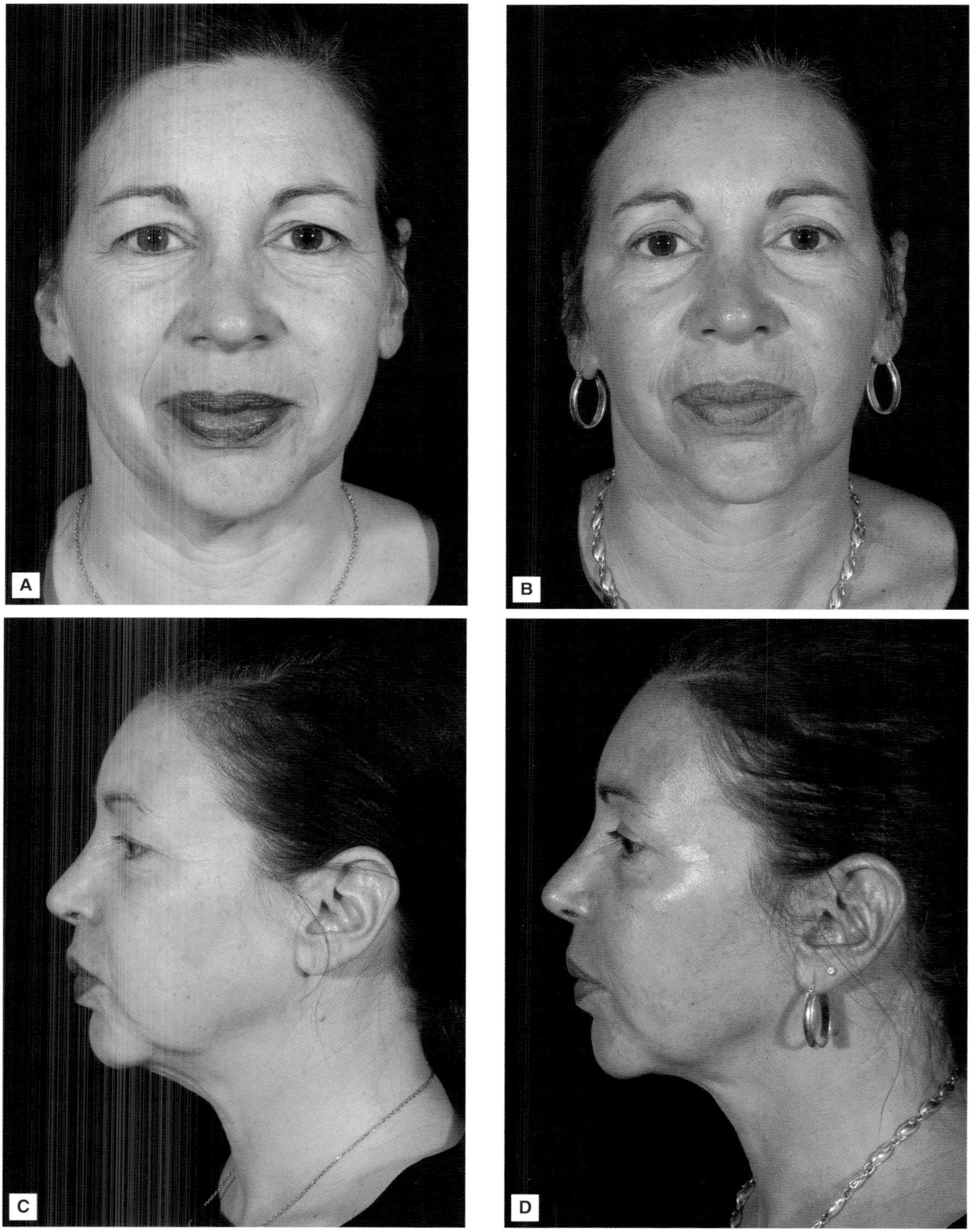

Figure 8–1. Preoperative and postoperative photographs of woman who has undergone limited incision face lift (LIFT). **A:** Preoperative frontal view. **B:** Postoperative frontal view. **C:** Preoperative lateral view. **D:** Postoperative lateral view. (Courtesy of Robert C. Silich, MD, FACS)

platysma, and muscles of facial expression may be thought of as a single anatomic unit. Deep to the SMAS-muscle layer in the face is the **parotid-masseteric fascia,** which temporally corresponds to the deep temporal fascia and, in the neck, the deeper layer of cervical fascia.

A few specialized soft tissue structures of the face deserve attention in understanding the aging face. The **malar fat pad** is a relatively discrete triangular shaped region of fat in the subcutaneous space medially above the zygomaticus muscles and laterally above the SMAS (Figure 8–2). Its inferior displacement, typical of midface aging, leads to infraorbital flattening and fullness lateral to the nasolabial fold. Anterior to the masseter lies the **buccal fat pad**, a segmented structure that lies in close proximity to the buccal branches of the facial nerve and the parotid duct.

A number of specialized retaining ligaments supporting the overlying skin have been identified. These ligaments attenuate with aging, allowing migration of the soft tissues of the face. In particular the **masseteric-cutaneous ligament** is largely implicated in jowl formation and the **zygomatic ligaments** are responsible for the above mentioned malar

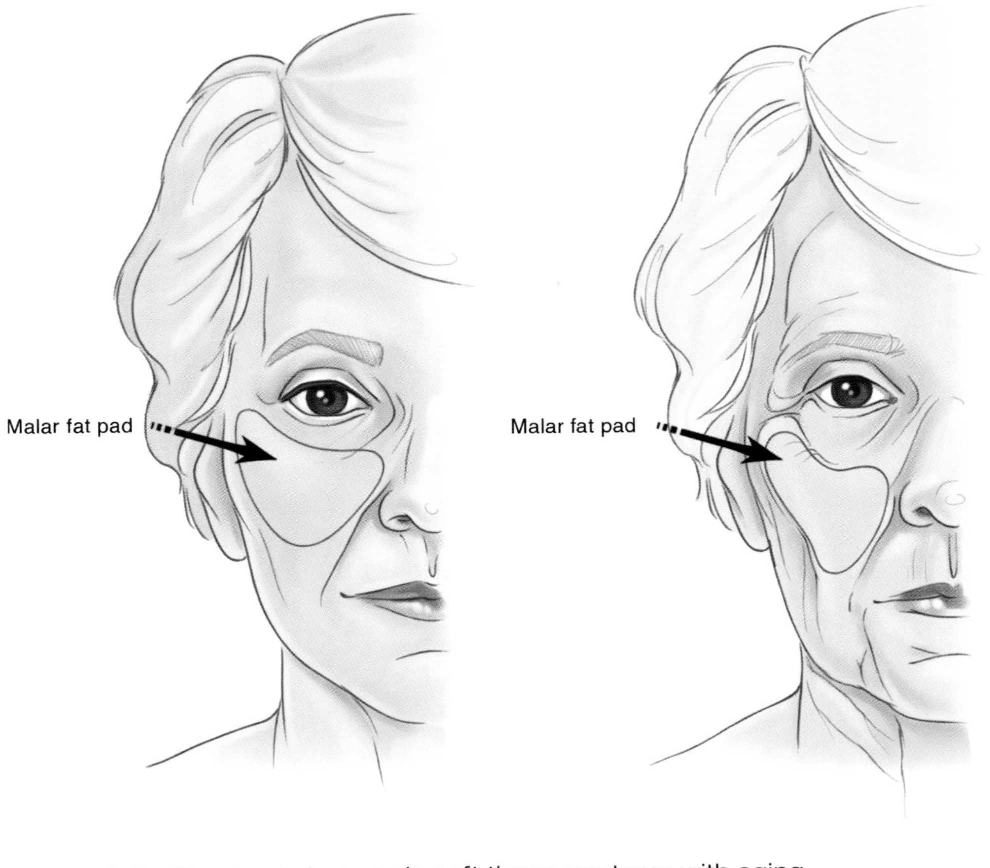

Figure 8–2. Structural changes in soft tissue anatomy with aging.

fat pad descent. The **mandibular ligament** supports the chin pad and sharply defines the anterior extent of jowling. Many surgeons do not see these as discrete anatomic structures and do not deal with them directly.

A thorough understanding of facial nerve anatomy and its relation to the concentric layers in the face will allow for safe dissection in face lift surgery. As the facial nerve plexus exits the skull at the sternomastoid foramen, it passes anterolaterally through the parotid gland, separated from it by a fascial invagination. The buccal and zygomatic branches consistently exit the parotid-masseteric fascia along the anterior border of the masseter in the cheek. In this sub-SMAS position within the cheek, the nerves terminate as branches innervating the levators and orbicularis oculi medially along its deep surface. The marginal mandibular branch also has a consistent position in the face. Exiting the parotid inferiorly, approximately 4 cm below the earlobe, the nerve passes along the mandible most commonly superior to the mandibular border and crosses superficial to the palpable facial artery and vein. The frontal branch or temporal branch of the facial nerve exits the parotid superiorly and is best approximated by a line connecting the tragus to a point 1.5 cm above the lateral end of the eyebrow. After crossing the zygomatic arch, the facial nerve traverses superomedially and always medial and inferior to the palpable frontal branch of the superficial temporal artery. Frontal branches should be considered a notable exception to the deep fascial course of the other nerve branches. After crossing the zygomatic arch, the frontal branch lies within sub-SMAS fat prior to penetrating the frontalis. The great auricular sensory nerve is mentioned since injury during cervical undermining can cause sensory loss over the region anterior and posterior to the ear. The nerve is classically described as overlying the mid-sternocleidomastoid muscle 6.5 cm below the ear canal. The nerve is protected with subcutaneous dissection in the neck because of its sub-SMAS/platysma position. Care should be taken to prevent exposure of any sternocleidomastoid muscle to prevent nerve injury.

The platysma muscle of the neck is contiguous with the SMAS layer of the face. The platysma mostly originates from the SMAS itself and is supported by fibrous attachments to the thyroid cartilage, the floor of the mouth, and a small attachment to the anterior mandible. The clinical changes in the neck with aging invariably include skin flaccidity with atrophy of subcutaneous fat.

PATIENT EVALUATION & SELECTION

The evaluation begins with a comprehensive review of the patient's medical history, including prior hospitalizations, surgical and anesthetic history, current medications, allergies, as well as pertinent social habits. The evaluation should focus on identifying those individuals suitable for general or local anesthesia with intravenous sedation. Patients with advanced age or any history of cardiopulmonary disease, diabetes, asthma, or thyroid condition should be evaluated by a specialist to support the safety of performing the planned procedure.

The history should focus on identifying risk factors for complications during face lift surgery, namely, bleeding, skin slough, nerve injury, and infection. Perioperative hypertension should be optimized before the procedure, since it puts the patient at increased risk for hematoma formation. In addition, the patient should be asked about any history of a bleeding disorder. A review of the patient's medications, including any herbal supplements, should be performed to confirm that none interfere with the normal clotting mechanism. Smoking has known adverse effects on wound healing and vascular perfusion, so cessation should be mandated for at least 3 weeks before and after the procedure. The viability of the distal skin flap and healing at areas of tension are at increased risk with smoking.

In addition, the surgeon must evaluate the psychological profile of the patient seeking face lift surgery. The ideal patient would have (1) practical motivations for wanting surgery, (2) realistic expectations, (3) stable interpersonal relationships, and (4) a healthy self-image. A poor surgical candidate would be (1) a patient who expects the physical changes of face lift surgery will make dramatic changes in his/her life, (2) a patient motivated for surgery based on fears of abandonment, or (3) a patient with a history of dissatisfaction after prior aesthetic procedures. There are few absolute psychological characteristics that contraindicate surgery. Rather, there is a series of "red flags" that require rethinking of the patient's motivation and potential happiness with surgery.

Thorough counseling and written documentation regarding the operative procedure in addition to preoperative and postoperative care, responsibilities, and possible complications are invaluable.

A comprehensive preoperative physical examination of the face and neck region is needed for optimal treatment planning. This evaluation should include current photographs, preferably taken by a professional, or at least consistently lit if done in the office. The examination of the face begins with assessing the skin for its texture and elasticity as well as soft tissues contour abnormalities. Textural changes of the face (including fine facial and periorbital rhytids) are generally unaffected by traditional face lifting procedures and may benefit from less invasive techniques such as chemical peels, laser resurfacing, chemical deinnervation, or injectable fillers. Malar fat pad descent with infraorbital flattening and deep nasolabial folds should be identified. Facial fat excess or atrophy, jowling, and the mandibular contour should be assessed. In the neck, findings of platysmal banding, cervicomental obliquity, and excessive subplatysmal fat are noted for appropriate planning of neck rejuvenation. Earlobe and hairline contour should be appreciated as the planned incisions are discussed with the patient.

PATIENT PREPARATION

The face lift procedure can be performed under general anesthesia or local anesthesia with intravenous sedation. Midazolam, fentanyl, and propofol are used in most instances.

On achieving full sedation, but before surgical preparation, the face is injected with 1% lidocaine with epinephrine in a 1:100,000 solution. A total of 30 mL is used off the field and augmented at surgery; this allows an additional 10 minutes for full effectiveness. Broad-spectrum antibiotics are routinely used prior to incision. These are adjusted in specific conditions, such as mitral valve prolapse. Preoperative hair shampooing and cleansing is not necessary.

TECHNIQUE

Although there are numerous variations to the modern face lift procedure, most incorporate some combination of deep and subcutaneous techniques. The approach for most procedures is similar and will be presented in a stepwise manner.

A. Incision Planning

With the head turned as far as comfortable, the temporal hair is combed back and managed with copious amounts of antibiotic ointment without the use of rubber bands. If a temporal scalp extension is planned, the hair is held in place with ointment without cutting, shaving, or banding. The ointment maintains a tidy field.

The LIFT procedure routinely begins with submental suction-assisted lipectomy for removal of fat and to facilitate the neck

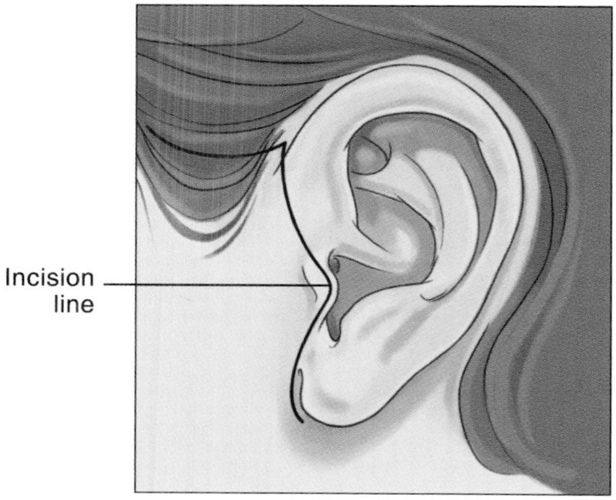

Figure 8–3. The incision for the limited-incision face lift technique (LIFT) begins at the sideburn and terminates in the dart beneath the lobule.

dissection. Subsequently, the most frequently performed incision begins at the sideburn, traversing a slightly retrotragal path and terminates in a dart beneath the lobule (Figure 8–3). This incision is indicated to address the cheek, nasolabial folds, jowls, submental laxity, and upper neck. Occasionally a pretragal position is better suited; the decision is dictated by the amount and position of adjacent hair-bearing skin and regional contours. In men, for example, advancement of hair-bearing skin onto the tragus would be unacceptable unless the patient was willing to accept postoperative laser hair removal.

Occasionally, a temporal extension is added if the operative plan is to address the forehead and eyebrow. To create this extension, the incision is carried from the temporal scalp into the non–hair-bearing preauricular skin to a posttragal position into the skin fold where the lobule meets the cheek. This continues behind the lobule where it terminates in a dart. In cases of great skin laxity, the standard incision is augmented by an infra-sideburn dart (Figure 8–4).

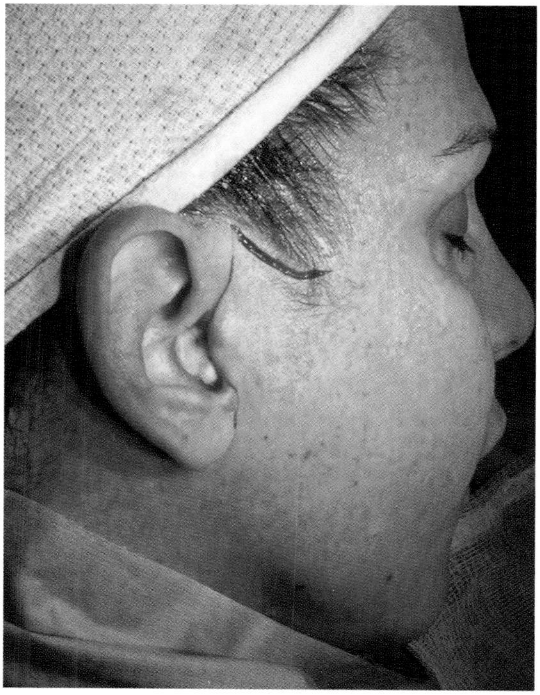

Figure 8–4. The limited incision is used without temporal extension when forehead or eyebrow surgery is not indicated.

This limited incision technique is successful under many circumstances. However, it is not indicated for treatment of significant skin laxity of the lower neck wherein a postauricular incision is added.

B. Dissection Technique

If a scalp incision is used, dissection begins in a superficial plane, keeping the undersurface of the hair follicles in view throughout. This does not result in hair loss and allows a smooth and safe transition over the zygomatic area, maintaining a plane considerably superficial to the temporal and zygomatic branches of the facial nerve.

Whether the sideburn dart alone or the temporal extension is used, undermining is carried medially 5 to 6 cm from the preauricular incision, throughout the cheek and over the mandible to the submental area, maintaining the safe superficial position throughout. When appropriate, this dissection continues in the supraplatysmal plane in the neck, taking care to fully free the skin across the midline. Where an open submental incision exists, this is fully joined to the facial flaps in the plane superficial to the platysma. Scrupulous hemostasis is achieved with electrocautery. Drains are never inserted in any face lift procedure.

When a temporal extension is used, the lowest hair-bearing scalp edge is grasped with toothed mosquito forceps and distracted upward. A notch is cut below the clamp at a place that will allow closure under tension with skin staples. After this first staple is placed and the resultant pull evaluated, the redundant skin is excised from the first staple upward. After securing the skin lift with several additional staples in the hairline, the upper limb of redundant scalp is excised and scalp closure proceeds from the apex downward, avoiding the possibility of terminal dog-ear. If a great deal of redundant skin exists, it would be unwise to elevate the hairline excessively; instead, a sideburn dart is used. If brow elevation is not contemplated, the sideburn dart alone is used. Closure begins by distracting the highest skin edge in a direction perpendicular to the nasolabial fold. Half-buried 3-0 nylon mattress sutures are taken from the hair-bearing skin through the dermis of the flap and tied within the hair to prevent visible suture marks. The dart of skin developed behind the lobule is rotated anteriorly and the crotch of the dart is placed at the tip of the lobule, which is sutured with a buried 4-0 polyglactin suture (Figure 8–5). Redundant preauricular skin is resected under minimal tension. Pretragal skin is defatted to dermis and the anterior incision is closed from post lobule to scalp with 4-0 nylon, first over and over until the lobule is secured, then intracuticularly throughout the anterior portion.

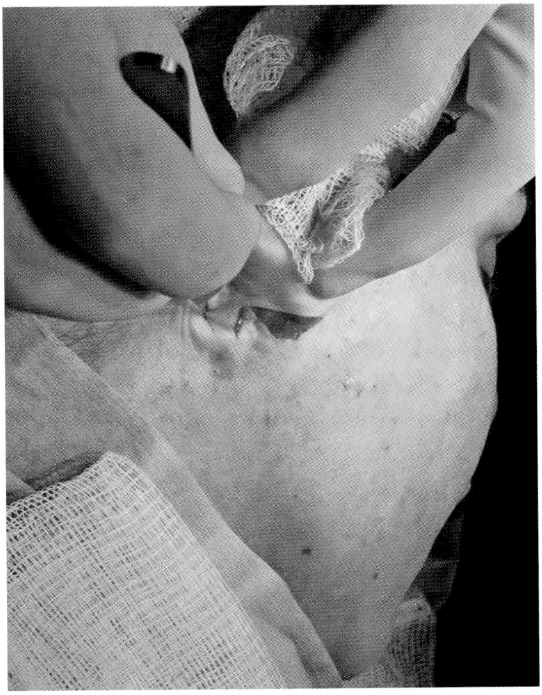

Figure 8–5. After undermining, point A is rotated anteriorly, and the lobule is inserted at point B.

C. SMAS Dissection

The modern conceptual goal for facial rejuvenation surgery is the restoration of facial volume to a youthful contour. It is well appreciated that a patient's youthful appearance cannot be fully restored by high-tension redraping of skin over lax soft tissue infrastructure. Various procedures on the SMAS, including traditional or extended SMAS dissection, composite SMAS-skin rhytidectomy, SMAS plication, and lateral SMASectomy were introduced to improve the results of skin-only face lifts.

To achieve the best results, a SMAS resection with a traditional subcutaneous dissection is recommended. The superficial preparotid fascia is inscribed roughly parallel to the nasolabial fold. Blunt dissection with the use of the spreading anterior-posterior action of face lift scissors (tips facing up) develops the sub-SMAS plane over the parotid gland; care is taken to avoid entering the gland. Medial dissection is carried out but not beyond the level of the zygomatic muscle. The SMAS is then developed distally toward the mandibular angle and often into its transition to pure platysma muscle. The fibrous SMAS edge is elevated and sutured under tension to the highest achievable point of the fibrous preauricular sheath. Redundant SMAS tissue is resected at the apex of the closure and along its posterior border. Plication is begun with two inverted permanent sutures at the highest area where most tension exists, and the remaining SMAS closure is performed with 3-0 polyglactin, taking care to invert knots.

D. Methods for Neck Contour Rejuvenation

Neck contour rejuvenation can be achieved as an isolated procedure or with face lift procedures that include deep plane techniques such as SMAS resection or plication.

Neck appearance can be categorized into three classes based on a treatment algorithm (Table 8–1). Class I includes the neck with minimal skin flaccidity and mild subcutaneous fat in the submandibular and subglandular regions without platysma flaccidity. These patients can be treated successfully with suction-assisted lipectomy alone. More advanced signs of neck aging within class II require a formal submental incision for management. This group is further subdivided into IIA (those patients not needing platysma plication) and IIB (those requiring platysma plication). The appearance of necks in class III includes severe skin flaccidity as well as platysma flaccidity and thick subcutaneous fat. This group is managed with the above techniques plus a postauricular neck lift.

As the first step in nearly every face lift procedure, via a submental stab wound, suction-assisted lipectomy with 2- and 3-mm cannulas is used to defat the jowl and submental areas. Special attention is given to the area between platysmal bands often adequately addressed by liposuction alone. Care is exercised to limit

▶ TABLE 8–1. NECK LIFT CLASSIFICATION AND MANAGEMENT

Neck Classification	Anatomic Features	Management
Class I	Minimal skin laxity Mild subcutaneous fat No platysma laxity	Micro-SAL only
Class IIA	Minimal skin laxity Mild to moderate subcutaneous fat No platysma laxity	Micro-SAL Submental incision; no platysma plication
Class IIB	Minimal skin laxity Mild to moderate subcutaneous fat Mild to moderate platysma laxity	Micro-SAL Submental incision with platysma plication
Class III	Severe skin laxity Extensive subcutaneous fat Moderate to extensive platysma laxity	Micro-SAL Submental incision with platysma plication Postauricular neck lift

SAL, suction-assisted lipectomy.

suction-assisted lipectomy to the superficial subcutaneous plane. In the presence of prominent platysmal bands visible in the erect position, a direct submental incision is performed. If required, dissection is carried out under direct visualization with use of a serrated fiberoptic lighted retractor. The skin elevation, much of which is accomplished with suction-assisted lipectomy, is completed with face lift scissors. Platysmal bands are either resected for extreme redundancy, or more usually plicated at the midline with interrupted sutures of 3-0 polyglactin. Plication begins distal to the hyoid and continues cephalad to the mentum.

To create the postauricular incision and lift for patients in class III, the previously described incision is carried superiorly along the conchal groove and then slants posteriorly along the natural hairline. The length of this incision depends on the amount of cervical neck resection that is anticipated. The dissection is again within the subcutaneous plane and joins the midline dissection. Vectors for planning skin resection are determined by trial and error after elevation of the flap. When proper tension is determined, resection begins from the distal limb toward the concha, leaving the inscribed limb as a tag for traction. Closure is carried out with intracuticular 4-0 nylon suture throughout. Post-conchal skin excision is a simple resection of redundancy and closed similarly.

E. Ancillary Techniques

Autologous fat transfer to the nasolabial folds, oral commissure, and glabellar frown lines are used in most cases to supplement the face lift procedure.

POSTOPERATIVE CARE

Most patients spend 2 hours in the recovery area prior to discharge. Patients generally have sutures removed by the eighth postoperative day and return to work thereafter. Exercise and strenuous activities are prohibited for 2 to 3 weeks.

COMPLICATIONS

The most frequent complications of rhytidectomy are hematomas, skin slough, alopecia, nerve injury, contour irregularities, unacceptable scarring, seromas, and infection. All of the above are minimized by limited incision techniques.

Hematoma is the most frequent complication of face lift surgery. Large hematomas generally present in the early postoperative period and have a direct toxic effect on the overlying skin flap, thus require early evacuation. The literature reports major hematomas have an incidence between 0.3% and 8%; the incidence of hematoma after LIFT is reported to be 0.6%. Hematomas are more frequent in males than in females. Most hematoma prevention is aimed at meticulous hemostasis and control of elevated blood pressure. Antiemetics can aid in reducing blood pressure fluctuations when necessary. Antihypertensives are not recommended, although some surgeons may use them. Pain, ecchymosis, and swelling are signs of hematoma formation, and in their presence, the surgeon should remove all dressings to adequately assess the skin flaps. Large hematomas require evacuation, irrigation, and a search for any bleeding vessels.

Facial nerve injury is a feared complication in face lift surgery. Motor nerve injury is probably less than 1%, and return of function is generally expected after blunt or traction nerve injuries as opposed to transection injuries. The buccal branch is the most commonly injured during the dissection of the loose areolar plane anterior to the parotid. Given the distal nature of the nerve injury and overlapping neural territories, recovery and accommodation is generally expected within 3 to 4 months. Injuries to the frontal branch generally occur where it takes a more superficial location crossing the zygomatic arch. These injuries are frequently longer lasting and occasionally need surgical correction for total frontalis paralysis. The marginal mandibular nerve branch also may be injured during anterior dissection or along the mandibular border. Injuries cause weakness of the lower lip depressors causing the affected side to become flattened and inwardly rotated. Some accommodation by the platysma, innervated by deep cervical branches of facial nerve, occurs. The most common sensory nerve injury that occurred with the classic face lift cervical dissection involved the sensory great auricular nerve; however, since the advent of limited incision techniques and conservative dissection, this injury is virtually unseen.

Skin slough is a direct result of compromised blood supply and is most common in the postauricular or mastoid areas. Tissue ischemia is worsened with high tension closures and in patients who smoke perioperatively or have comorbid vascular conditions, such as atherosclerotic disease or diabetes. Skin flap ischemia also can be attributed to hematoma formation. If full thickness necrosis with eschar ensues, management involves conservative topical antibiotics and possible need for periodic debridement.

Alopecia can occur in the temporal region with superficial dissection and damage to the hair follicles. Infections after rhytidectomy are less than 1%.

REFERENCES

Baker DC. Lateral SMASectomy. *Plast Reconstr Surg.* 1997 Aug;100(2):509–13. [PMID: 9252623]

Baker TJ et al. Personal technique of face lifting. *Plast Reconstr Surg.* 1997 Aug;100(2):502–8. [PMID: 9252622]

Hamra ST. The deep-plane rhytidectomy. *Plast Reconstr Surg.* 1990 Jul;86(1):53–61. [PMID: 2359803]

Imber G et al. Limited-incision face lift technique. *Aesthetic Surg J.* 2001 May;21(3):216–26. [PMID: 19331896]

Owsley JQ. Face Lift. *Plast Reconstr Surg.* 1997 Aug;100(2):514–9. [PMID: 9252624]

Skoog T. *Plastic Surgery: New Methods.* Philadelphia: Saunders; 1974.

CHAPTER 9

Blepharoplasty

Jeffrey D. Hoefflin, MD, Roy Foo, MD, & Henry M. Spinelli, MD

The correction of the deformities associated with aging eyes is based on the principles of the facial subunits. There are many different techniques reported in the plastic surgery literature. In this chapter, the basic principles of aesthetic surgery of the eyes will be presented, and it is hoped that this will be a platform from which the many different proposed techniques and points of contention of blepharoplasty can be evaluated and understood.

▶ ANATOMY

A fundamental concept in viewing the eyelid is that it is composed of three distinct anatomic layers: the external coverage or skin, a middle support layer, and an internal lining (Figure 9–1). Together, they form a tri-lamellar structure supported and anchored across the orbital rim by the medial and lateral canthal tendons. The outermost layer of this tri-lamellar structure consists of the outer coverage of skin, which is especially thin over the tarsus and preseptal areas with minimal to no subcutaneous fat. The middle, or supportive layer, includes the orbicularis muscles, with the pretarsal portion lying in front of the tarsal plate. Finally, the deepest layer is the preorbital portion of this tri-lamellar structure, which lies anterior to the orbital septum.

The tarsal plate is a rigid cartilaginous-like structure that measures 4 to 6 mm in the lower lid and 8–10 mm in the upper lid (see Figure 9–1). This structure is pierced by glands that drain or open posterior to the eyelashes. The tarsal plates are the end point for retractor insertion and provide lid stability and orientation. It is an especially important structure for vertical support and eyelid rigidity.

The orbicularis oculi muscle is in the same contiguous layer as the frontalis, the occipitalis, and the superficial musculo-aponeurotic system of the midface. It has a medial and lateral raphé and is divided into three divisions: preorbital, preseptal, and pretarsal. It functions as a sphincter. The orbicularis muscle is innervated by the facial nerve (cranial nerve VII) and, hence, with facial nerve paralysis, the cornea and globe are typically exposed owing to an atonic eyelid.

The orbital septum is confluent with the periosteum of the skull and the orbit. Analogously, the inferior orbital septum is intimately linked to the periosteum and the capsulopalpebral fascia.

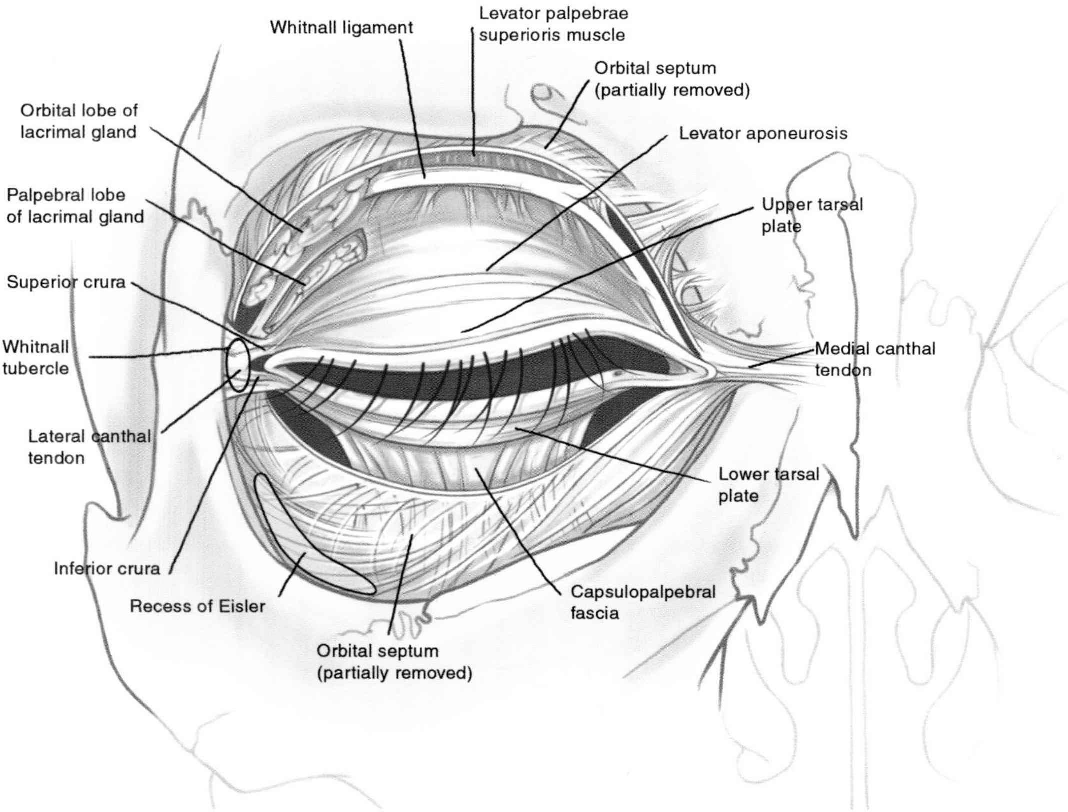

Figure 9–1. **The anatomy of the periorbital region.** The upper and lower eyelids are suspended in space, tethered medially and laterally by the canthal tendons and, in turn, are lined to Whitnall and Lockwood ligaments. The orbital and palpebral lobes of the lacrimal gland are divided by Whitnall ligament. The orbital septum inserts at the orbital rim, except inferolaterally where it inserts beyond the rim forming Eisler recess. (Reproduced, with permission, from Spinelli H. *Atlas of Aesthetic Eyelid and Periocular Surgery. Copyright Elsevier 2004.*)

The main retractors of the upper eyelids possess a voluntary or primary retractor, namely, the levator palpebrae superioris muscle and a secondary sympathomimetically innervated muscle called Müller muscle. This muscle is the so-called fight or flight response muscle and is responsible for approximately 2 mm of lid elevation. The levator muscle sends some fibers to the dermal surface of the upper lid skin, creating an upper eyelid fold. The lower lid retractors, namely, the capsulopalpebral fascia, are intimately linked to the inferior extraocular muscles. The inferior rectus and inferior oblique muscles send out extensions by way of the capsulopalpebral fascia, and these insert onto the inferior edge of the tarsal plate of the lower eyelid.

Whitnall ligament suspends the levator muscle from the superior orbit, allowing the muscle to change vector forces from anterior to posterior and superior to inferior, thus serving as a pulley. The lateral canthal tendon is formed by two crurae, which are continuous with the tarsal plates. This common canthal tendon inserts at Whitnall tubercle 2 to 3 mm inside the lateral orbital rim. Whitnall tubercle serves as a common insertion point for a number of structures, which cumulatively are known as the lateral retinaculum. These include the orbital septum, canthal tendon, Lockwood ligament, and Whitnall ligament, along with the deep head of the orbicularis and check ligament of the lateral rectus muscles.

▶ PATIENT EVALUATION & SELECTION

The initial consultation should begin with a detailed history. The surgeon should ask the patient about the presence of dry eyes or the use of ophthalmic lubricants and artificial tears, contact lens wear and the type of lenses used, thyroid or Graves disease, previous refractive surgery, recurrent acute or chronic blepharitis, history of herpes zoster, and other ocular or periocular conditions that are relevant. Such conditions may predispose the patient to surgical complications. It is also important to have the patient describe his or her aesthetic complaints while looking in a mirror.

A detailed history and physical examination assists the surgeon in choosing the most appropriate procedure for the patient. This information will help the surgeon tailor the surgical procedure to the needs of the individual patient.

During the physical examination, a significant amount of information can be obtained by simply studying the particular anatomy of the patient's eyelids and periocular region.

At the start of the examination, the general periocular region, including the upper and lower eyelids, is evaluated. It is important to assess the presence or absence of the proper anatomic position of the upper and lower eyelids. The upper lid should divide the width of the upper iris in half. The distance between the corneoscleral junction and the pupillary aperture should be bisected by the upper lid. The lower lid should lie above or at the corneoscleral junction. The upper and lower eyelids should have a smooth sweeping arch or contour. The highest point or maximal arch of the upper lid should lie at the most medial aspect of the pupillary aperture. Inflammatory changes and crusting along the eyelid margins or within the eyelashes are indications of blepharitis.

Although the surgical approaches may be the same, an appreciation of the differences between blepharochalasia and dermatochalasia should be made. **Blepharochalasia** is the presence of redundant upper lid tissue secondary to an underlying pathophysiology, such as recurrent edema due to renal failure, cardiac disease, or angioneurotic edema. **Dermatochalasia** is the commonly found redundancy of upper eyelid tissue secondary to the senescent process with or without ptotic eyebrow changes.

Documenting visual acuity, whether using a standardized Snellen chart at a distance or a hand-held Snellen card is important. A visual acuity assessment is obtained for both eyes with and without correction. It is not uncommon for patients to complain of visual acuity changes postoperatively, and it is therefore, important to document presurgical visual acuity.

Next, extraocular muscle motion and pupillary function are assessed. Any asymmetry in motion and function is carefully noted. The lower lid snap back test is used to ascertain delays or asymmetries in the tone of the lower lid. The snap back of the lower lid skin can be graded as weak, moderate, or brisk. A youthful and intact lower eyelid should position itself against the globe and revert to an appropriate height within 1 second of distraction. In planning a procedure on a patient with anything but a brisk snap back test, the surgeon must either increase intrinsic support factors or at least not increase extrinsic distraction forces.

Palpating and visualizing the orbital rim and malar eminence can determine the level of zygomatic and malar support. In patients with lower eyelid malposition, the surgeon should try to determine which lamella (anterior, middle, or posterior) is deficient. This will serve to assist the surgeon in planning complimentary procedures as adjuncts to a canthopexy, such as a cheek or midface suspension, to optimize aesthetic results if needed.

All patients should be assessed for the quantity and quality of tears produced. The Schirmer test, which uses topical anesthesia and precut standardized No. 41 filter paper strips, can assess quantitative tear production. It may be beneficial to place the patient in a dark room while testing to obviate the effect that ambient light has on tear production. The results of the Schirmer test can be graded into three categories: low tear production (0–9 mm), moderate tear production (10–20 mm), or high tear production (21–30 mm). In high tear producers, the diagnosis of nasolacrimal obstruction should be considered.

The tear film break-up time is a simple method of evaluating tear film quality. Fluorescein is introduced onto a topically anesthetized eye and, after the patient is allowed to blink and disperse the agent, the eyelids are then held apart and the uniform tear film is visualized over the corneal surface through a cobalt blue filter. The time period between holding the patient's eye open and the deterioration of the tear layer (tear film break-up) is an assessment of tear film break-up time and is usually over 20 seconds.

The importance of evaluating the history and physical examination in each patient is to first identify the problem and second to tailor the surgical procedure according to the specific physical findings. It is important to obtain definitive historical and physical signs that will help direct the surgeon choose an appropriate surgical procedure for the individual patient.

▶ UPPER LID BLEPHAROPLASTY

The key steps to upper lid rejuvenation are illustrated in Figure 9–2.

In the patient undergoing upper lid blepharoplasty, it is extremely important to assess eyebrow position and note the presence or absence of brow ptosis. The surgeon who attempts to correct significantly eyebrow ptosis by means of an upper lid blepharoplasty alone will meet with unsatisfactory results and usually have a dissatisfied patient.

It is usually the lateral one-third of the eyebrow that is most important from a cosmetic standpoint. Redundancy in this area can be eliminated in one of two ways: either the surgeon may elevate the lateral one-third of the eyebrow and then perform a more conservative blepharoplasty, or a very aggressive lateral blepharoplasty extending beyond the orbital rim is necessary in addressing this hooding. The constraint for the surgeon is that incisions that extend beyond the lateral orbital rim become proportionaly more noticeable the more laterally they extend the incision. Therefore, the surgeon must balance the extent of lateral hooding against the desire to minimize lateralization of the upper lid blepharoplasty scar.

TECHNIQUE

The key points in planning and executing the upper lid blepharoplasty are as follows:

- Determination of the endogenous lid crease or height at which to create a new lid crease. The level of this crease will serve as the lower limb of the blepharoplasty incision and the height of the supratarsal fixation, should that be necessary.
- The width or extent of skin excision is determined by pinching the lid skin

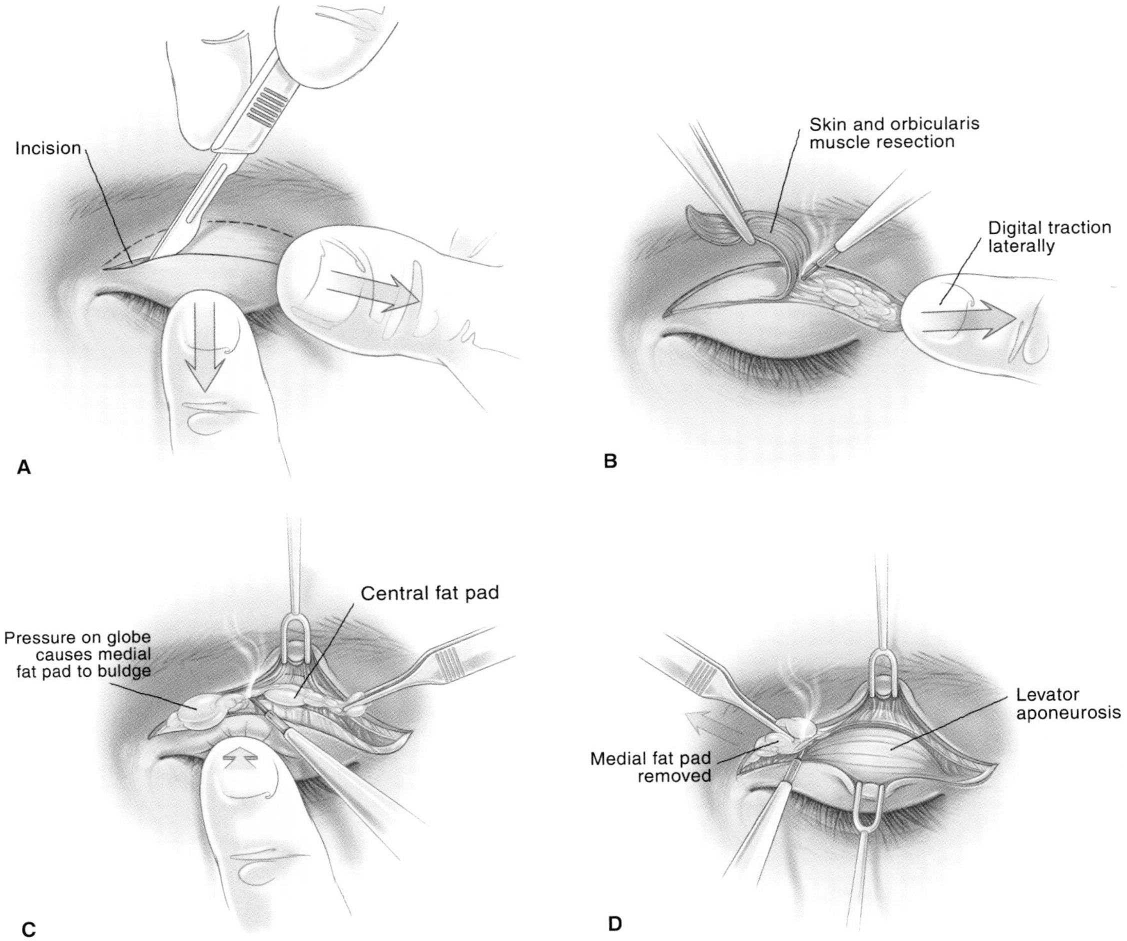

Figure 9–2. **The steps of an upper lid blepharoplasty. A:** Slightly more pressure must be exerted on the scalpel laterally as the skin thickens around and lateral to the orbital rim. **B:** The skin may be elevated with the orbicularis muscle in one maneuver using an instrument on the skin-muscle section to be resected and pulling this superonasally while providing digital traction laterally. **C:** The underlying levator aponeurosis is protected by opening the septum as cephalad as possible, because the levator and septum diverge as the surgeon moves superiorly. **D:** The medial fat pad may require some digital pressure to expose and grasp; however, care should be taken not to overly resect fat when using digital pressure techniques. Excessive traction and manipulation of fat could cause a deep orbital hemorrhage and should, therefore, be avoided. **E:** Closure may then be performed and 6-0 nylon interrupted sutures laterally and 5-0 nylon intracuticular sutures medially are preferred. (Reproduced, with permission, from *Spinelli H. Atlas of Aesthetic Eyelid and Periocular Surgery.* Copyright Elsevier 2004.)

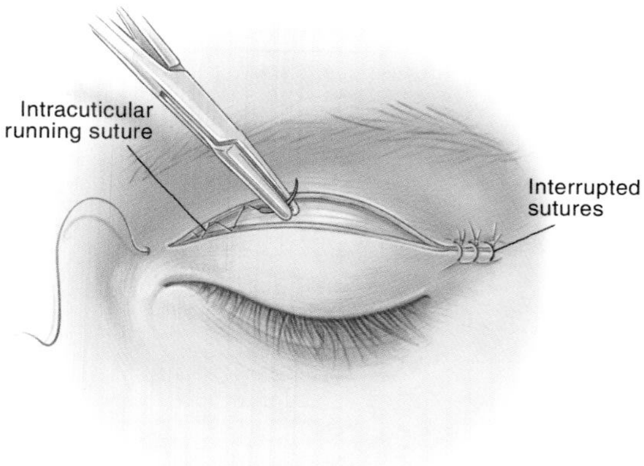

Figure 9–2. (Continued)

between the forceps using slight lash line eversion as the end point. This superior point will determine the location for the superior limb of the incision.

- The degree of lateral hooding will dictate the point of the lateral extension needed to treat the hooding. The greater the hooding, the more lateral the extent of the incision. In general, extensions beyond the orbital rim are not well tolerated.
- The upper blepharoplasty incision lines are marked with ink.
- Using digital traction and light pressure, the incision is performed with a scalpel.
- The skin and the orbicularis muscle may be elevated in one maneuver. Using a fine-needled tipped insulated cautery may be most advantageous, especially in avoiding any hemostasis problems.
- The orbital septum is then widely opened, exposing the preaponeurotic space.
- The underlying levator aponeurosis is protected by opening the septum as cephalad as possible. The levator and septum diverge as the surgeon moves superiorly. Note that the orbital septum must be violated to gain access to the superior orbit, the levator, and the preaponeurotic fat.
- Modifications in the levator or at the levator-tarsal junction can be easily performed with this exposure.
- Digital pressure may be required to expose the medial and central upper eyelid fat pads. However, care should be taken not to overly resect fat when using digital pressure techniques. Excessive traction and manipulation of fat could cause a deep orbital hemorrhage. When fat excision is performed, it should be conservative to avoid a hollowed-out appearance.
- Skin closure is performed with 6-0 interrupted sutures laterally and 5-0 nylon intracuticular sutures medially.
- Skin should be redraped, with the line between the nasojugal groove and the lateral canthus kept in mind, inducing a lateral cephalic vector.
- Careful skin eversion lateral to the canthus is important to avoid a depressed incision line.

▶ LOWER LID BLEPHAROPLASTY

In assessing the choices for lower lid blepharoplasty, the importance of evaluating the patient for the degree of horizontal lid laxity; position of the lateral and medical canthal angles; conditions such as scleral show, entropion, and ectropion; or other pathologic processes cannot be overstated. Choices for lower lid rejuvenation include the following: either the transcutaneous or transconjunctival approach; a canthal procedure, such as a tarsal tuck or tarsal strip procedure; or common canthoplasty (repositioning of the entire lateral canthus). Decisions about how to address the skin or fat, or both, are equally numerous.

An appreciation of midface position is as important in lower lid blepharoplasty as is appreciation of brow position in upper lid blepharoplasty.

▶ TRANSCUTANEOUS LOWER LID BLEPHAROPLASTY

The transcutaneous lower lid approach is a powerful technique for addressing lower lid cosmetic abnormalities. A number of adjuvant procedures can be performed easily at the same time. Its disadvantages include greater technical demands; more time; more extensive dissection; and hence, greater secondary fibrosis. However, it is more powerful because the surgeon may address fat alone, address skin or muscle separately, and approach lower lid tightening by way of a direct approach to the lateral lower lid tarsus or inferior crus of the lateral canthal tendon.

The decision to use the transcutaneous route rather than the transconjunctival route should be predicated on the amount of skin redundancy and whether a canthal tightening procedure is indicated. The transconjunctival route alone does not in general provide adequate exposure to the midface and does not allow appropriate cephalic and lateral elevation of the cheek unit. Therefore, should the surgeon want to address the midface (cheek suspension), then an access incision either by way of lateral lower eyelid, lateral upper eyelid, or face lift approach is usually necessary.

TECHNIQUE

Key points for performing the transcutaneous lower lid blepharoplasty include the following:

- The primary incision should be in a desired fold or potential fold at and lateral to the lateral canthus. This is usually inferiorly declined and mirrors an existing skin crease. In the more youthful patient, the incision may only extend a few millimeters lateral to the canthus, and in the older patient, it may extend much farther.
- Curved Stevens scissors are introduced and used to undermine in the preseptal suborbicularis potential space. This plane is developed in a lateral to medial fashion.
- Once this plane is developed, the myocutaneous flap can be mobilized with ease by withdrawing the scissors and reintroducing only one blade into the preseptal postorbicularis plane; the scissors are then beveled toward the eyeball to include less skin and more muscle.
- Orbicularis muscle should be preserved when raising a skin muscle flap.
- Orbicularis muscle suspension through the transcutaneous access route is the simplest but also is the least effective method of increasing lower lid support.
- The second incision is completed lateral to medial with the assistance of inferior digital traction, ending just lateral to the lower lid punctum.
- Superior lid traction with a small hook will assist in providing exposure.
- The flap should be mobilized to the orbital rim without violating the septum.
- The septum may then be elevated widely or with small serial stab incisions.
- The inferior oblique muscle should be visualized and protected during conservative fat pad resection.
- Digital pressure on the upper lid can cause the lateral orbital fat pad to anteriorly bulge.
- Over resection of fat, especially in the lateral compartment, can lead to less than acceptable results.

- Orbital fat may be repositioned throughout or in selected pockets and combined with resection techniques depending on the needs of the patient.
- Redrape the skin in a cephalic and lateral direction. Interrupted sutures are used for a lateral closure, and a running suture is placed in a medial to lateral fashion.
- The amount of skin resected and the degree of cephalic lateral suspension should be judged on the patient's history, physical examination, and appearance.
- In patients who have a minimal tolerance for over resection, the surgeon might want to evoke distraction tests, such as forcibly opening the patient's mouth or having the patient look up, before finally trimming the skin muscle flap.

▶ TRANSCONJUNCTIVAL LOWER LID BLEPHAROPLASTY

The transconjunctival approach to the retroseptal space may be accomplished in one of two ways: preseptal or retroseptal. The preseptal route is by far the most controlled and anatomically consistent method. In either case, an insulated retractor (eg, Desmarres) is extremely useful. The retroseptal route entails simply incising the conjunctiva and cutting through the lower lid retractors into the postseptal space. The preseptal route requires entry into the post orbicularis preseptal space above the fusion of the lower lid retractors and the orbital septum. This will allow direct visualization of the septum, and each fat pad can be addressed separately in a controlled fashion. To expediently achieve this, a few simple steps are necessary. A protective lens may be used. The key steps of the transconjunctival lower lid blepharoplasty are illustrated in Figure 9–3.

TECHNIQUE

The key points of the procedure include the following:

- Once the patient is appropriately sedated, topical anesthesia (tetracaine) may be instilled into the conjunctival sac.
- Care must be taken at the initial part of the procedure to protect the cornea and eyeball during the local anesthesia infiltration and the initial dissection.
- Local anesthetic of choice containing epinephrine may be infiltrated with a small needle, preferably by way of the transconjunctival route with the lower lid either everted with slight digital pressure placed on the inferior tarsus or with light traction with an instrument such as the Desmarres retractor.
- A protective contact lens may then be placed, or the surgeon may chose to use an autologous contact lens created by the elevated conjunctival flap.
- Once adequate time for hemostasis is allowed to elapse, the conjunctiva and lower lid retractors are grasped near the central cul de sac or fornix with a tooth forceps and engaged with a traction suture.
- The lower lid is everted with a small eyelid hook, and a transconjunctival incision is made just below the tarsal plate with the conjunctiva and lower lid placed on cephalic traction.
- Once the lower lid retractors are disinserted from the tarsal plate, the eyelid hook is removed and a Desmarres retractor inserted to engage the lower edge of the tarsal plate.
- Traction is placed cephalad and anteriorly, and dissection is carried out in front of the orbital septum, in the preseptal postorbicularis plane, down to the orbital rim.

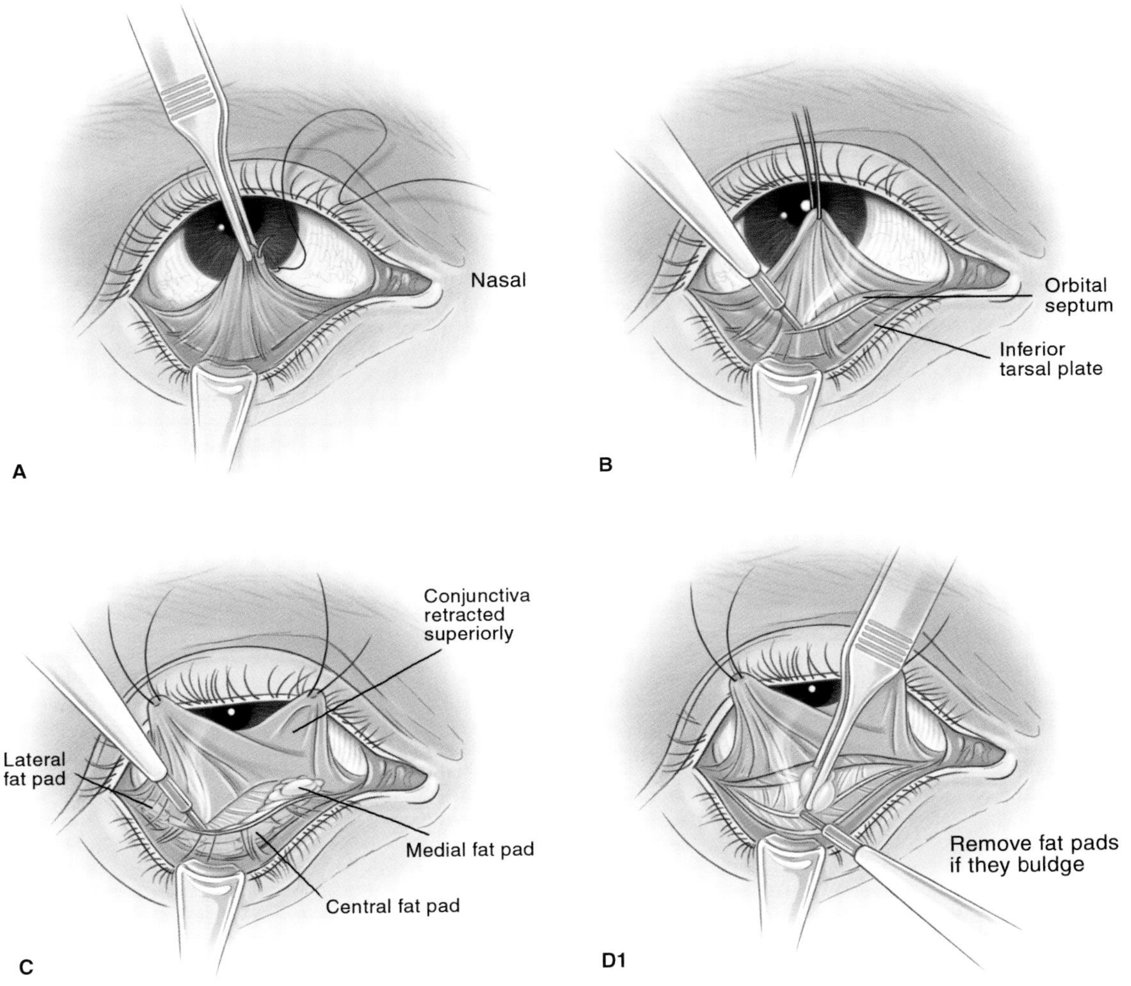

Figure 9–3. **Transconjunctival lower lid blepharoplasty. A:** A conjunctival stay suture is placed deep in the fornix and traction is applied superiorly while the lid margin is everted. This causes the inferior edge of the tarsal plate to rise toward the surgeon. **B:** The conjunctiva and lower lid retractors are incised just below the tarsal plate entering the post orbicularis preseptal space. This plane is developed in the orbital rim with the assistance of the traction suture and a nonconductive instrument. **C:** The orbital septum may then be widely incised or punctured and the inferior oblique muscle identified and preserved **D1 and D2**, the fat pads may be addressed individually in keeping with preoperative plans with either resection, repositioning, conservation or any combination of these techniques. In repositioning, a supraperiosteal tunnel with a temporary transcutaneous stay suture is preferred to maintain the proper location. **E:** A single absorbable closure suture is useful in avoiding Tenon inclusion cysts. It should be placed laterally to avoid postoperative complaints of corneal irritation.(Reproduced, with permission, from Spinelli H. *Atlas of Aesthetic Eyelid and Periocular Surgery.* Copyright Elsevier 2004.)

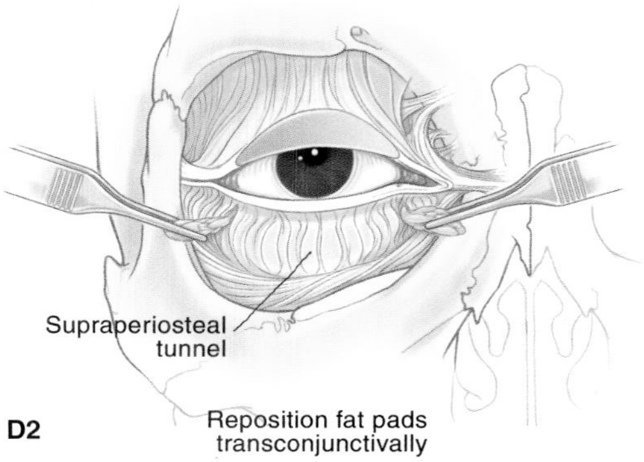

D2

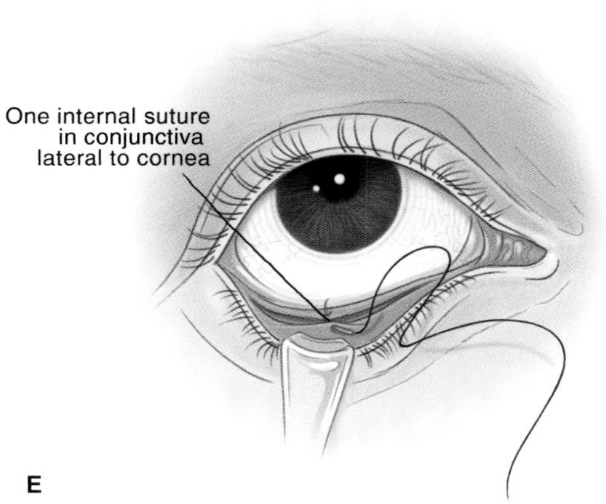

E

Figure 9–3. (Continued)

- The orbital septum is then widely incised by a wide transverse incision at the midseptum, or three distinct openings in the orbital septum may be created to access underlying fat compartments. A total transverse septal incision is preferred, especially in fat redraping, to avoid tethering or strangulation of the fat pedicle through a narrowed orbital septal opening.
- Conservative resection of the spontaneously herniated tissue is most appropriate.
- The inferior oblique muscle, lying between the medial and central fat pads, should be visualized and protected.
- Hemostasis is usually spontaneous and complete when this procedure is executed appropriately.
- The conjunctiva may be apposed with a single interrupted small absorbable suture lateral to the corneal surface. Reapproximate the conjunctiva because this eliminates Tenon cysts or pyogenic granulomas.
- The surgeon may then initiate a skin tightening procedure such as a laser or marginal skin trim.
- It is advantageous to use a topical antibiotic drop containing a corticosteroid (eg, dexamethasone and tobramycin [Tobradex] or prednisolone/sulfacetamide [Blephamide]) in the postoperative period when not contraindicated by corticosteroid-responsive glaucoma or other conditions.

▶ COMPLICATIONS

The increase in popularity of blepharoplasty procedures in the United States has coincided with an increased number of early and late complications. These may include, but are not limited to, visual loss due to hemorrhage, perforation of the globe during anesthesia, damage to extraocular muscles, lower lid malposition, loss of lashes, dryness, infection, incisional scarring, excessive upper lid fat resection, and inappropriate lower lid fat resection.

VISION LOSS DUE TO HEMORRHAGE

Retrobulbar hematoma is one of the most commonly feared complications of blepharoplasty. The overall incidence of retrobulbar hemorrhage is thought to be 1 in 25,000 cases. It can occur during or after the procedure. Bleeding is believed to result from inadequate hemostasis during the removal of superficial orbital fat pads or secondary to disruption of deep orbital vessels from manipulation of superficial fat pads, because these pads are linked to deep orbital fat. Patient-related factors include hypertension, certain coagulopathies as well the use of medication (such as aspirin or vitamin E). The potential for blindness can result without expedient treatment. It is important to recognize the signs of retrobulbar hemorrhage as early as possible to avoid permanent visual compromise. On the operating room table, these include sudden pupillary changes, proptosis, visual loss, and loss of ocular motility.

All surgeons should be familiar with how to perform tonometry and basic technique for assessing the globe. Should retrobulbar hemorrhage occur during the procedure, the status of the globe (including intraocular pressure) and the optic nerve should be assessed.

Mild hemorrhage can be controlled by head elevation and close observation. For more severe hemorrhage, a stepwise approach must be undertaken to decompress the globe. These include the lysis of one or both crura of the lateral canthal ligament. In addition, the elevated intraocular pressure can be reduced by means of topical medications (ie, timolol 0.5%, dorzolamide 2%, or brimonidine) or systemic administration of hyperosmolar agents.

The sequence of treatment in the event of orbital hemorrhage should usually be canthotomy with concomitant medical treatment: systemic corticosteroids, hyperosmolar agents, and carbonic anhydrase inhibitors. Finally, paracentesis of the anterior chamber is very effective in decreasing intraocular pressure.

PERFORATION OF THE GLOBE DURING ANESTHESIA

Perforation of the globe during anesthesia is a rare but potentially devastating complication. It is best avoided by protecting the globe with a corneal shield before injecting the anesthetic agent and by directing the needle away from the globe. Some indicative signs are sudden change in vision or a change in the position or circular symmetry of the pupil.

DAMAGE TO EXTRAOCULAR MUSCLES

Damage to the extraocular muscles during local anesthetic injection, or surgical maneuvers, can result in temporary or permanent strabismus. A muscle that is at theoretical highest risk of damage during blepharoplasty is the inferior oblique muscle. This most commonly occurs from failure to adequately identify the muscle during lower lid blepharoplasty. The muscle is best visualized between the medial and central fat pads and has a pink/purple coloration, which is easily indistinguishable from the surrounding tissue.

DAMAGE TO THE CORNEA

One of the most common complications during blepharoplasty is trauma to the corneal epithelium. Although most abrasions heal spontaneously within 24 hours or less, this is a cause of significant discomfort to the patient and a potential source of infection. It is usually caused from abrasive movements of instruments and sutures as well as traumatic insertion and removal of protective lenses. Close attention to maneuvers and handling of instruments can be protective. Should an abrasion occur, antibiotic ointment can be prescribed and the patient should be observed daily until healing occurs.

WOUND DEHISCENCE

Wound dehiscence may occur acutely immediately after the surgery or subacutely within days to weeks postoperatively. This is most commonly caused by the formation of a hematoma. This may occur slowly as vessels recover from the effects of the epinephrine used in anesthesia, or may occur from the lysis of the coagulum.

LOSS OF LASHES

This is more common in patients undergoing combined cases of blepharoplasty and ptosis repair where the anterior tarsal surface is exposed.

REFERENCES

Castro E et al. Upper lid blepharoplasty. *Facial Plast Surg.* 1999;15(3):173–81. [PMID: 11816080]

Della Rocca R, Nesi F, Lisman R. *Ophthalmic Plastic and Reconstructive Surgery.* St. Louis: CV Mosby; 1997, vol 1.

Goldberg RA. Transconjunctival orbital fat repositioning: transposition of orbital fat pedicles into subperiosteal pocket. *Plast Reconstr Surg.* 2000 Feb;105(2):743–8. [PMID: 10697189]

Lisman RD et al. Complications of blepharoplasty. *Clin Plast Surg.* 1988 Apr;15(2):309–35. [PMID: 3349744]

Spinelli H. *Atlas of Aesthetic Eyelid and Periocular Surgery.* Philadelphia: W.B. Saunders Company; 2004.

Zarem HA et al. Expanded applications for transconjuctival lower lid blepharoplasty. *Plast Reconstr Surg.* 1999 Mar;103(3):1041–3. [PMID: 10077100]

CHAPTER 10

Rhinoplasty

Gregory S. LaTrenta, MD, FACS & Jessica Erdmann-Sager, MD

▶ ANATOMY

The nose is an osteocartilaginous vault that is divided into two chambers by the median septum. Its inner surfaces are lined by mucous membranes and its outer surfaces are covered with skin. The important external landmarks include the glabella, nasion, dorsum, lower tip including the tip, nostrils, columella, nasolabial angle, alae and alar grooves (Figure 10–1). The quality of the skin is a major factor in determining the final appearance after rhinoplasty. Skin varies in its thickness, presence of sebaceous glands, and subcutaneous fat. The vestibule is the inferior cavity of the nose. It is lined with hair follicles called vibrissae and sebaceous glands. In the vestibule, the stratified squamous epithelium of the nares transitions to mucosa. It is in this region of the nose that air filtration, warming, and humidification are begun.

Rhinoplasty has both aesthetic and physiologic implications because the nose serves several functions, including air modification, immune defense, olfaction, and phonation. For instance, the nose modulates the temperature of inspired air, filters, and humidifies it. In the unoperated nose, the majority of air flows over the inferior turbinate. The temperature of the mucosa is regulated by vasodilation or vasoconstriction. Filtration occurs via the vibrissae, which are small hairs that exclude particulate matter (such as soot, plant debris, and insects). Dust, pollen, and powder are trapped on the mucosal surface. A mucociliary elevator then moves them toward the posterior pharynx. They are eventually swallowed. IgA is secreted along the mucosal surface and helps protect the person against infection by bacteria and viruses. Olfaction occurs in the root of the nasal vault along the olfactory membrane well clear of the area of dissection during the usual rhinoplasty. The nose also greatly affects vocalized sounds, exemplified by how different one sounds when suffering from the common cold.

OSSEOUS STRUCTURES

A. Nasal Bones

A paired set of nasal bones form the superior aspect of the dorsum of the nose. Each one is trapezoidal in shape. Superiorly, they descend from the nasal process of the frontal bone. Laterally, they attach to the nasal process of the maxilla. Inferiorly, they attach to the upper lateral cartilages (Figure 10–2). Together, the

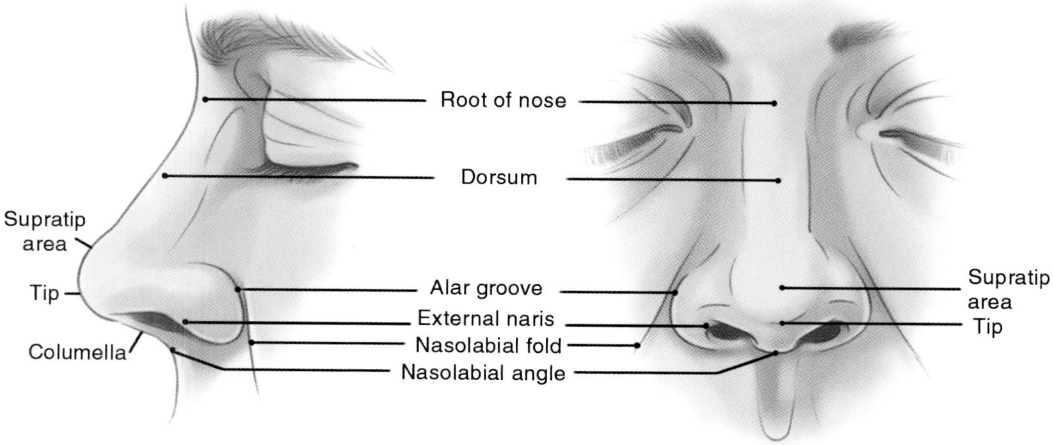

Figure 10–1. The external landmarks of the nose. (Reproduced, with permission, from Rees TD, LaTrenta GS, eds. *Aesthetic Plastic Surgery,* 2nd edition, Volume I. Philadelphia: W.B. Saunders Company; 1994:40.)

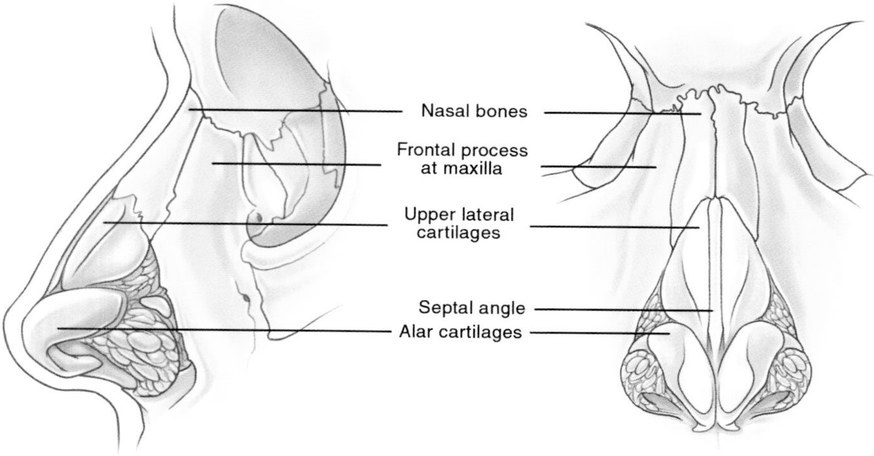

Figure 10–2. The nasal bones attach superiorly to the frontal bone, laterally to the nasal process of the maxilla, and inferiorly to the upper lateral cartilages. (Reproduced, with permission, from Rees TD, LaTrenta GS, eds. *Aesthetic Plastic Surgery,* 2nd edition, Volume I. Philadelphia: W.B. Saunders Company; 1994:40.)

paired nasal bones and the nasal processes of the maxilla form the piriform aperture. The nasofrontal angle is where the frontal bone meets the dorsum of the nose. The nasofrontal angle is also known as the nasion. Altering the nasion is difficult given the thick nature of the frontal bone.

B. Lacrimal Groove

The lacrimal groove, which contains the lacrimal duct, is formed by the posterolateral border of the frontal process of the maxilla and part of the lacrimal bone. It is to be considered when performing lateral osteotomies.

C. Osseous Septum

The septum divides the nasal cavity into two chambers. It is made of bone and cartilage. Underneath the "hood" of the nasal bones, it is bone. The bony septum arises from the perpendicular plate of the ethmoid bone. Where the nasal bones attach to the upper lateral cartilages, the septum transitions from osseous to cartilaginous.

D. Turbinates

Turbinates consist of bone covered with highly vascular mucosa. They project from the lateral wall of the nasal cavity. There are three turbinates: superior, middle, and inferior. The majority of airflows occurs through the base of the nose by the inferior turbinate. If the tip of the nose plunges significantly, airflow is redirected superiorly toward the superior turbinate.

CARTILAGE

A. Cartilaginous Septum

Superoposteriorly, the septal cartilage attaches to the osseous portion of the septum. The septal cartilage becomes thicker where it joins the perpendicular plate of the ethmoid bone. Posteroinferiorly, the septal cartilage attaches to the vomer. Anteriorly, it protrudes from the piriform aperture. The caudal portion extends over the nasal spine (Figure 10–3). Anteriorly, it connects to the membranous septum, which in turn attaches to the columella. The septum in part determines the shape of the columella.

B. Nasal Cartilages

The nasal cartilages lie anterior to the piriform aperture. The paired upper lateral cartilages are an extension of the bony "hood." Superiorly, they attach to the nasal bones. The perichondrium of the nasal cartilages attaches to the periosteum of the nasal bones, which makes the four structures function as one unit. Medially, the upper lateral cartilages fuse with the septal cartilage, contributing to the dorsum

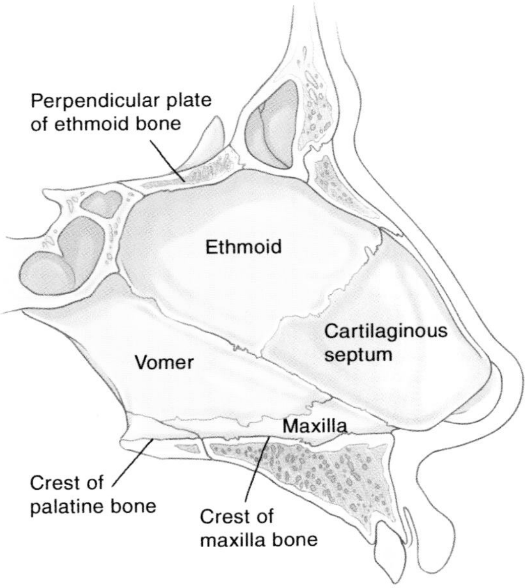

Figure 10–3. The cartilaginous septum. (Reproduced, with permission, from Rees TD, LaTrenta GS, eds. *Aesthetic Plastic Surgery,* 2nd edition, Volume I. Philadelphia: W.B. Saunders Company; 1994:42.)

of the nose. Laterally, they attach to the frontal process of the maxilla and the nasal bones. Inferiorly, they loosely connect to the alar cartilages, which flare up over the inferior aspect of the upper lateral cartilages.

C. Alar Cartilages

The alar cartilages define the shape of the tip, columella, and ala. Each alar cartilage is roughly shaped like a "c," and together they form an "m" (Figure 10–4). They are divided into medial, middle, and lateral crura (Figure 10–5). They are connected to the septum by dense connective tissue. The shape of the alar cartilages is highly variable, and impacts not only appearance but also airflow. The medial crura vary in base separation as well as curvature. The lateral crura diverge from the midline in a posterolateral direction. The lateral portion of the alar cartilage forms a good portion of the nostril rim.

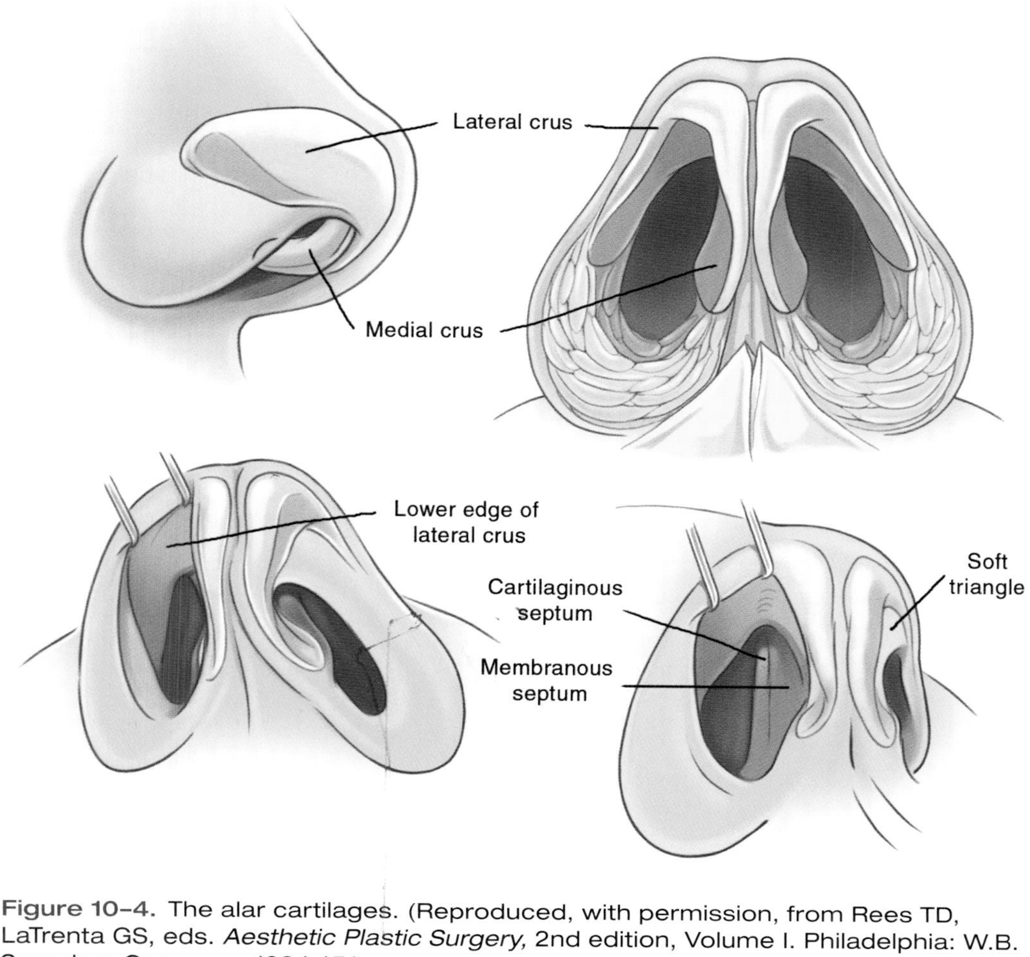

Figure 10–4. The alar cartilages. (Reproduced, with permission, from Rees TD, LaTrenta GS, eds. *Aesthetic Plastic Surgery,* 2nd edition, Volume I. Philadelphia: W.B. Saunders Company; 1994:45.)

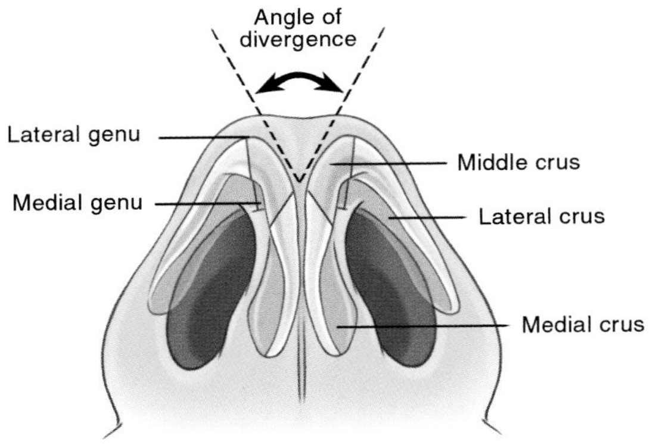

Figure 10–5. There are three divisions of the alar cartilages: medial, middle, and lateral. (Reproduced, with permission, from Rees TD, LaTrenta GS, eds. *Aesthetic Plastic Surgery,* 2nd edition, Volume I. Philadelphia: W.B. Saunders Company; 1994:43.)

D. Columella

The width of the columella is determined by the distance between the medial crura of the alar cartilages. The medial crura, with the inferior aspect of the septum, give rise to the shape of the columella. The nasolabial angle is the angle formed by the lip and the base of the columella.

E. Nasal Hump

Many people erroneously believe that the nasal hump is primarily bony in nature. In fact, the hump is made up primarily of cartilage—the dorsal border of the septal cartilage with the upper lateral cartilages *as well as* the nasal bones. Figure 10–6 depicts a patient who underwent closed rhinoplasty with reduction of her hump.

MUSCLES

The procerus muscle is a continuation of the frontalis muscle. It descends midline to insert on the superior aspect of the piriform aperture (Figure 10–7A). The pars transversa of the nasalis muscle runs perpendicular to the procerus. It arches over the dorsum of the nose just cephalad to the alar cartilages. Along the dorsum, these two muscles form an aponeurosis and belong to the superficial musculoaponeurotic system. Soft tissue skeletonization of the osteocartilaginous structures should be deep to this plane in order to camouflage any bony imperfections. The levator labii superioris runs parallel and lateral to the procerus, to insert on the nostril and orbicularis oris. This muscle flares the nostrils. The pars alaris and depressor septi nasi, which are components of the nasalis, depress the lobule (Figure 10–7B). The zygomaticus major and minor start at the lateral aspects of the orbicularis oris, and insert onto the zygoma. Contraction of these muscles creates the smile, and activates the nasalis. This action causes the nasal tip to plunge.

NERVES

The fifth cranial nerve supplies sensory innervation to the external nose. The dorsum and tip are supplied by V1. This branch of V1 is occasionally divided during surgery, resulting in hypoesthesia, which is rarely permanent. V2, via the infraorbital nerve, provides sensory innervation to the lateral nasal walls, lateral alar walls, and the columella. Sensation of the internal nose is provided by branches of the anterior ethmoid nerve and V2 via the sphenopalatine ganglion. The sphenopalatine foramen is accessible behind the posterior end of the middle turbinate. The seventh cranial nerve provides innervation of the musculature of the nose.

VESSELS

The arterial supply of the external nose is twofold. This includes the facial and infraorbital

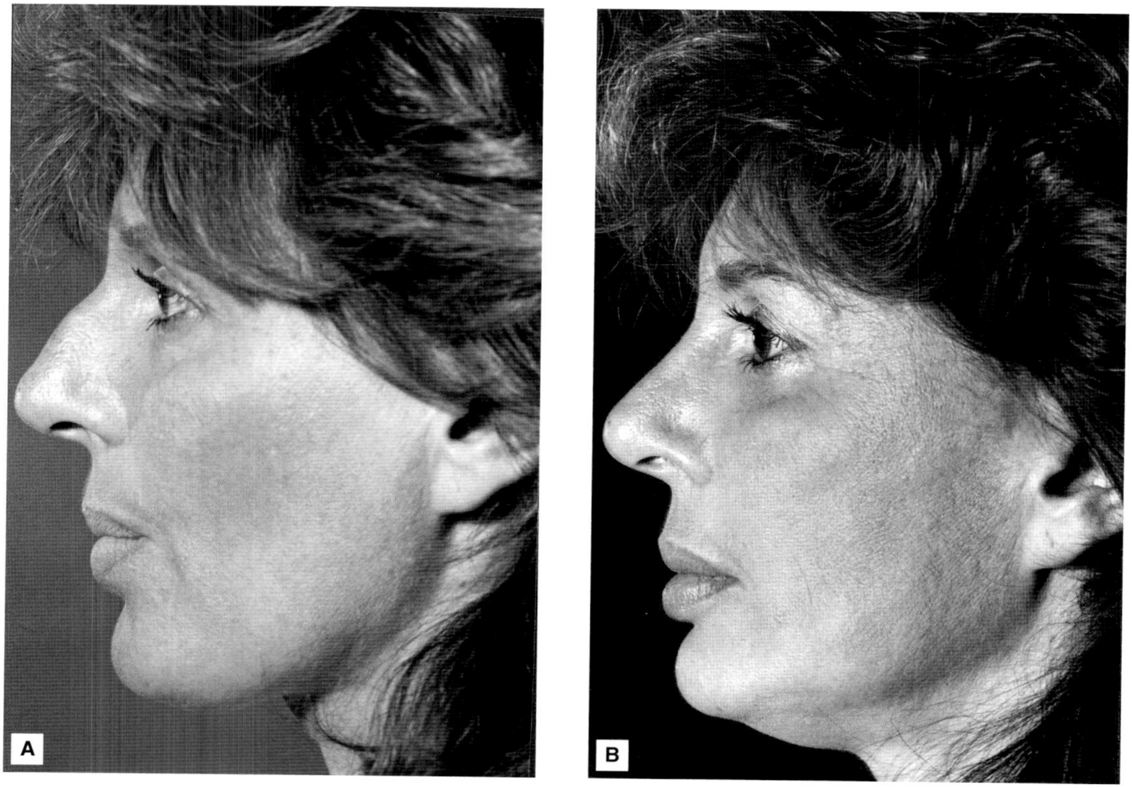

Figure 10–6. Preoperative **(A)** and postoperative **(B)** photographs of a patient who underwent closed rhinoplasty with reduction of the dorsal hump. (Reproduced, with permission, from Rees TD, LaTrenta GS, eds. *Aesthetic Plastic Surgery,* 2nd edition, Volume I. Philadelphia: W.B. Saunders Company; 1994.)

arteries, from the external carotid artery. The radix is supplied by the supraorbital branch of the ophthalmic artery, which is a branch of the internal carotid (Figure 10–7C). The arterial supply of the internal nose consists of the sphenopalatine, the major palatine, the septal branch of the superior labial artery, and the anterior and posterior ethmoid arteries. The venous system of the nose parallels its arterial supply. Of great importance, however, is that the ophthalmic vein drains into the cavernous sinus and that the ethmoid vein drains directly into superior sagittal sinus. Hence, infection or thrombosis of these sinuses is an extremely rare complication of rhinoplasty.

▶ PATIENT EVALUATION & SELECTION

During the consultation, the surgeon should elicit what the patient desires to achieve with their rhinoplasty. A past medical history of facial/nasal trauma, allergic rhinitis, and visual impairment are particularly important to elicit during the rhinoplasty consultation. In general, reduction of one or more parts of the nose is the most common reason for corrective rhinoplasty. Other complaints usually include impeded nasal airflow and a perpetually "stuffy nose." Impeded airflow is usually caused by hypertrophied turbinates

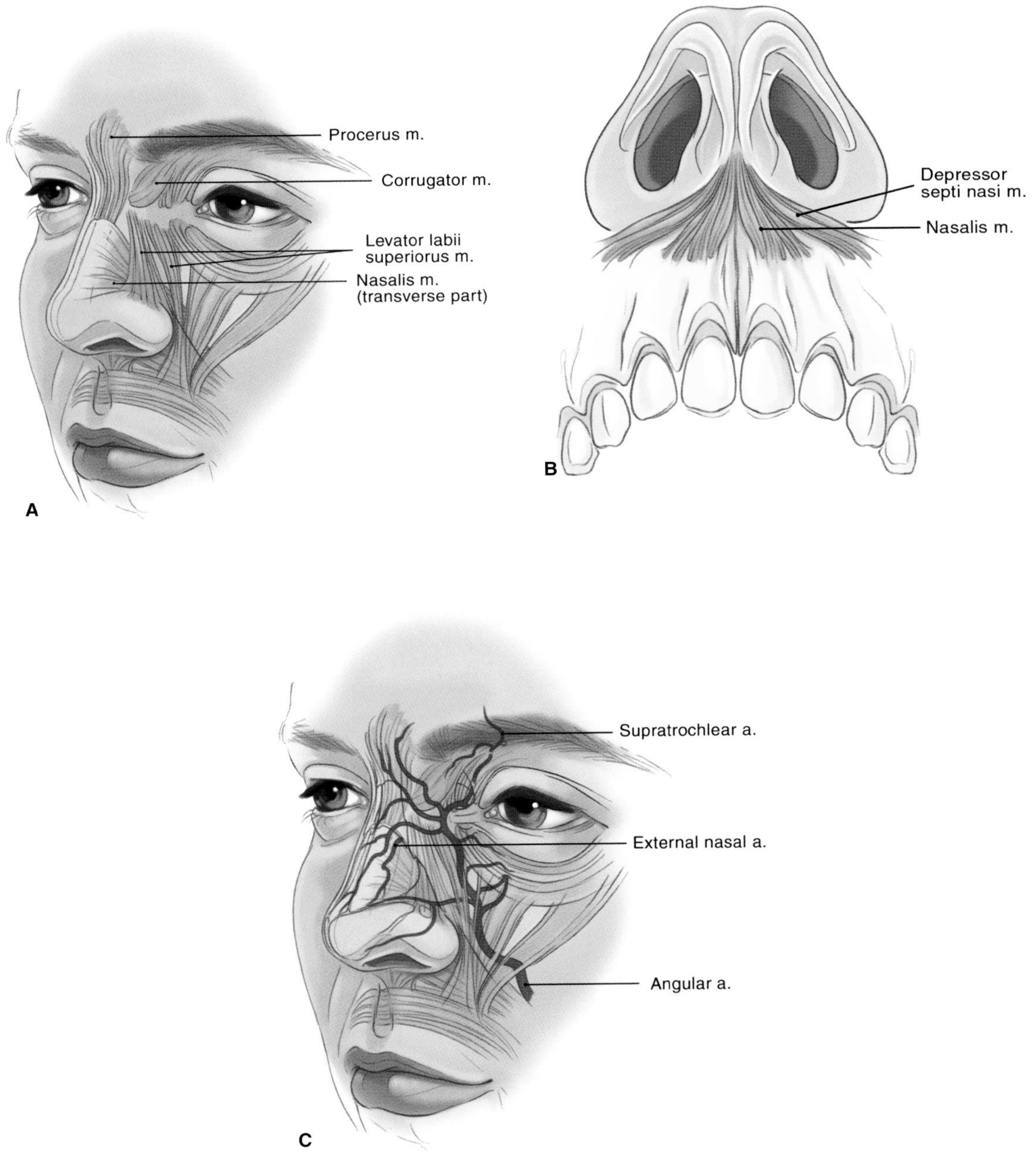

Figure 10–7. **A** and **B:** Muscles of the nose. **C:** Vessels of the nose. (Reproduced, with permission, from Rees TD, LaTrenta GS, eds. *Aesthetic Plastic Surgery,* 2nd edition, Volume I. Philadelphia: W.B. Saunders Company; 1994;49, 52.)

or a structurally abnormal septum, or both. A patient who is realistic and well-informed preoperatively is more likely to avoid postoperative disappointment and frustration. Reality shows on television and Internet sources can fuel unrealistic expectations. It is imperative to address these issues during the initial patient interview.

As with all surgeries, the surgeon should elucidate a surgical history during the consultation. This includes all prior surgeries, adverse reactions to anesthesia, and a history of easy bruising or bleeding. A list of current medications, especially aspirin, warfarin, clopidogrel, nonsteroidal anti-inflammatory drugs (NSAIDs), and psychiatric drugs, should be obtained; a history of nonprescription medicine (vitamins, minerals, herbal remedies, and diet pills) use should also be noted. As with most surgeries, aspirin, warfarin, and clopidogrel should be stopped 10 to 14 days prior to surgery. Preoperative blood tests, electrocardiogram (ECG), chest radiographs are ordered according to the patient's age, gender, and comorbidities.

Physical examination then includes the following:

- Determining the nasofrontal angle and the depth of the radix.
- Evaluating the anterior septum, noting its thickness and location. External evidence of deviation of the septum is often noted in the curvature of the nose. This will become more evident after removal of the dorsal hump. Therefore, it behooves the surgeon to explain to the patient why correction of this is paramount to achieving an aesthetically attractive nose.
- Examining the position, size, and angulation of the nasal tip cartilage.
- Observing the alae during respiration, to look for collapse or flaring.
- Appraising the thickness, texture, color, and elasticity of the skin. Facial asymmetry should be noted as well as how well the nose interfaces with the eyes, lips, and mouth.
- Assessing the patency of each nasal passage by occluding one side at a time and asking the patient to breathe through the nose.
- Noting the nasolabial angle, since it has a profound effect on the overall appearance of the nose. The ideal angle is said to be 100 degrees.

Preoperative photographs are essential. The standard frontal, lateral, three quarter, and basal views should be taken with hair pulled back, minimal makeup, and without jewelry. Some surgeons find the digital photographic manipulation helpful in conveying to patients what changes can be achieved by rhinoplasty. In a retrospective study of 120 consecutive rhinoplasties, 83% of patients rated the surgical outcome as identical or similar to the computer images. The authors were careful to emphasize to patients that the computer image was a goal to aim for and not a guarantee. Others maintain that digital imaging gives false hopes and could be construed as a guarantee of postoperative outcome. Of interest, Dr. Joseph drew on black-on-white photographs in the 1880s to convey his proposed alterations to patients.

Patients who are younger than 18 years are often brought in for evaluation. Minors should have completed their growth prior to surgery. This generally happens around age 15 but can vary from individual to individual.

▶ PATIENT POSITIONING & PREPARATION

The break in the bed should be positioned at the lower back. This facilitates elevation of the head above heart level, which diminishes bleeding. Arms are tucked, and pressure points are padded. If overhead lighting is inadequate, a headlight or lighted retractor can be used. Eye protection is placed. The skin and external nares are prepared with antiseptic, and nasal hairs are trimmed. The entire face is draped into the sterile field. A prophylactic dose of appropriate antibiotics should be given preoperatively.

► ANESTHESIA

Rhinoplasty can be performed under local anesthesia with intravenous sedation or under general anesthesia. The choice of anesthesia is surgeon-based after consulting with the patient. In general, anesthesia of the nose is achieved with field blocks first of the dorsum, then the infraorbital nerves where they exit the maxilla, then the membranous septum and the columella, and finally the base of the nose (Figure 10–8). The tip is anesthetized on the field immediately prior to surgery in order to minimize distortion.

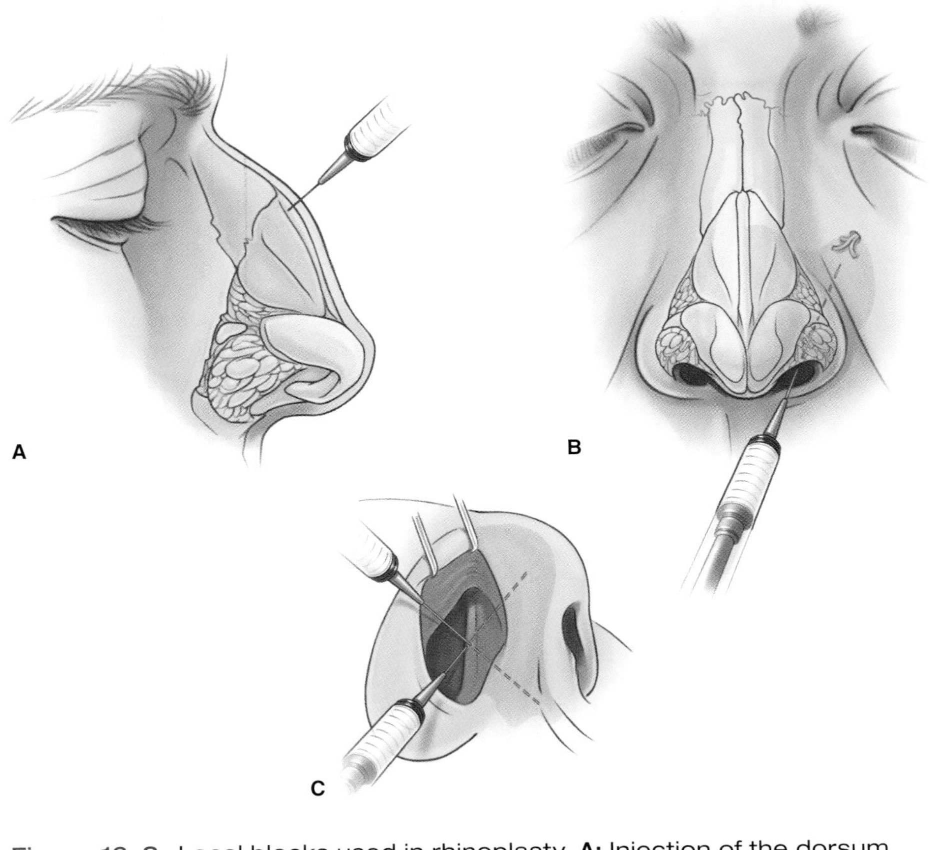

Figure 10–8. Local blocks used in rhinoplasty. **A:** Injection of the dorsum. **B:** Injection of the infraorbital nerve. **C:** Injection of the membranous septum. (Reproduced, with permission, from Rees TD, LaTrenta GS, eds. *Aesthetic Plastic Surgery,* 2nd edition, Volume I. Philadelphia: W.B. Saunders Company; 1994:37.)

▶ TECHNIQUE

The individual steps of standard rhinoplasty can be performed in any order depending on the surgeon's preference. The steps vary little in primary or secondary rhinoplasty. The steps are as follows:

- **Exposure:** Intercartilaginous incisions and raising soft tissue flaps for the closed approach or a mid-columellar incision and nasal degloving for the open approach.
- **Modification of dorsum:** By altering the dorsal borders of the upper lateral cartilages and the dorsal border of the cartilaginous septum, and then reducing the osseous dorsum.
- **Lateral osteotomies:** If needed.
- **Tip plasty:** For reducing and altering the lateral crura of the alar cartilages or shortening the caudal border of the upper lateral cartilages. This requires an intracartilaginous incision for closed rhinoplasty.
- **Refinement techniques:** Such as grafts.

EXPOSURE

The two major approaches are closed or open. For the **closed technique,** the nostril is retracted by a double-pronged retractor and the intercartilaginous groove is incised. This groove lies between the upper lateral cartilage and the upper border of the lateral crus of the alar cartilage (Figure 10–9). The incision is carried from lateral to medial toward the septal angle and through the membranous septum. The intercartilaginous incisions on both sides are joined by raising a subdermal flap over the lateral cartilages and to the inferior border of the nasal bones. Elevation of the perichondrium over the dorsum of the nose is accomplished using a Joseph double-edged subperiosteal elevator (Figure 10–10). The soft tissues are elevated laterally only so far as the hump is going to be excised. The periosteum is not elevated off of the entire portion of the nasal bones in case of inadvertent comminution of the bones during osteotomy. The periosteum prevents the comminuted bones from collapsing into the nasal vault. In most cases, the upper lateral cartilages are then dissected away from the septum. It is important to remember that the intersection of these two cartilages form the internal valve of the nose, an essential component for breathing. The alar cartilages remain with the soft tissue flap when performing closed rhinoplasty (Figure 10–11). The intercartilaginous incision is connected to a transfixion incision, which separates the medial crura from the caudal septum and concludes the exposure for the closed approach.

For the **open technique,** an incision is made in the mid-columella. The most popular transcolumellar incisions are an upside-down V, stair-step, and straight line. The major advantage of the open approach is its excellent exposure, especially for difficult tips, tips with inadequate projection, and for secondary rhinoplasty. Figure 10–12 shows a patient in whom the open technique was chosen for a secondary rhinoplasty. Rarely is the scar problematic, even in keloid formers. After the incision has been made in the open approach, dissection down to the medial crura is performed. It is very important at this point to stay on the cartilage for degloving. A rim incision is then carried out bilaterally for full dissection of the alar cartilage. The upper lateral cartilages are then degloved along with the nasal bones, maintaining a thick degloved flap. Hemostasis is performed, aided by a Colorado-tip electrocautery.

With either the open or closed technique, extreme care should be used when raising the skin and superficial soft tissue. Dissection below the superficial musculoaponeurotic system preserves the neurovascular system. Creating a thick flap also camouflages any

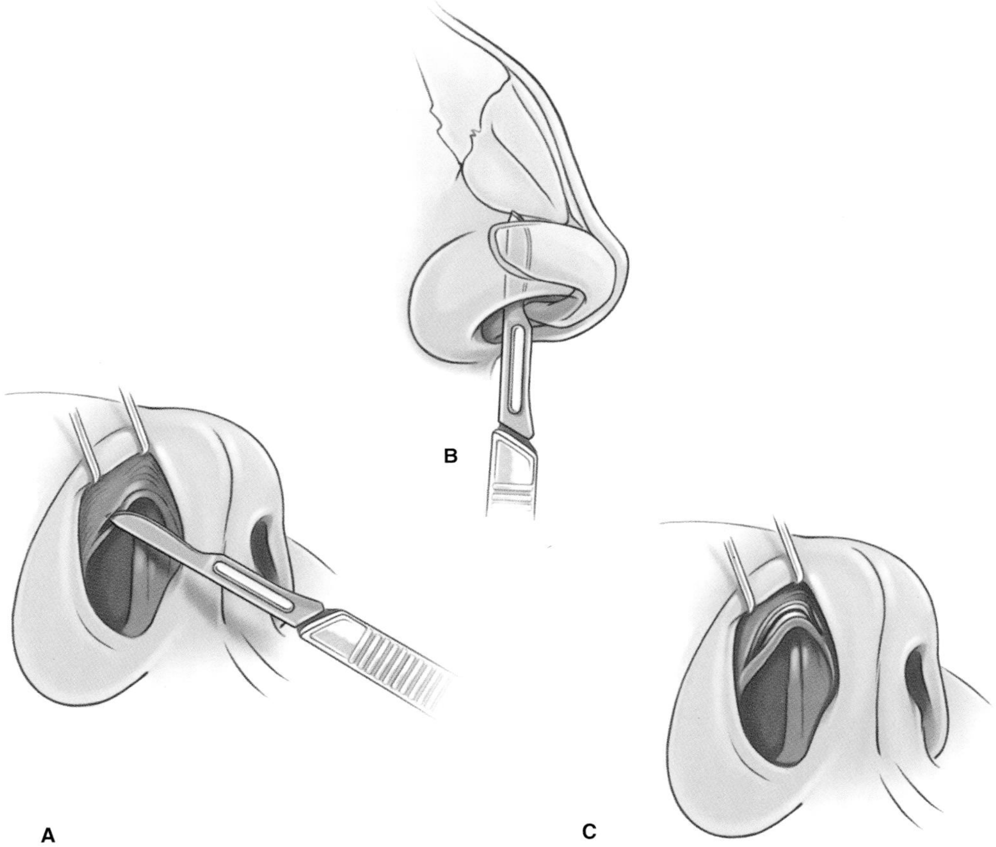

Figure 10–9. The intercartilaginous groove is incised in the closed technique. (Reproduced, with permission, from Rees TD, LaTrenta GS, eds. *Aesthetic Plastic Surgery,* 2nd edition, Volume I. Philadelphia: W.B. Saunders Company; 1994:82.)

osteocartilaginous irregularities that exist at the end of the case. Later in the procedure, defatting of the superficial soft tissue flap to thin the dorsum can be performed if required.

MODIFICATION OF THE DORSUM

Small dorsal humps are mostly cartilaginous. The cartilaginous hump is first reduced using sharp-angled scissors or scalpel (Figure 10–13). It is best to begin the reduction conservatively; additional cartilage can always be taken later. Conservative reduction of the upper lateral cartilages is then performed making certain never to violate the mucosa in the area. Every effort should be made to preserve the internal valve of the nose for breathing. The osseous dorsum is reduced either with a McIndoe chisel (Figure 10–14A) or osteotome (Figure 10–14B). In general, the osseous dorsum is

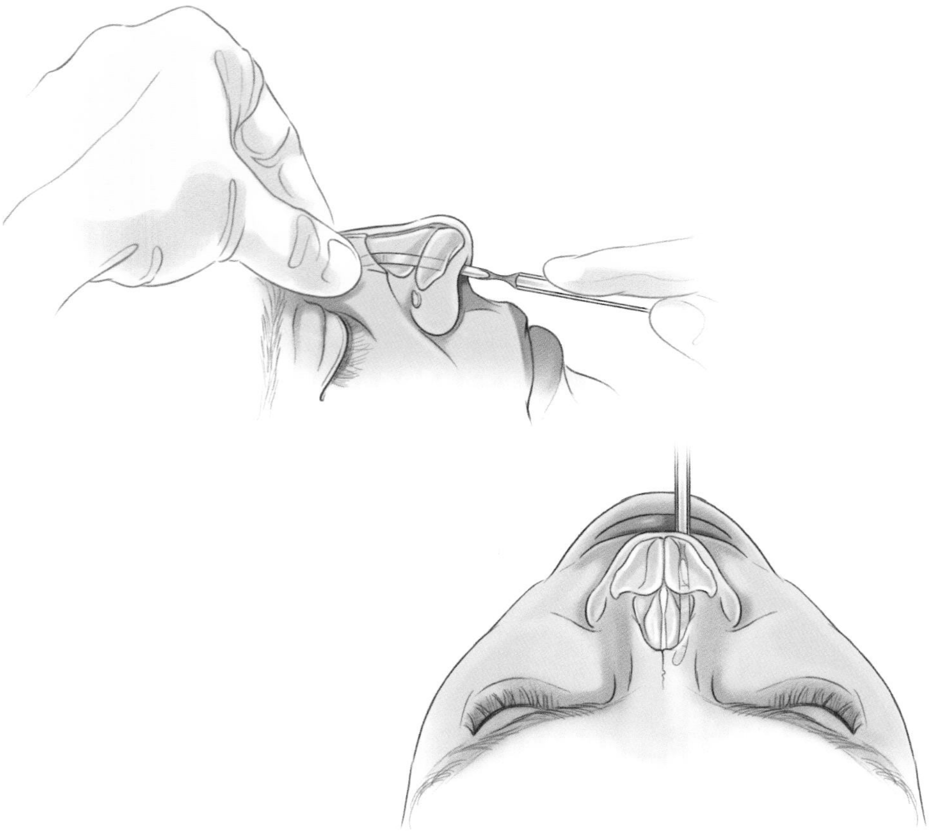

Figure 10–10. A subperiosteal elevator is used to elevate the perichondrium off the dorsum of the nose. (Reproduced, with permission, from Rees TD, LaTrenta GS, eds. *Aesthetic Plastic Surgery,* 2nd edition, Volume I. Philadelphia: W.B. Saunders Company; 1994:84.)

reduced with rasps after the cartilaginous dorsum. Alternatively, the osseous dorsum can be rasped before the cartilage is reduced.

After the bony dorsum is removed, the nasal bones and upper lateral cartilages may not meet in the midline. This results in an open roof deformity (Figure 10–15). Large humps that require reduction of the bony dorsum inevitably result in such a defect. An intact bony dorsum means that there is no open roof deformity, therefore no osteotomy is necessary. Every open roof deformity requires closure, or at a minimum camouflage, or else the dorsal nose will appear wide and open. One unique way to address an open roof deformity is using grafts. Sheen spreader grafts are long narrow strips of cartilage that can be harvested from the cartilaginous septum and inserted between the septum and the upper lateral cartilage (Figure 10–16). These are far easier to place via the open approach.

A new roof can also be fashioned as an onlay graft using the existing cartilage that has been removed, as described by Skoog.

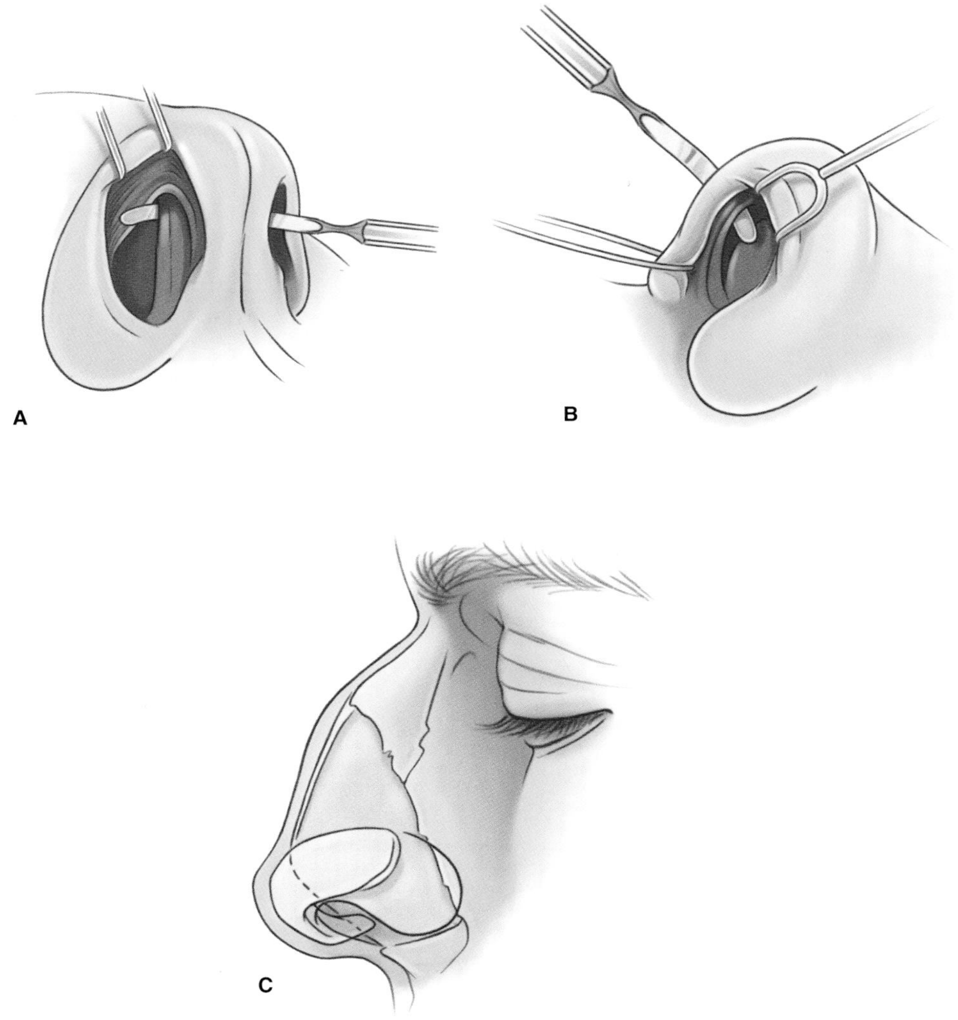

Figure 10–11. The alar cartilages are dissected off the septum. This provides mobility of the tip during the procedure. (Reproduced, with permission, from Rees TD, LaTrenta GS, eds. *Aesthetic Plastic Surgery,* 2nd edition, Volume I. Philadelphia: W.B. Saunders Company; 1994:86.)

After reducing the hump with an osteotome, the bony and cartilaginous hump is removed from the patient, trimmed, and the periosteum is removed. The smaller hump piece is then slid back into the nose to create the desired contour (Figure 10–17). The key to the Skoog technique is that cartilage matches up with cartilage, and bone to bone. The newly sculpted hump thus functions as a lid that closes an open roof deformity. If the septum is significantly deviated, the deviation must be corrected before the open roof

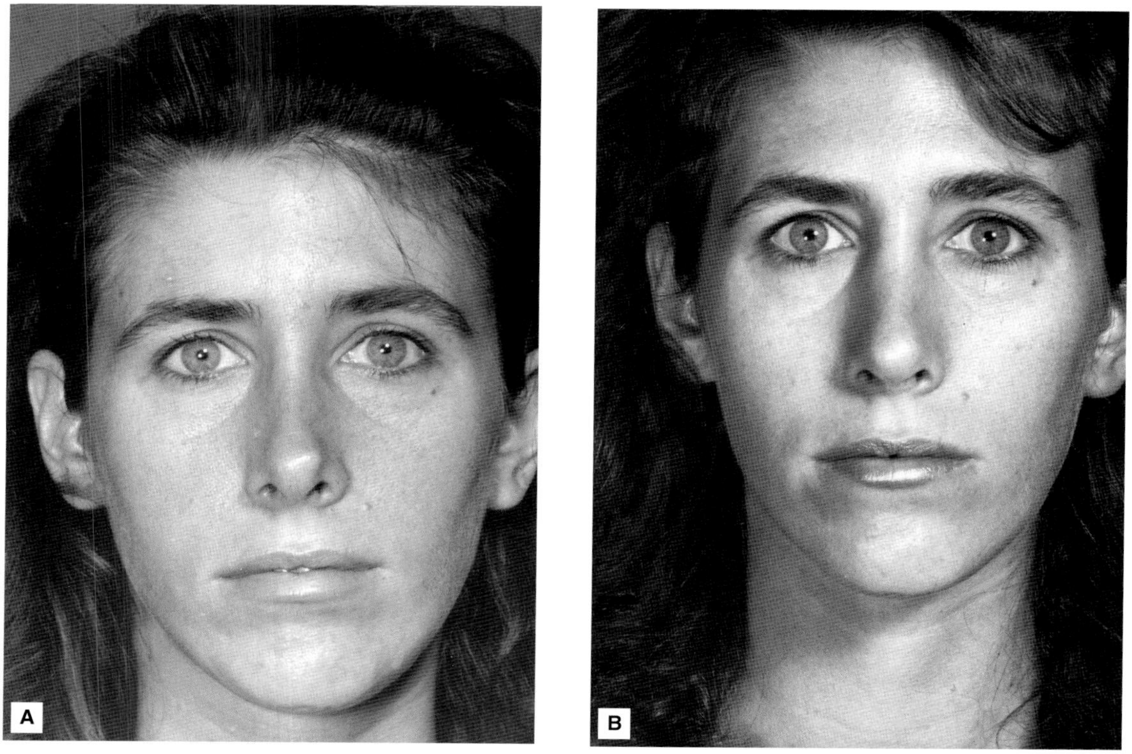

Figure 10–12. Preoperative **(A)** and postoperative **(B)** photographs of a patient who underwent a secondary rhinoplasty via open technique. (Reproduced, with permission, from Rees TD, LaTrenta GS, eds. *Aesthetic Plastic Surgery,* 2nd edition, Volume I. Philadelphia: W.B. Saunders Company; 1994.)

deformity is addressed, or camouflaged with an onlay graft.

LATERAL OSTEOTOMIES

The wide nose can be narrowed by breaking the nasal process of the maxilla and allowing the two nasal bones to slide more medially. It is generally performed toward the end of the procedure, since the osteotomy can result in irksome oozing. There are two methods: infracture and outfracture. For infracture, a small stab incision is made in the lateral nose after injecting the area with a local anesthetic. The incision is carried down through the periosteum. A linear vertical osteotomy is then made through the nasal process of the maxilla using a 2- or 3-mm osteotome (Figure 10–18). According to Rees and LaTrenta, the osteotomy should be extended superiorly to above the level of the inner canthus. The lacrimal duct is generally too posterior to be injured; however, the surgeon should be mindful of it depending on where exactly the osteotomy is performed. After the osteotomies are complete, digital pressure on the bones moves them medially. If the lateral osteotomy is performed too superficially, then a ridge becomes visible (Figure 10–19). This is known as a stair-step

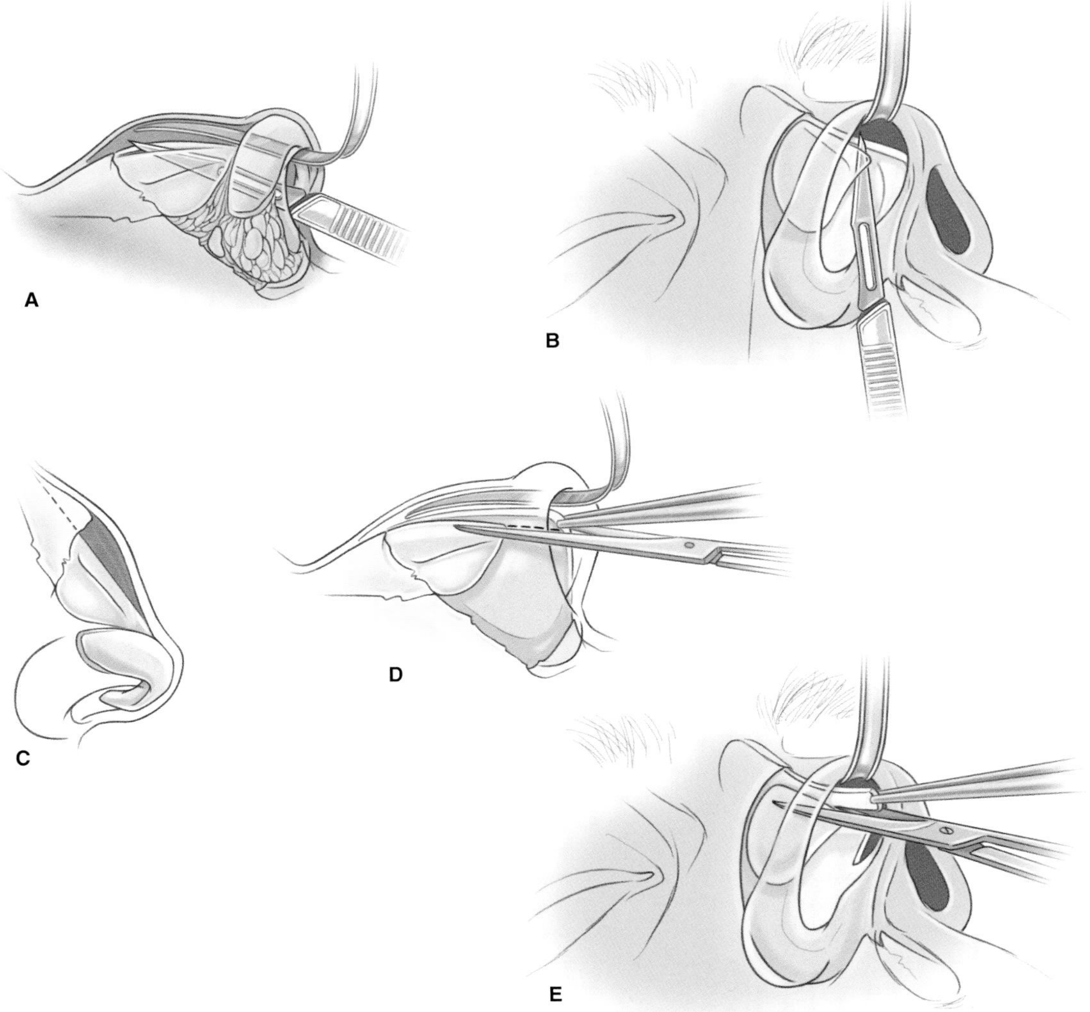

Figure 10–13. Small humps are mostly cartilaginous. **A and B:** The upper lateral cartilages are dissected off the septum using a scalpel. **C:** The planned resection. **D–E:** The cartilaginous septum is reduced using sharp scissors. (Reproduced, with permission, from Rees TD, LaTrenta GS, eds. *Aesthetic Plastic Surgery,* 2nd edition, Volume I. Philadelphia: W.B. Saunders Company; 1994:88–9.)

deformity. Lateral osteotomy and infracture does not affect the movement of air through the internal valve.

The most common method used to close an open roof is infracturing. Lateral osteotomies and infractures should be performed to close a small open roof defect if the nasal bones are long enough. Infracture is generally performed with an osteotome and mallet by beginning and the piriform aperture via stab incision and

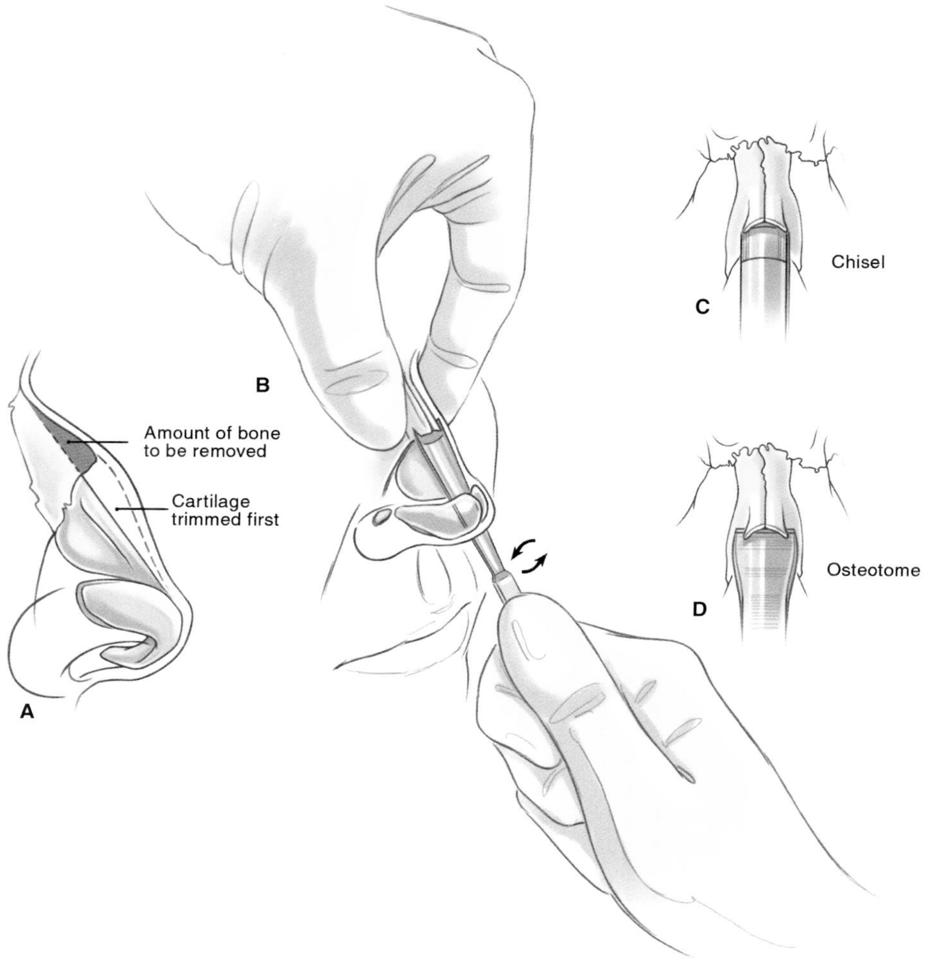

Figure 10–14. The osseous dorsum can be reduced using either a chisel or with an osteotome. (Reproduced, with permission, from Rees TD, LaTrenta GS, eds. *Aesthetic Plastic Surgery,* 2nd edition, Volume I. Philadelphia: W.B. Saunders Company; 1994:90, 94.)

hugging the maxilla up to the frontal bone complex. Manually assisted lateral infractures complete the closure of the open roof.

TIP PLASTY

Reduction of tip projection can be achieved by transecting the medial crura and allowing the tip to telescope posteriorly on itself (Figure 10–20). This preserves the roundness of the tip. Tip plasty usually begins with trimming of the caudal septum. The caudal margin should be gently curved, to preserve the natural curve in the columella. Conservativism is essential in tip plasty. Rees and LaTrenta suggest that correction of tip deformity before hump removal avoids a saddle nose deformity

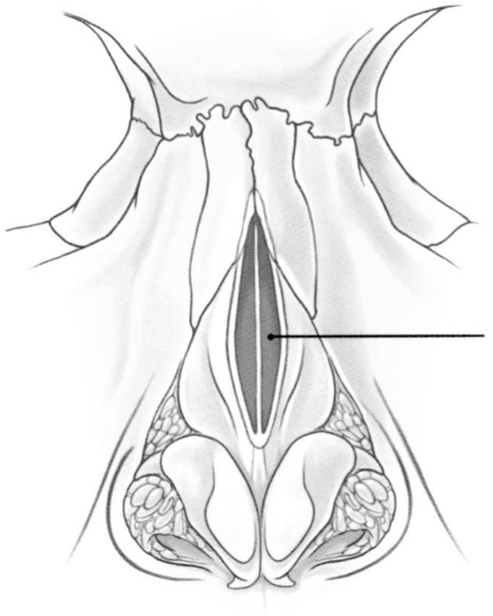

Figure 10–15. An open roof deformity. (Reproduced, with permission, from Rees TD, LaTrenta GS, eds. *Aesthetic Plastic Surgery,* 2nd edition, Volume I. Philadelphia: W.B. Saunders Company; 1994:138.)

due to overaggressive reduction of the hump. Figure 10–21 shows a patient who had a closed rhinoplasty with alteration of her bridge and tip.

The width of the tip is determined by the degree of divergence between the two genu of the alar cartilages as well as their size. There are various ways to reduce the width of the tip. If the angle of divergence is acceptable, resection of the superolateral portion of the alar cartilage is the simplest and most effective way to modify the tip. An incision parallel to the sides of the alar cartilage can be made, and one-third to one-half of the width of the alar cartilage can be removed. Crosshatching to weaken the strength of the alar cartilage without actually dividing it fully can also be used. When the angle of divergence is wide, the splayed domes can also be brought together by mattress sutures through the medial crura at the genua and the base of the columella after weakening the dome (Figure 10–22). For patients with a flat tip and wide ala, the surgeon may chose to suture the medial crura together to improve tip projection as well as to graft the resected portions of the superolateral tip cartilages to the remaining alar cartilages. A third maneuver is to graft a midline strut of the septum and suture the alar complex at a higher level to increase tip projection.

In the case of a plunging tip, tip rotation in a cephalad direction is essential. The exact technique depends on the magnitude of the problem. For a small correction, the caudal margins of the septum and upper lateral cartilages are trimmed. The cartilage is then transfixed to the septum using mattress sutures through the medial crura and septum to hold the tip in a more cephalad location. This is called a "tongue-in-groove" or sandwich method. For larger deformities, the superior aspects of the lateral crura are trimmed to allow for cephalad rotation. Grafting to augment the tip is often required. In cases where the tip plunges only with animation due to activation of the depressor septi nasi, division of muscle usually improves it.

At the conclusion of a rhinoplasty, the overall appearance of the nose is checked. Excess length of the upper lateral cartilages is assessed by applying caudal traction. If there is excess length, the caudal portion of the upper lateral cartilages need to be trimmed. As stated, the resection should be extremely conservative because of the role of the cartilages in the internal valve. Special attention is given to any contour irregularities, to the removal of debris, and to hemostasis. Gentle pressure on the lateral nose with the thumb and forefinger will reduce tissue edema and reapply the soft tissue flap to the underlying osteocartilaginous structures. For closed rhinoplasty, interrupted 4-0 chromic sutures are used to close the mucosa. For open rhinoplasty, interrupted 5-0 or 6-0 nylon sutures are used to close the skin incisions. Nasal packing may be inserted if extensive submucosal

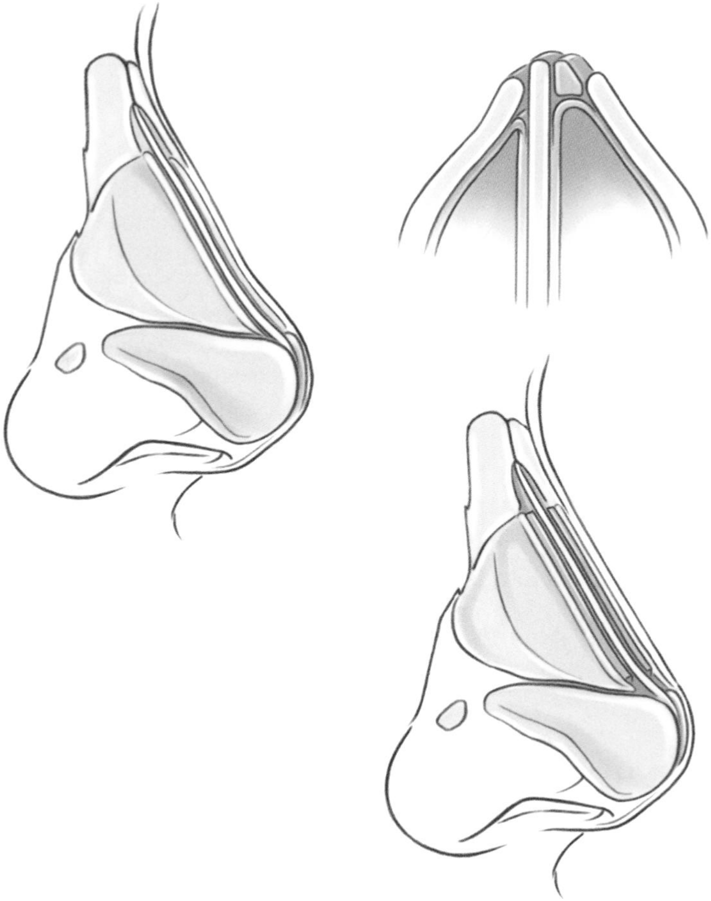

Figure 10–16. Sheen Spreader grafts. A strip of cartilage is placed in the defect between the upper lateral cartilages and the septum. (Reproduced, with permission, from Rees TD, LaTrenta GS, eds. *Aesthetic Plastic Surgery,* 2nd edition, Volume I. Philadelphia: W.B. Saunders Company; 1994:141.)

resection has been performed. Paper tape may be applied to minimize dead space. An external splint is placed to prevent hematoma and to protect against trauma. The splint is left on for 3 to 10 days, depending on the surgeon's preference. Postoperatively, the patient is advised not to blow or pick the nose for 10 to 14 days. Intense physical activity can be resumed after 2 to 3 weeks. Contact sports should be avoided for 4 to 6 months.

REFINEMENT TECHNIQUES

The placement of autogenous grafts is one of the most important ancillary techniques. These

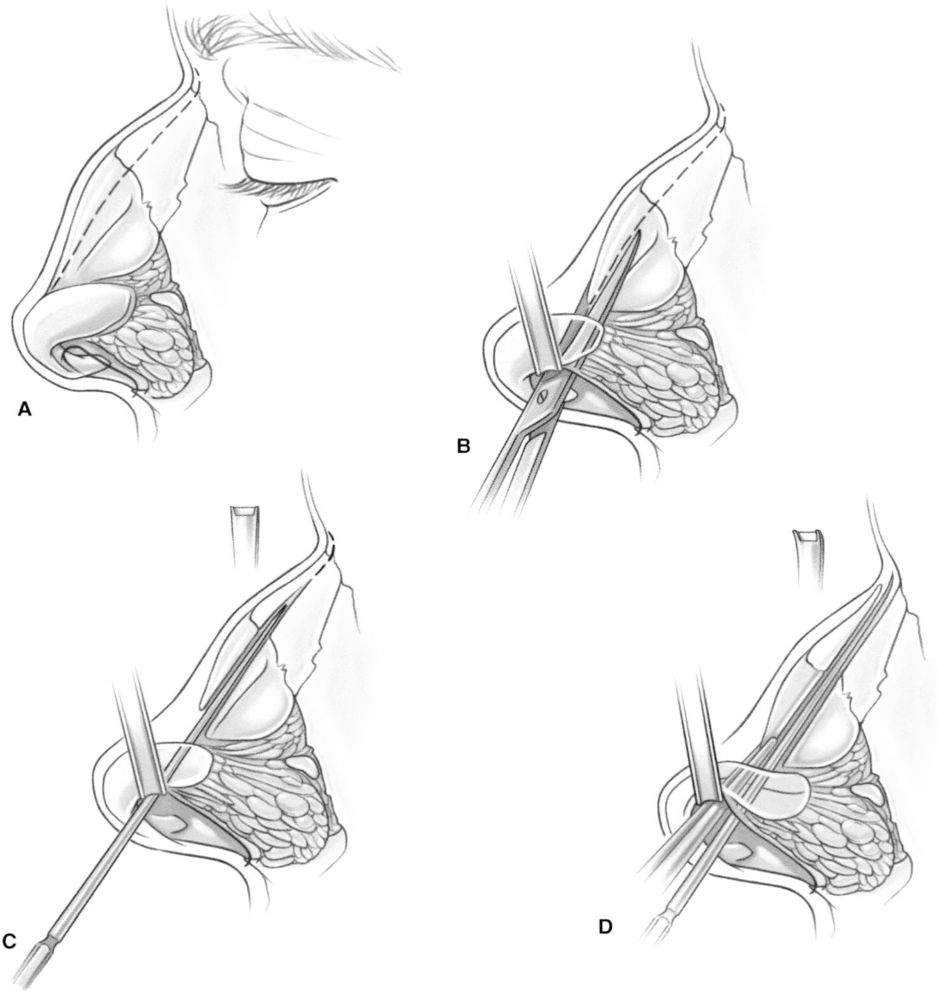

Figure 10–17. The Skoog technique. After removing the hump, it is refined and replaced as an onlay graft. (Reproduced, with permission, from Rees TD, LaTrenta GS, eds. *Aesthetic Plastic Surgery,* 2nd edition, Volume I. Philadelphia: W.B. Saunders Company; 1994:112.)

grafts are harvested ideally from discarded remains of cartilage or from the septum. If neither is available, conchal cartilage is used. Fixation can be achieved with direct intracartilaginous sutures or by a loose transcutaneous suture that affixes the graft to the soft tissue (Figure 10–23). Figure 10–24 shows a patient who had septal spreader grafts as well as an onlay graft. Cartilage grafts can be used to augment the dorsum, improve tip projection, or alter the labio-columellar angle. Grafts to increase tip projection can include a single

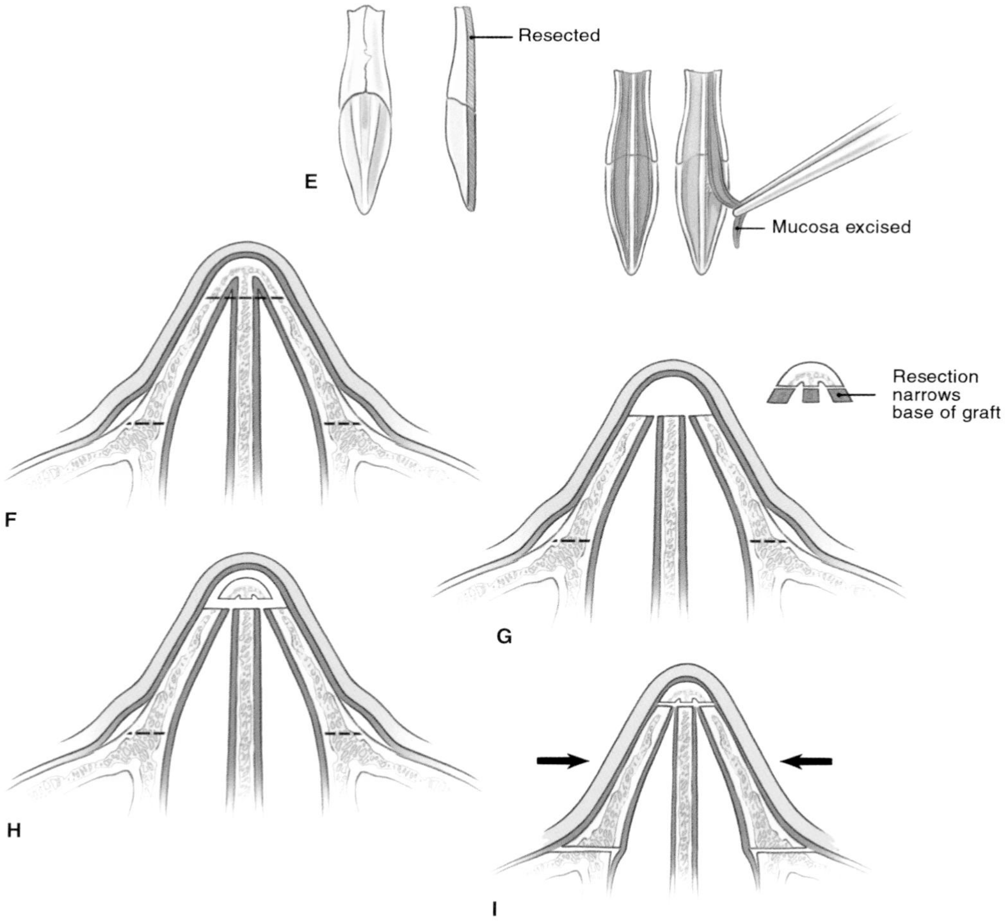

Figure 10–17. (Continued)

piece of cartilage, or multiple layers sutured together, and then placed between the medial crura. Tip grafts are often used in secondary rhinoplasty when the alar cartilages have been over-resected.

Alar base resection is used to decrease flaring or the width of the nostrils, or both. The basic principles are to narrow the base of the ala by excising a wedge of the nostril sill, which causes minimal scarring and contour deformity of the rim. The shape of the wedge determines whether the width, flare, or both are reduced. There are numerous variations of alar base resections. This is especially important for the correction of ethnic noses.

Altering the nasion is another ancillary technique. Augmentation of the nasion is especially useful for patients with an excessively deep nasofrontal angle, as in the Asian patient. The primary solution for a patient with a recessed nasion is augmentation of the nasion (Figure 10–25). Augmentation can be

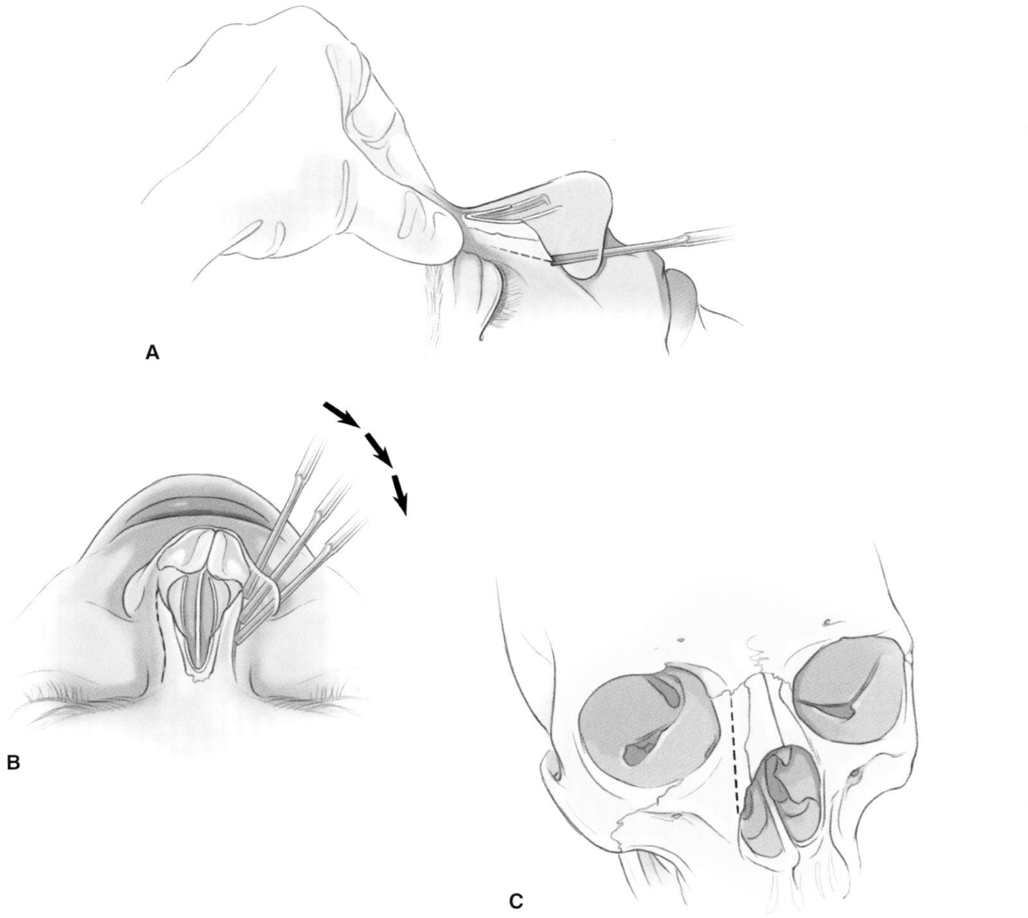

Figure 10–18. Performing lateral osteotomies. (Reproduced, with permission, from Rees TD, LaTrenta GS, eds. *Aesthetic Plastic Surgery,* 2nd edition, Volume I. Philadelphia: W.B. Saunders Company; 1994:118.)

accomplished by using dermal grafts, temporal fascia grafts, cartilage grafts, bone grafts, or implants. Again, layering of cartilage grafts may be necessary to achieve projection. In contrast, some patients have too shallow of a nasofrontal angle. Often, the frontal bone is not bossed, and this makes the nasion appear shallow. Removing bone, muscle, or other soft tissue deepens the nasofrontal angle.

▶ COMPLICATIONS

Postoperative complications are categorized as early or late. The most common early complication is epistaxis, or nasal hemorrhage. The timing of epistaxis is bimodal, occurring either in the first 48 hours or 10 to 14 days later. Septoplasty and submucosal resection are particularly prone to cause bleeding in the

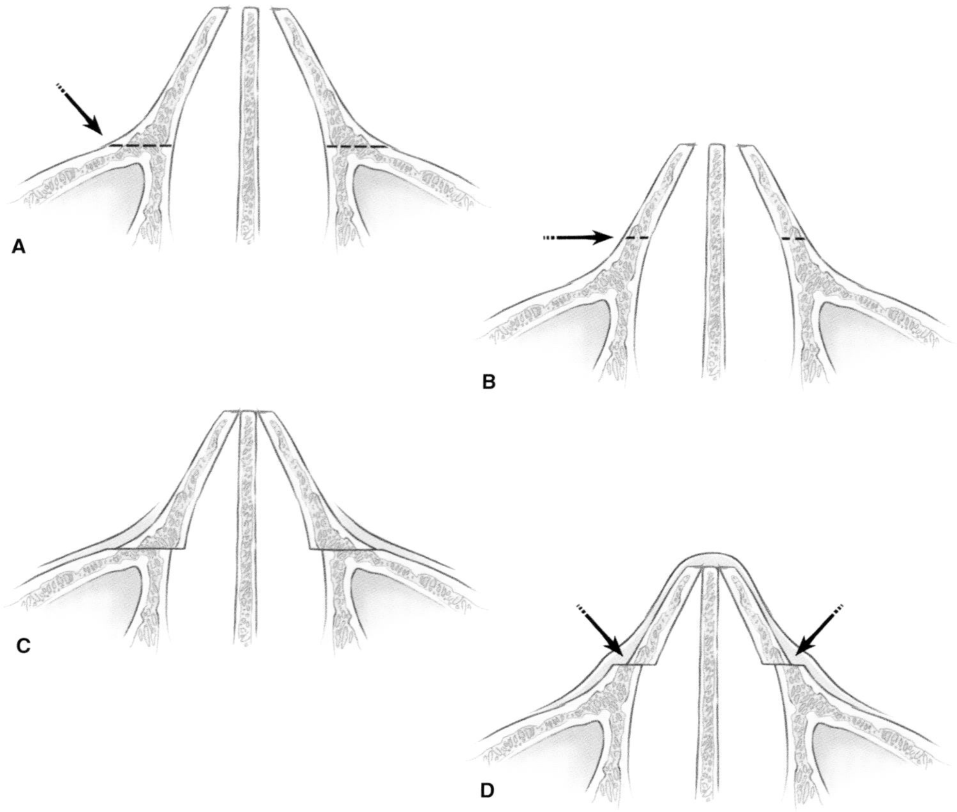

Figure 10–19. Stair-step deformity from an anterior osteotomy. **A:** The desired level of osteotomy. **B:** An osteotomy too high on the nasal vault. **C:** No deformity results when the nasal bones are mobilized medially when the correct site of infracture was selected. **D:** Stair-step deformity results when the bones move medially after the infracture was performed too high. The defect is visible. (Reproduced, with permission, from Rees TD, LaTrenta GS, eds. *Aesthetic Plastic Surgery,* 2nd edition, Volume I. Philadelphia: W.B. Saunders Company; 1994:122.)

first 48 hours. Bleeding also classically occurs between postoperative days 10 and 14, when separation of eschars from incisions can result in hemorrhage. Epistaxis can, however, occur up to several weeks postoperatively. Bleeding can be controlled with epinephrine-soaked pledgets and nasal packing. To avoid postoperative hemorrhage, patients should be queried preoperatively for personal and family histories of bleeding and bruising tendencies. If the history suggests a bleeding diathesis, the appropriate laboratory tests can be ordered. Medications including NSAIDs, antiplatelet agents (such as aspirin and clopidogrel, heparin [unfractionated and low-molecular-weight], and warfarin) should be discontinued 10 to 14 days prior to surgery.

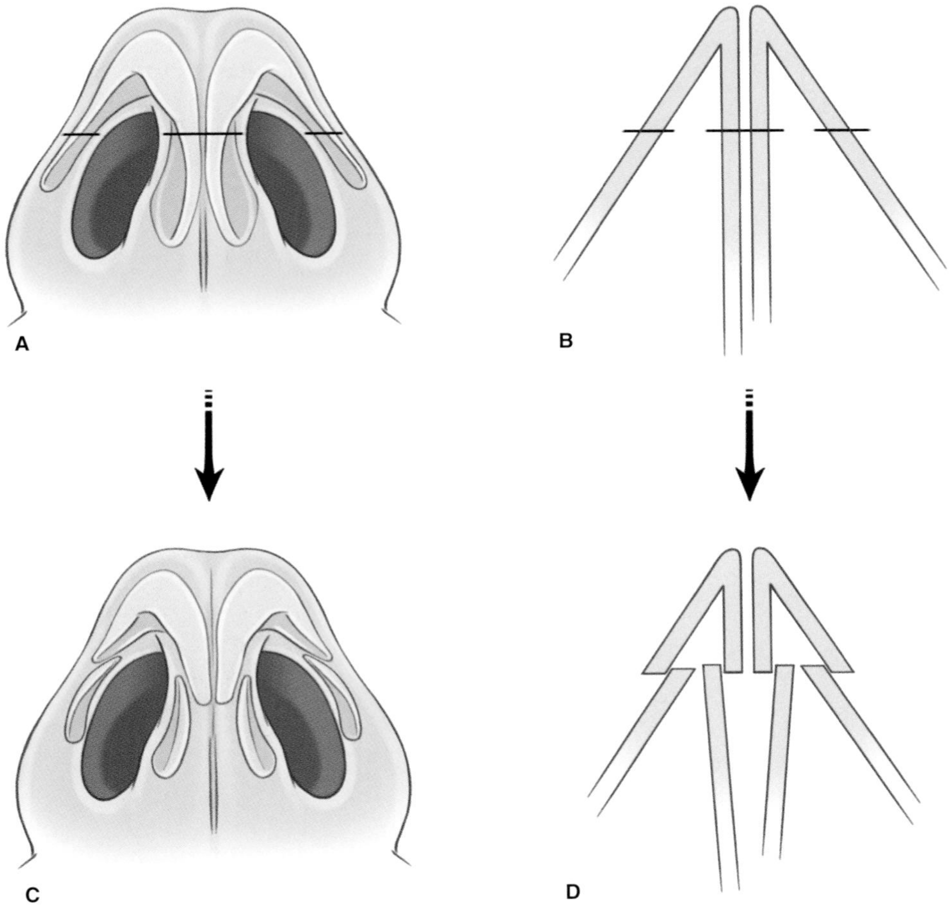

Figure 10–20. Transecting the alar cartilages allows the tip to telescope in on itself, thus reducing projection. (Reproduced, with permission, from Rees TD, LaTrenta GS, eds. *Aesthetic Plastic Surgery,* 2nd edition, Volume I. Philadelphia: W.B. Saunders Company; 1994:236.)

Other early complications include hematomas, septal perforation, infection, lacrimal duct injury, and delayed wound healing. Hematomas distort the final nasal appearance. Appropriately applied dorsal splints are used to avoid dorsal hematomas. Septal hematomas can cause nasal obstruction and septal perforation. Careful monitoring and early evacuation is the treatment of choice for septal hematomas.

The rate of infection after rhinoplasty is around 1%. The most common pathogen is *Staphylococcus aureus*. Soft tissue infections and periostitis can usually be treated with antibiotics. All abscesses must be incised and

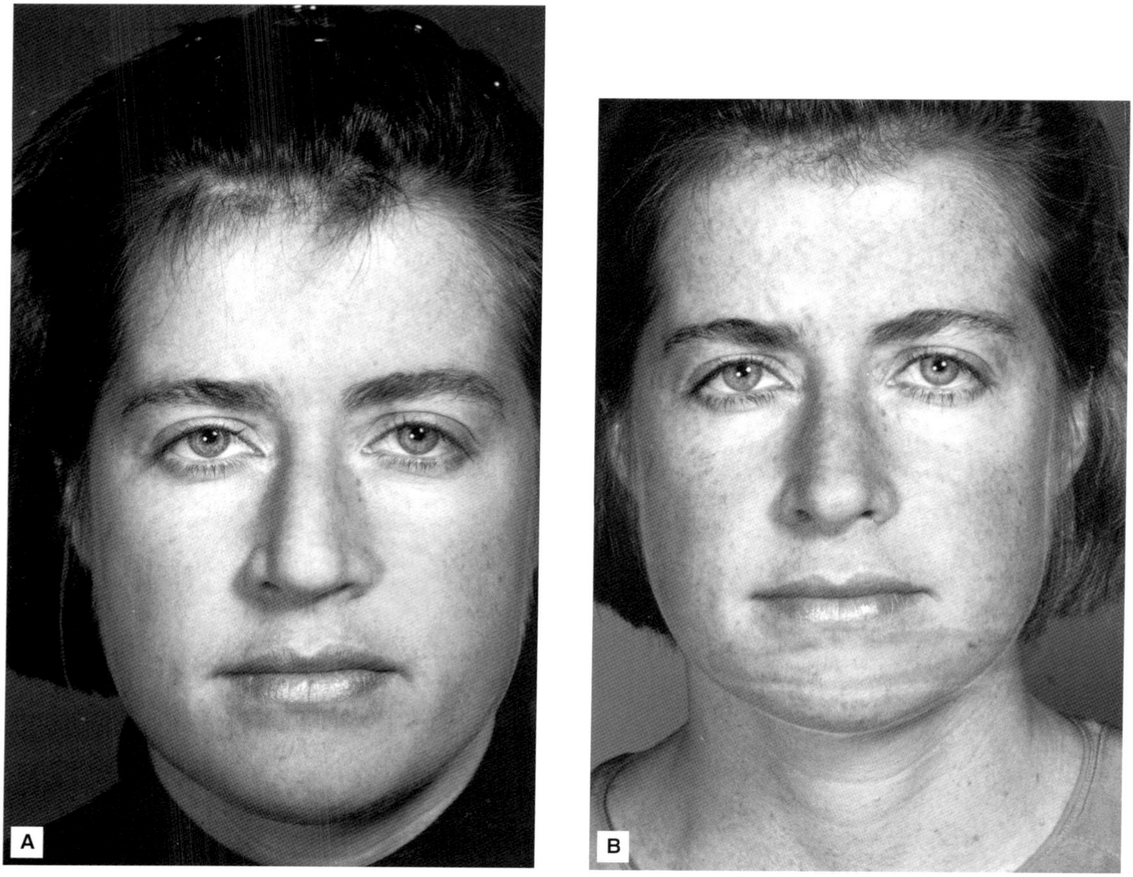

Figure 10–21. Preoperative **(A)** and postoperative **(B)** photographs of a patient who had a closed rhinoplasty with alteration of her bridge and tip. (Reproduced, with permission, from Rees TD, LaTrenta GS, eds. *Aesthetic Plastic Surgery,* 2nd edition, Volume I. Philadelphia: W.B. Saunders Company; 1994.)

drained. Bone fragments and dust can serve as a nidus of infection and thus should be evacuated during the operation. A rare but catastrophic sequela of unrecognized infection is septic cavernous sinus thrombosis, which can lead to cerebral abscess and even death.

Injury to the lacrimal system is uncommon. Symptoms usually last for only a short time and usually resolve spontaneously. Skin necrosis, either partial or full thickness, rarely occurs. Management is conservative until the necrosis has clearly demarcated. Reconstructive attempts with either full thickness skin graft or regional flap are rarely required.

Patients who have undergone grafting of cartilage are prone to untoward graft sequelae. Grafts can become malpositioned, especially if transcutaneous sutures are not used. Visible

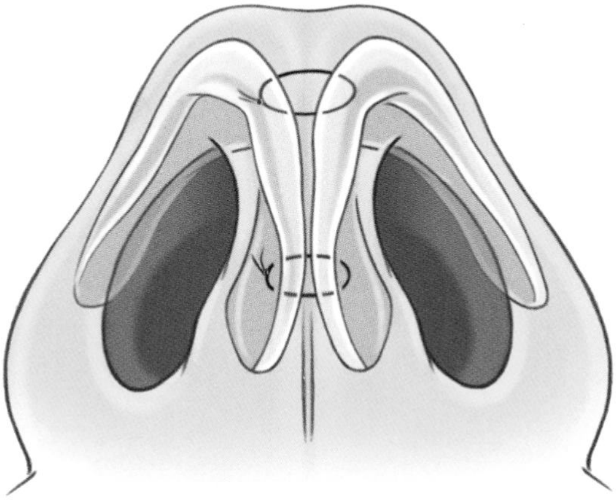

Figure 10–22. Sutures through the medial crura narrows the tip and improves projection. (Reproduced, with permission from, Rees TD, LaTrenta GS, eds. *Aesthetic Plastic Surgery,* 2nd edition, Volume I. Philadelphia: W.B. Saunders Company; 1994:219.)

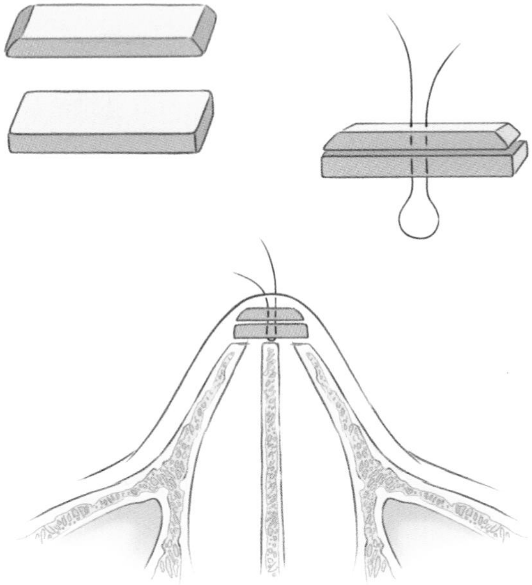

Figure 10–23. The graft is fixed in place with a transcutaneous suture. (Reproduced, with permission, from Rees TD, LaTrenta GS, eds. *Aesthetic Plastic Surgery,* 2nd edition, Volume I. Philadelphia: W.B. Saunders Company; 1994:147.)

graft edges are another undesirable outcome and occur more commonly in patients with thin skin. This can be avoided by the morcellation of cartilage grafts. Autogenous cartilage grafts can also become infected. Perioperative antibiosis and soaking the graft in antibiotic solution intraoperatively are ways that surgeons try to minimize the risk of graft infection.

More serious intraoperative complications are extremely rare but can be catastrophic. Traumatic brain injury due to misguided infractures have been reported. A recent death of an 18-year-old woman undergoing rhinoplasty in New York City was reported in the lay press but the cause was not identified. One published case describes a 23-year-old woman who underwent rhinoplasty for asymmetric nostrils and a dorsal hump. After the osteotomy, she began to hemorrhage and her neurologic condition deteriorated. Computed tomography showed air in the anterior cranial fossa, an irregular defect in the floor of the anterior cranial fossa, third and fourth ventricular hemorrhage, and subarachnoid hemorrhage in the posterior fossa. Autopsy revealed hemorrhage in the frontal lobe and fracture of the cribiform plate. These events occur but fortunately are extremely rare.

▶ OUTCOMES ASSESSMENT

The most common undesirable outcome is patient dissatisfaction. Even in expert hands, revision rates of 8% to 15% are commonly

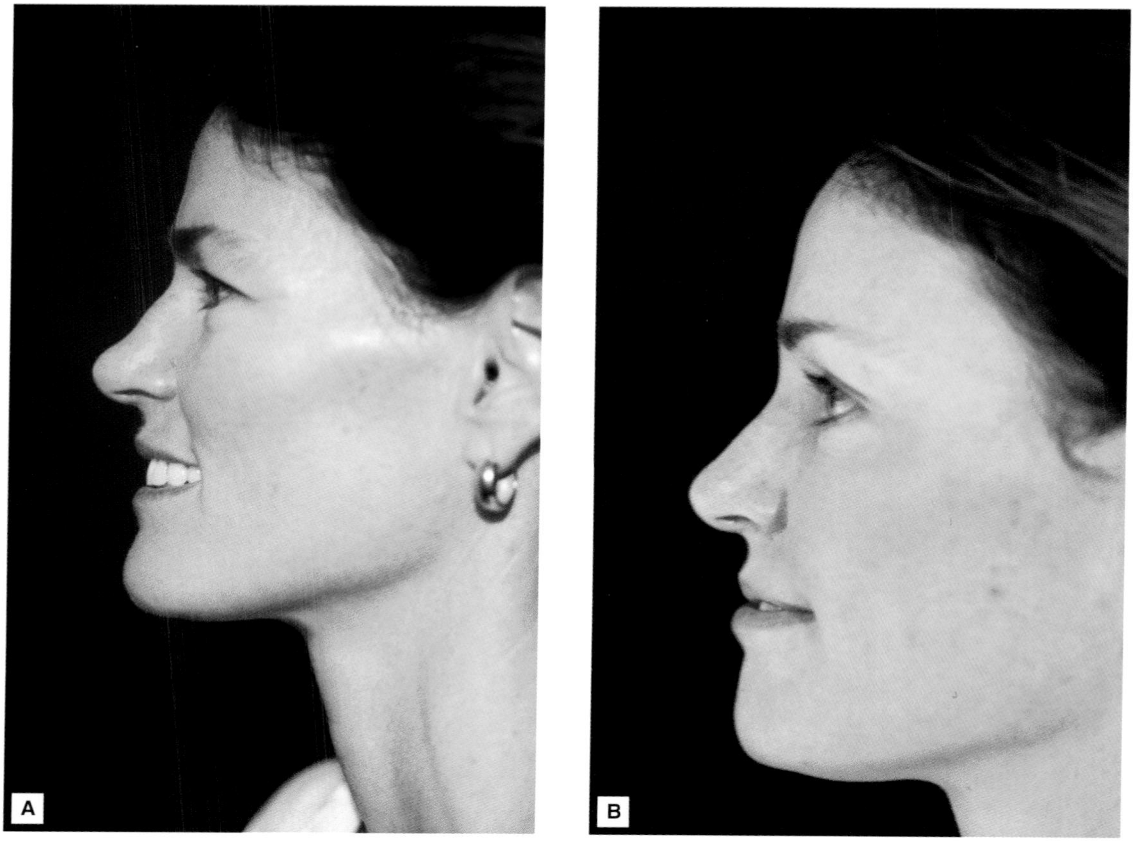

Figure 10–24. Preoperative **(A)** and postoperative **(B)** photographs of a patient who had spreader grafts as well as an onlay graft. (Reproduced, with permission, from Rees TD, LaTrenta GS, eds. *Aesthetic Plastic Surgery,* 2nd edition, Volume I. Philadelphia: W.B. Saunders Company; 1994.)

quoted. In a retrospective review of 315 revision rhinoplasties, the most frequent deformities prompting revision were asymmetry, excessive resection of the dorsum, open roof deformity, and supratip deformity. Postoperative nasal obstruction is also a frequent complaint. Patients with allergic or vasomotor rhinitis are prone to postoperative nasal obstruction. Underlying causes of nasal obstruction included uncorrected septal deviations, inferior turbinate hypertrophy, alar collapse, and internal valve stenosis.

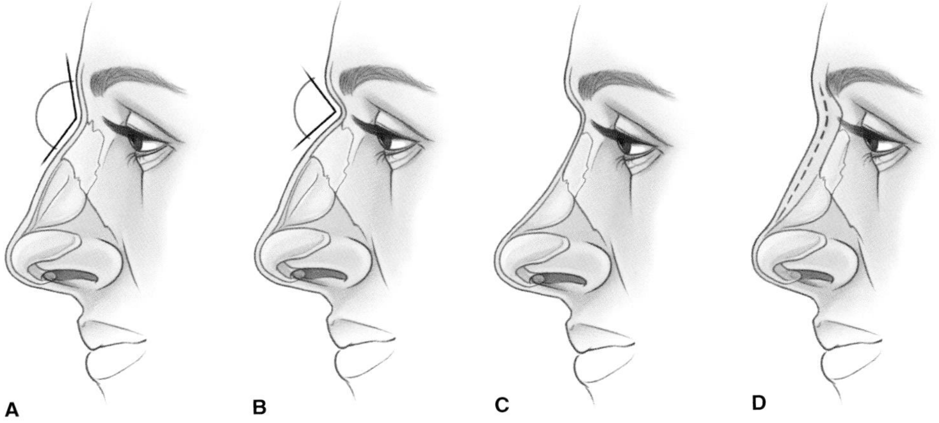

Figure 10–25. Augmentation of the nasion. **A:** A moderate hump with a normal nasofrontal angle. **B:** A moderate hump with a recessed nasofrontal angle. Correction requires reducing the hump and augmenting the angle. **C:** The profile that would result if only the hump depicted in **B** were reduced. **D:** The profile that would result from hump reduction and nasion augmentation. (Reproduced, with permission, from Rees TD, LaTrenta GS, eds. *Aesthetic Plastic Surgery,* 2nd edition, Volume I. Philadelphia: W.B. Saunders Company; 1994:105.)

REFERENCES

ABC News via 7online.com. Parents search for answers in death of daughter. Website: http://abclocal.go.com/wabc/story?section=local&id=4846253. Published: 12/13/06. Accessed on July 13, 2009.

American Society of Plastic Surgeons, Plastic Surgery Statistics 2006, http://www.plasticsurgery.org/media/statistics/2006-Statistics.cfm

Bracaglia R et al. Secondary rhinoplasty. *Aesthetic Plastic Surg.* 2005 Jul–Aug;29(4):230–9. [PMID: 16044235]

Davis RE. Rhinoplasty and concepts of facial beauty. *Facial Plast Surg.* 2006 Aug;22(3):198–203. [PMID: 17048161]

Mühlbauer W et al. Computer imaging and surgical reality in aesthetic rhinoplasty. *Plast Reconstr Surg.* 2005 Jun;115(7):2098–104. [PMID: 15923861]

Rees TD, LaTrenta GS, eds. *Aesthetic Plastic Surgery,* 2nd edition, Volume I. Philadelphia: W.B. Saunders Company; 1994.

Sanaei-Zadeh H et al. Death related to the septorrhinoplasty procedure. *Eur J Plast Surg.* 2004;25:276–8.

Skoog T. *Plastic Surgery: New Methods.* Philadelphia: Saunders; 1974.

CHAPTER 11

Otoplasty

Melissa A. Doft, MD & Anthony N. LaBruna, MD

Ear deformities cause anxiety and self-consciousness in many patients, possibly leading to behavioral problems, social avoidance, and psychological distress. Although the deformity is often corrected during childhood, subtle irregularities may not be realized until adulthood when the patient is more conscious of his or her appearance.

Otoplasty is a common cosmetic procedure. There is a 5% incidence of ear deformities in the white population. Eight percent of these patients will inherit the deformity as an autosomal dominant trait. In 2006, according to a survey by the American Society for Aesthetic Plastic Surgery, there were 20,417 otoplasties performed in the United States. It is, therefore, crucial that plastic surgeons understand the anatomy of a normal ear, the pathology of ear deformities, and the possible corrective surgical procedures. There are many proposed techniques to correct the complex three-dimensional nature of the deformed ear including resection, suturing, molding, scoring, and repositioning, indicating that there is no one technique appropriate for all patients. By understanding the multitude of techniques and evaluating each ear individually, the surgeon may use these fundamental principles to correct all ear deformities and provide gratifying results.

HISTORY

Interest in the appearance of a child's auricle is recorded in ancient times. A newborn's ear was believed to foretell his future character. Although Sushruta and Tagliacozzi described otoplasty techniques, the modern era of otoplasty is credited to Dieffenbach, who in 1845 used the term "otoplastick" for the correction of microtia. In 1881, Ely described a technique to electively correct congenitally prominent ears. His treatise details the procedure being performed on a 12-year-old boy who was psychologically crippled by his deformity. In a two-staged operation, Ely first corrected the right ear and then corrected the left 6 weeks later. He excised both skin and cartilage to alter ear shape via a postauricular elliptical incision and then used horsehair sutures to reapproximate the cartilage and skin.

In 1910, Luckett modified Ely's procedure by introducing the need for antihelical restoration, which he achieved by a single skin and cartilage incision along the length of the neo-antihelical fold. He secured the new fold with horizontal mattress sutures. This procedure leads to a sharp and unnatural appearing antihelix. To soften the contour of the antihelix, Becker introduced the idea of conical antihelical tubing in which parallel incisions are cut along the neo-antihelical fold, excising a strip of cartilage. The band of cartilage is placed in the position of the desired antihelix and then the edges of the cartilage are rolled to form a tube-like antihelix. Mustardé modified the concept of antihelical tubing by adding permanent conchoscaphal mattress sutures to bend and secure the cartilage to maintain an antihelical fold without cartilage excision.

To further mold the cartilage, Chongchet and Stenstroem applied Gibson and Davis' concept of cartilage manipulation. Gibson and Davis discovered that altering the costal cartilage by scoring caused the release of "interlocked stresses" within cartilage, allowing the cartilage to bend in the opposite direction. Chongchet and Stenstroem used this technique to bend auricular cartilage to soften the antihelix. Through histologic evidence, Weinzweig discovered that a fibrocartilaginous cap develops after cartilage scoring that promotes and stabilizes cartilage bending.

After delineating the antihelix, attention turned to modifying the shape of the concha, which is often hypertrophied in the prominent ear. Furnas and Spira popularized the use of conchal reduction. Furnas described setting back the conchal bowl by suturing it to the mastoid periosteum to reduce conchal projection and decrease the concha-scaphoid angle.

EMBRYOLOGY

The external ear is derived from the first (mandibular) and second (hyoid) brachial arches. The pinna develops in utero around 4 weeks gestation from six mesenchymal proliferations or hillocks that surround the first pharyngeal cleft. The hillocks fuse into an anterior fold (mandibular origin) and a posterior fold (hyoid origin) (Figure 11–1). The posterior fold forms the helix, scapha, concha, antitragus, lobule, and the superior and inferior crura, which combine to form the antihelix. The mandibular-derived anterior fold contributes to the tragus and helical crus. Thus, abnormal development of the second brachial arch can cause malformation or absence of the majority of the external ear.

By the fifth month of gestation, the ear has developed into its adult configuration. By the age of 3, the ear is 85% of its adult size. The length of the ear is full size by age 13 in boys and age 12 in girls, and the width matures by age 7 in boys and 6 in girls. As the child ages, cartilage stiffens, becoming more calcified.

ANATOMY

A complex, convoluted composite of cartilage and skin, the ear has five main anatomic elements: the helix, antihelix, concha, tragus, and lobule (Figure 11–2). The lateral auricular skin tightly adheres to the cartilage while the postauricular and medial skin has looser connective tissue, facilitating dissection from the underlying scapha and concha. The vascular supply to the external ear is from the posterior auricular and superficial temporal arteries, which are both terminal branches of the external carotid artery. The venous drainage mirrors the arterial supply. Consistent with its embryologic origin, the innervation of the first brachial arch structures (tragus and helical crus) is the anterior and posterior branches of the great auricular nerve, a branch of the cervical plexus. The structures derived from the second brachial arch (helix, antihelix, concha, antitragus, scapha, posterior sulcus, lobule, and external acoustic meatus) are innervated by the auriculotemporal nerve (V3). A portion of the concha and the posterior canal wall is innervated by the Arnold nerve, a branch of the vagus nerve. The glossopharyngeal

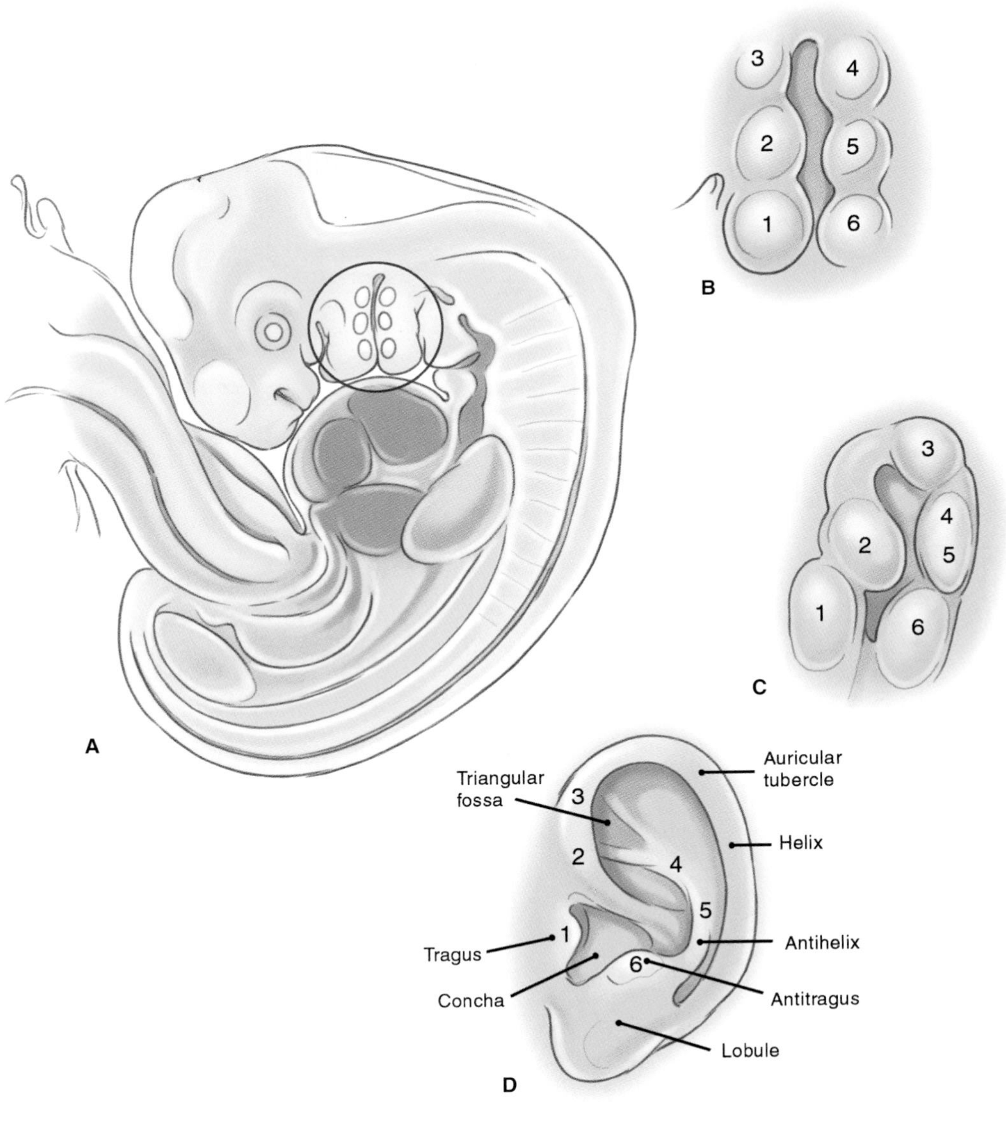

Figure 11–1. The ear is derived from the six hillocks of His during the fifth week of fetal development. The above diagram follows each hillock from early fetal life (A) to the fully developed ear (D). The tragus is derived from the mandibular arch and the remainder of the ear from the hyoid arch. Key: 1, tragus; 2, crus of helix; 3, ascending helix; 4, upper helix, scapha, and antihelix; 5, descending helix, middle scapha, and antihelix; 6, inferior helix, antitragus, and lobule.

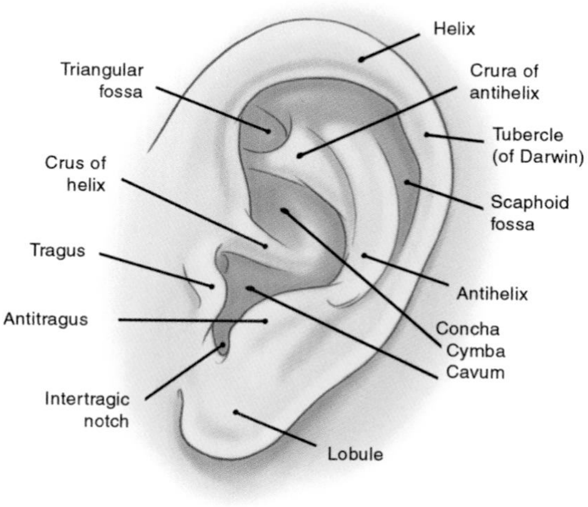

Figure 11–2. Anatomy of the ear.

nerve also supplies innervation to the external auditory meatus. The pinna has intrinsic and extrinsic muscles supplied by the facial nerve. These muscles serve no function other than allowing patients to wiggle their ears.

A. Definition of a Normal Ear

It is difficult to define an ear as normal. Every auricle is unique, even between identical twins. Historically, the individuality of the auricle inspired kidnappers to slice off the ear of their victims as proof of their captivity. Although all ears are different, several anthropometry studies of "normal" ears have lead to the following proportions for an aesthetically pleasing ear:

1. The axis of the ear is defined as the line passing through the longest dimension of the ear. The axis should incline posteriorly approximately 20 degrees from vertical.
2. The ear's axis does not parallel the bridge of the nose but is instead angled 15 degrees.
3. A normal ear forms an angle of about 23 degrees with the temporal surface of the head and is at a 1.5–2 cm distance from the scalp. A more obtuse angle gives the allusion of a prominent ear on frontal view.
4. The ear is approximately one ear length from the lateral orbital rim. The top of the ear is level with the eyebrow and the bottom is level or slightly lower than the columella.
5. The height of the ear ranges from 5.5 cm to 7.5 cm and the width from 3.0 cm to 4.5 cm or 55% of the height.
6. The lobule and antihelix are parallel to each other and form an acute angle with the mastoid process.
7. The helix and antihelix are separated by 2 to 5 mm.

B. Etiology of Ear Prominence

There are four main causes of ear prominence: effaced or deficient antihelical fold, conchal hypertrophy, deformity of the skeletal anatomy, and macrotia (generalized overgrowth of the ear). These deformities can combine to form complex pathologies. There are also several uncommon named deformities. Understanding these pathologies will allow the surgeon to tailor the corrective procedure.

1. Antihelical fold—

This is the most commonly discussed deformity. There is a large range of irregularities from loss of definition at one end of the fold, to effacement, to complete deficiency of the fold.

2. Conchal size and shape—

The concha is often overdeveloped or the cup is excessively deep. Conchal enlargement projects the ear away from the mastoid surface. Excess concha creates a firm strut that pushes the ear outward and forward. Abnormal protrusion can affect lobule position, the lower third of the ear, and antitragal prominence. To diagnose a conchal hypertrophy, the surgeon can manipulate the antihelical fold into normal position. This will make an abnormal concha easier to visualize.

3. Concha and antihelical fold—

A combination of an overdeveloped concha and a deformed antihelix is common.

4. Underlying skeleton—

The ear is positioned on the bony base of the underlying temporal bone. Asymmetries or bony anomalies may affect one or both ears.

5. Macrotia—

In the above anomalies, the prominent ear appears to have an increased height and width; however, these dimensions are usually normal. Although there is a large spectrum of normal sized ears, some patients have ears that are out of proportion to their other facial features. Macrotia may be the result of an isolated congenital overgrowth or facial hemihypertrophy. It may be secondary to a vascular anomaly or neurofibromatosis. Sometimes only sections of the ear are enlarged; for example, an enlarged lobule is common and causes the lower third of the ear to project from the face.

6. Other auricular deformities accompanied by protrusion—

Although a protruding ear is the most commonly treated ear deformity, there are several other named deformities. There are two constricted types of ear deformities: a "lop" and a "cup." The lop ear is a deformity where there is an acute downward folding of the helix and scapha. The cup ear is a combination of both a lop ear and a prominent ear. Stahl deformity is defined as a triad of a third crus, flattened helix, and malformed scaphoid fossa. More common in the Asian population, cryptotia occurs when the root of the helix invaginates into the temporal skin.

PATIENT EVALUATION & SELECTION

Many children are brought into the surgeon's office by parents who are concerned about the prominence of their child's ears. Parents are anxious to spare their children from embarrassment and harmful teasing.

The appropriate age for surgical correction is 5 years. The prevailing thought is that once a child has reached that age, he is able to communicate the extent of teasing and whether he wants to undergo surgery. Moreover, younger children are less likely to be compliant with postoperative instructions such as activity limitations or dressing changes.

A. Preoperative Assessment

Patients are often seen once for a preoperative evaluation to review the procedure and their general health. As in all elective cosmetic procedures, it is paramount that the patient or the patient's parents have a realistic expectation of the procedure's results and how these results will affect their perception of themselves. Each patient is asked to describe the bothersome aspects of the deformity, their motivation to have the deformities corrected, and their expectations for the procedure.

All patients require a thorough history and physical examination, including pertinent laboratory tests. Preoperative photographs are taken. The specific ear deformity is evaluated as well as existing asymmetries. It is important to assess the depth and possible excess of the conchal bowl, degree of antihelical folding, angle of the ear protuberance, quality and spring of the auricular cartilage, and lobule deformity shape and plane. The procedure is discussed in detail as well as anesthesia, dressings, and postoperative care. The risks of hematoma, infection, chondritis, keloid or hypertrophic scar formation, and the possibility for additional surgery are reviewed.

B. Contraindications

Other than serious comorbidities, there are few contraindications to otoplasty. When the procedure is appropriate, it is usually well tolerated. Otitis externa, otitis media, and scalp infections must be eradicated well in advance of surgery.

In the pediatric population, it is necessary that the child not strongly resist the idea of surgery. If the child is acting out or extremely concerned during preoperative visits, it is often best to delay surgery until the child is older and requests to have the procedure.

In the adult population, it is paramount that the patient understands the realistic outcome of the operation and does not have unrealistic expectations. A surgeon must be alert to the adult patient who magnifies a small defect that may be deemed near normal by others.

PATIENT PREPARATION

General endotracheal tube anesthesia is advisable for pediatric patients. Monitored anesthesia care (MAC) may be used as an alternative for adults. The operating room table is turned 180 degrees to the anesthesiologist to allow ample room for the surgical team. Prior to incision, antibiotics (eg, a first-generation cephalosporin) are administered to reduce the risk of postoperative infection. The patient must be thoroughly prepared with povidone-iodine or chlorhexidine. Preparation should include the external meatus, external auditory canal, hair, and surgical site. A head drape is wrapped so that both ears are simultaneously visualized.

Local anesthesia is injected into the surgical site starting in the area of the great auricular nerve, then the posterior crease and concha, and then the lateral skin overlying the antihelical fold. While injecting the lateral skin, the anesthetic is used to hydro-dissect skin from cartilage to facilitate dissection and hemostasis. For children, 0.5% lidocaine with 1:200,000 parts epinephrine is injected, since a more dilute mixture is appropriate for their body weight. The vasoconstrictive local anesthetic will render the surgical field a blanched white. At the end of the case, great auricular nerve blocks are performed using 0.25% bupivacaine for postoperative analgesia.

TECHNIQUE

There are many proposed operative techniques and no uniform opinion among surgeons as to which is best. Surgeons must remember that each deformity is complex and different, and thus, knowledge of many corrective measures is necessary to appropriately repair the anomaly.

The goal of correction is to delineate the antihelical fold and correct a hypertrophied concha. The basic goals of otoplasty were further delineated by McDowell and Wright in 1968 and 1970, respectively, to include the following:

1. All trace protrusion of the upper third of the ear must be corrected.
2. From the frontal view, the helix of both ears should be visualized beyond the antihelix.
3. The helix must form a smooth and regular line throughout.
4. The postauricular sulcus should not be markedly decreased or distorted.
5. The ear must be the correct distance from the head so that the helix to mastoid distance is 10 to 12 mm in the upper third of the ear, 16 to 18 mm in the middle third, and 20 to 22 mm in the lower third.
6. There must be facial symmetry so that the lateral ear edge matches bilaterally to within 3 mm at any point.

LaTrenta adds that there must be a smooth, rounded, and well-delineated antihelical fold, the conchoscaphal angle should be

90 degrees, and a reduction of either the concha or the conchamastoidal angle is necessary. Furthermore, the lateral projection of the helical rim should exceed the lobule.

A. Open Operative Technique

Attention is focused on the most prominent or deformed ear first. The other ear is then tailored to match.

The location of the antihelix is delineated using a 22-gauge needle dipped in methylene blue. The blue dots mark both the skin and cartilage. This is very useful for posterior auricular incisions because the markings serve as a map on the posterior surface.

An elliptical incision is made on the posterior auricular surface, allowing the surgeon to remove redundant skin and providing necessary exposure. Meticulous hemostasis with cautery is crucial because it prevents formation of postoperative hematomas.

The posterior perichondrium is exposed and posterior landmarks are identified, including the scapha, helical sulcus, and helical tail. The initial methylene blue markings are now visible. The initial incision may need to be extended for improved exposure. It is important not to strip the perichondrium from the cartilage. This decreases the risk of recurrent deformities, since the sutures will not cut through the cartilage as easily with a thick perichondrium in place.

The antihelical fold is corrected first. The four methods that have been described to correct the antihelix involve rasping alone, suturing alone, rasping and suturing, and cartilage cutting techniques. Some surgeons advocate for the Gibson technique, during which the cartilage is scored or abraded on the anterior surface of the auricular to facilitate posterior bending. Stenstroem used a rasp to sharply score the lateral scaphal cartilage to form the antihelix.

Furthermore, the upper third of the ear easily retains its original shape because elasticity and memory are stronger in the upper third than in the middle or lower thirds of the ear, and therefore, suture support is necessary. Mustardé mattress sutures secure the antihelical fold. This works particularly well in the upper third of the ear. In this technique, a 4.0 polydioxanone (PDS) suture is passed from the scaphoid fossa or the triangular fossa to the concha to include the full thickness of the cartilage and anterior perichondrium but not the anterior skin. The sutures are tied with increasing tension to form the correct fold. A minimum of three sutures is necessary to form the helical fold. Sometimes a fourth is used to reposition the antitragus (Figure 11–3).

To maintain the correct temporal-helical angle, the auricular cartilage is sutured to the temporal fascia. Mattress sutures penetrate the full thickness of the triangular or scaphoid fossa cartilage or both and then pass through the temporal fascia, anchoring the auricle.

Often the earlobe continues to project after these first major steps. Excess posterior lobular skin is excised. It is helpful to suture the fibro-fatty tissue of the lobule to the concha or aponeurosis of the sternocleidomastoid. To reposition the earlobe medially, the causa helicus is sutured to the posterior wall of the concha.

In many patients with prominent ears, hypertrophied posterior auricular musculature has been noted. Without excising the auricularis posterior muscle, the ear will continue to protrude. By removing the bulk of the auricularis muscle to the level of the mastoid fascia, the surgeon creates a space for the repositioned concha to rest.

Conchal hypertrophy can be corrected through the posterior incision to avoid scarring and potential keloid formation. A conchal incision is made from the cymba concha along the cavum concha to below the antitragus. If the incision in the concha is too high, there is a decrease in control of the antihelical fold. By starting at the cymba concha, the antihelix will spring forward during antihelical shaping. A crescent of cartilage is excised. The cut

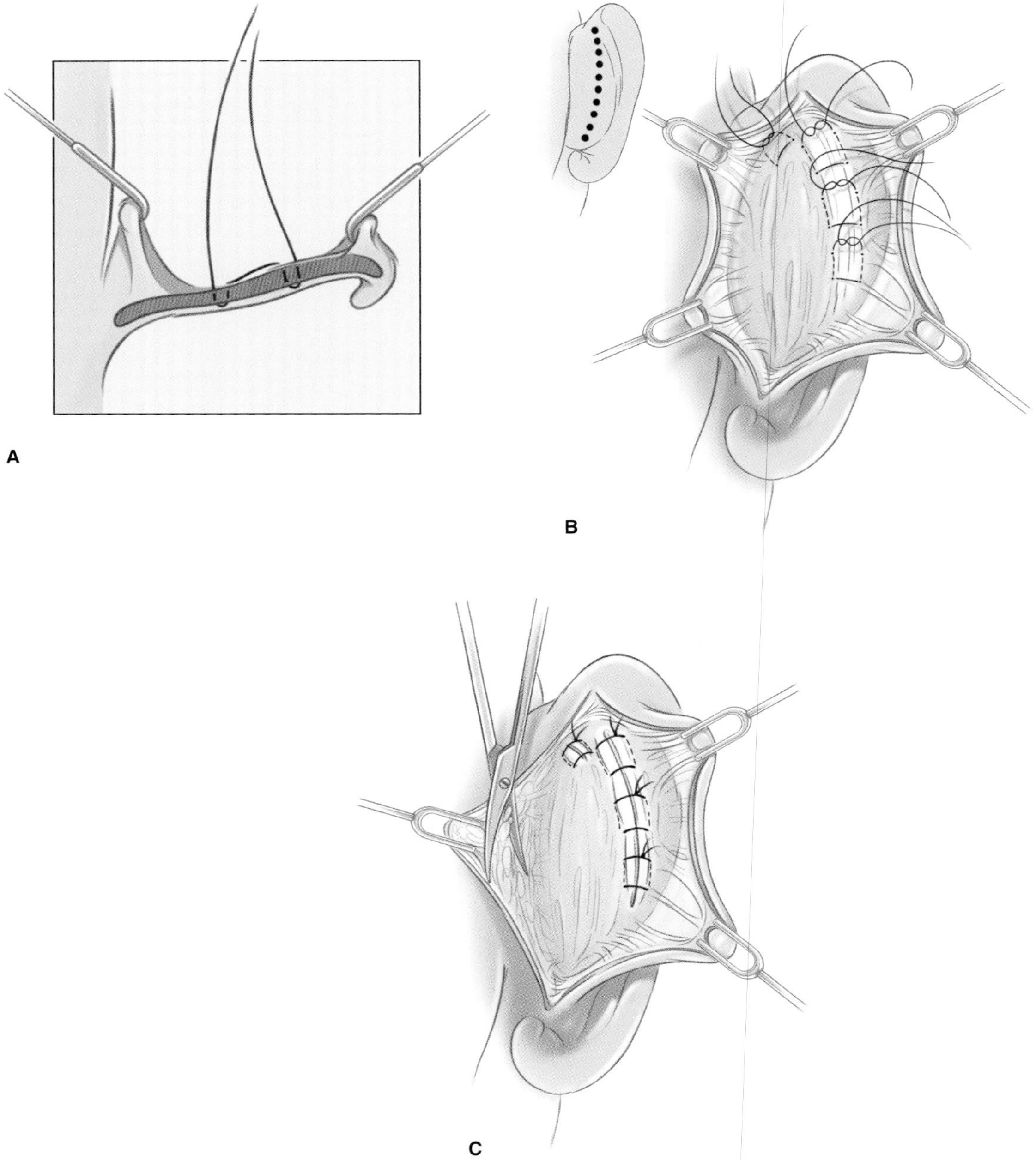

Figure 11–3. **A:** An example of Mustardé mattress suture used to secure the antihelical fold using 4.0 polydioxanone (PDS). **B:** Three Mustardé mattress sutures are placed in the upper third of the ear from the scaphoid fossa or the triangular fossa to the concha to include the full thickness of the cartilage and anterior perichondrium but not the anterior skin. The dots indicate the location of the antihelix. They were made using a 22-gauge needle dipped in methylene blue while viewing the anterior surface of the ear. **C:** The sutures are tied with increasing tension to form the correct fold. A minimum of three sutures is necessary to form the helical fold. Sometimes a fourth is used to reposition the antitragus.

conchal edges are approximated and sutured together with 4.0 monocryl. Additional sutures are placed between the concha and the mastoid fascia. The auricle is lowered into the newly excavated space where the posterior auricular muscles used to rest and anchored with a 4.0 PDS to the mastoid prominence.

The skin incision is closed with 4.0 chromic sutures in the pediatric population and 5.0 nylon in adults.

To reduce the prominence of the antitragus or correct the helical rim, adjunctive procedures are necessary. Each is accomplished through a small incision parallel to the edge of the prominence to allow direct exposure for cartilage resection.

Bacitracin ointment and xeroform gauze are packed into the convolutions of the auricle to preserve the external architecture. This is covered by a fluff dressing and secured with a stretch head wrap. The dressing is changed the morning after surgery, and the ear is examined for hematoma formation. A new dressing may be applied. Once the dressing is removed on postoperative day 3, a stretch terry sport headband is worn at night for up to 6 weeks.

B. Minimally Invasive Techniques

As minimally invasive technology expands, the fundamental doctrines have been applied to otoplasty to help reduce dissection, postoperative edema, and hematoma formation; eliminate the need for postoperative drain placement; and decrease scarring and keloid formation. The minimally invasive or incisionless otoplasty has been evolving since its induction in 1992. Graham and Gault report an endoscopic-assisted otoplasty in which they approach the correction posteriorly through a port in the temporal scalp. The posterior auricular cartilage is weakened by abrasion and the antihelical fold is created and supported by nonabsorbable scaphal-mastoid sutures placed via small postauricular stab incisions. The authors report excellent aesthetic results and zero recurrences in 18 patients. Fritsch adds that a combined cartilage scoring procedure and a percutaneously placed retention suture procedure creates a predictable and permanent correction of the absent or deformed antihelical fold with rare complications. The surgery is not performed on infants because their cartilage is too malleable allowing the retention sutures to cause an accordion-like folding instead of a smooth bend.

C. Nonoperative Otoplasty in Infants

During the first few days of infancy, the ear cartilage is abnormally plastic due to increased circulating maternal estrogen. Estrogen levels peak during the first 3 days of life and return to normal by 6 weeks. During this time, a prominent ear may be molded with tape and soft dental compound to correct the deformity. Tan demonstrated that if auricular molding is performed during the first 3 days of life and continued for up to 6 months, the ear is permanently altered. Unfortunately, poor results occur if the surgeon waits until after the first 3 days of infancy to start molding. Furthermore, many deformities may not be realized at birth. Matsuo observed that the percentage of protruding ears increases from 0.4% at birth to 5.5% by age 1. Therefore, many protruding ears are an acquired deformity.

COMPLICATIONS

A complication from any surgery is a dreaded event, and thus, meticulous surgical technique is paramount. Many surgeons will change the head dressing on the first postoperative day to evaluate for hematoma formation, malpositioning of the ear, or excessive pressure. Malposition of the ear is often fixed by exterior struts like headbands, postauricular props, or dental wax. Hematoma formation may be secondary to the effects of preoperative epinephrine wearing off and poor hemostasis. If a patient complains of sudden, severe, persistent pain or unilateral pain in a bilateral otoplasty case, immediate evaluation and evacuation of clot is necessary.

Although wound infections occur in less than 5% of patients regardless of the surgical technique, they can lead to chondritis and residual deformity. Early identification of infection and prompt treatment are key, since the loss of auricular cartilage may result. Cellulitis is usually caused by staphylococci or streptococci and occasionally *Pseudomonas*. If infection is suspected, intravenous antibiotics and topical mafenide acetate should be started. If the patient has chondritis, the devitalized cartilage should be promptly debrided to avoid a deformity.

Long-term complications resulting from the surgery, including a sharply ridged antihelical fold, irregular contours, sinus tracts, and overcorrection, may necessitate a second surgery. Residual deformities are seen in 10% to 30% of cases but less than 10% of these require further surgery. This may be attributed to the high satisfaction rate among patients. The surgical goal of most patients is not to achieve a perfect form but to decrease ear prominence.

There are several defined deformities that occur weeks to months after surgery. Overcorrection of the mid-portion of the ear with undercorrection of the lobule and superior third of the ear can cause a telephone deformity. Other new deformities, such as a protruding lobule, an obliterated external ear canal, contour deformities on the antihelical fold, and post-perichondritis deformities, are all well documented in the surgical literature and often require a second procedure.

Secondary to thin postauricular sulcal skin and the use of tension-free closures, keloid formation and hypertrophic scarring are rare complications. Close observation in the postoperative period is necessary to diagnose a keloid early. If one is found, an intralesional injection of 10 mg/mL triamcinolone mixed with lidocaine is placed every 2 to 4 weeks to truncate keloid growth and potentially lead to resolution. For large keloids, excision and primary closure with intraoperative triamcinolone injection may be necessary.

OUTCOMES ASSESSMENT

Otoplasty surgery leads to a 96% satisfaction rate among patients. Surgeon satisfaction is only 92%, demonstrating that physicians are often more critical of the results than patients or patients' parents. The social and psychological outcomes from otoplasty have been well documented. Bradbury found an improved well-being in 90% of children 12 months postoperatively. After otoplasty, children experienced a significant reduction in peer ridicule and an increase in self-esteem. Otoplasty has been shown to have a positive impact on the quality of life of adult patients as well. Overall patient satisfaction is extremely high. Recurrence rates are less than 10% in most studies.

REFERENCES

Adamson JE et al. The growth pattern of the external ear. *Plast Reconstr Surgery.* 1965 Oct;36(4):466–70. [PMID: 5831865]

Adamson PA et al. Otoplasty techniques. *Facial Plast Surg.* 1995 Oct;11(4):284–300]. [PMID: 9046617]

Becker OJ. Correction of the protruding deformed ear. *Br J Plast Surg.* 1952 Oct;5:187–96. [PMID: 12987613]

Bradbury ET et al. Psychological and social outcome of prominent ear correction in children. *Br J Plast Surg.* 1992 Feb–Mar;45(2):97–100. [PMID: 1562855]

Calder JC et al. Morbidity of otoplasty: A review of 562 cases. *Br J Plast Surg.* 1994 Apr;47(3):170–4. [PMID: 8193854]

Chongchet V. A method of antihelix reconstruction. *Br J Plast Surg.* 1963 Jul;16:268–72. [PMID: 14042756]

Dieffenbach JE. Die Ohrbildung Otoplastik. In: *Die operative Chirurgie*. Leipzig FA. Brockhause; 1845:395–7.

Ely ET. An operation for prominent auricles. *Arch Otolaryngol*. 1881;10:97.

Farkas LG. Anthropometry of the normal and defective ear. *Clin Plast Surg*. 1990 Apr;17(2):213–21. [PMID: 2189638]

Farkas LG et al. Anthropometric growth study of the ear. *Cleft Palate Craniofac J*. 1992 Jul;29(4):324–9. [PMID: 1643061]

Fritsch MH. Incisionless otoplasty. *Facial Plast Surg*. 2004 Nov;20(4):267–70. [PMID: 15778913]

Furnas DW. Correction of prominent ears by conchamastoid sutures. *Plast Reconstr Surg*. 1968 Sep;42(3):189–93. [PMID: 4878456]

Georgiade GS et al. Prominent ears and their correction: a forty-year experience. *Aesthetic Plast Surg*. 1995 Sep–Oct;19(5):439–43. [PMID: 8526160]

Gibson T, Davis W. The distortion of autogenous cartilage grafts: Its cause and prevention. *Br J Plast Surg*. 1958;10:257.

Graham KE et al. Endoscopic assisted otoplasty: a preliminary report. *Br J Plast Surg*. 1997 Jan;50(1):47–57. [PMID: 9038515]

Janis J et al. Otoplasty. *Plast Reconstr Surg*. 2005 Apr;115 (4):60e–72e. [PMID: 15793433]

LaTrenta GS. Otoplasty. In: Rees TD, LaTrenta GS, eds. *Aesthetic Plastic Surgery,* 2nd ed. Philadelphia: Saunders; 1994:891–921.

Luckett WH. A new operation for prominent ears based on the anatomy of the deformity. *Surg Gynecol Obstet*. 1910;10:635.

Matsuo K et al. Nonsurgical correction of congenital auricular deformities in the early neonate: a preliminary report. *Plast Reconstr Surg*. 1984 Jan;73(1):38–51. [PMID: 6691074]

Matsuo K et al. Nonsurgical correction of congenital auricular deformities. *Clin Plast Surg*. 1990 Apr 17(2):383–95. [PMID: 2189652]

McDowell AJ. Goals in otoplasty for protruding ears. *Plast Reconst Surg*. 1968 Jan;41(1):17–27. [PMID: 5639206]

Mustardé JC. The correction of prominent ears using simple mattress sutures. *Br J Plast Surg*. 1963 Apr;16:170–8. [PMID: 13936895]

Pirsig W. The auricle in the visual arts. *Facial Plast Surg*. 2004 Nov;20(4):251–66. [PMID: 15778912]

Richards SD et al. Otoplasty: a review of the surgical techniques. *Clin Otolaryngol*. 2005 Feb;30(1):2–8. [PMID: 15748181]

Spira M et al. Correction of the principal deformities causing protruding ears. *Plast Reconstr Surg*. 1969 Aug;44(2):150–4. [PMID: 5799297]

Stenstroem SJ. A "natural" technique for correction of congenitally prominent ears. *Plast Reconstr Surg*. 1963 Nov;32:509–18. [PMID: 14078273]

Tan ST et al. Molding therapy for infants with deformational auricular anomalies. *Ann Plast Surg*. 1997 Mar;38(3):263–8. [PMID: 9088465]

Tolleth H. A hierarchy of values in the design and construction of the ear. *Clin Plast Surg*. 1990 Apr;17(2):193–207. [PMID: 2189636]

Weinzweig N et al. Histomorphology of neochondrogenesis after antihelical fold creation: a comparison of three otoplasty techniques in the rabbit. *Ann Plast Surg*. 1994 Oct;33(4):371–6. [PMID: 7810952]

Wright WK. Otoplasty goals and principles. *Arch Otolarygol*. 1970 Dec;92(6):568–72. [PMID: 4922432]

CHAPTER 12

Alloplastic Facial Implants

Juliet C. Park, MD, Jeffrey Ascherman, MD, & Ferdinand Ofodile, MD

► AUGMENTATION OF CHEEKS, CHIN, & NOSE

Alloplastic implant augmentation of the face offers a simple and effective technique for correcting acquired or congenital facial deformities and enhancing aesthetic appearance with low morbidity in appropriately selected patients.

Aesthetic implant augmentation surgery of the face is guided by principles of aesthetic facial analysis. Earlier implant approaches to facial anatomy regarded the aesthetic units of the face as discrete units that did not overlap or relate to each other. Implants were small and designed to address only the specific area of deficit. Except for the mildest defects, augmentation with small implants resulted in inadequate correction with palpable and sometimes visible step-offs, capsular scar contractures, and implant migration.

Over the last three decades, aesthetic understanding of the face has evolved into a more sophisticated analysis pioneered by Terino. In this analysis, aesthetic units of the face are extended beyond their traditional boundaries and divided into zones. The chin is evaluated in continuity with the jawline and the cheek is evaluated in continuity from the paranasal region to the lateral extent of the zygomatic arch. Terino calls this concept "zonal anatomy" (Figure 12–1). Furthermore, the overall harmony of the face is balanced between the upper two-thirds of the face and the lower third, rather than considering each third of the face separately and of similar contribution to the overall aesthetic impression.

Recognition of the aesthetic significance of the extended zonal anatomy of the face has led to the development of modern-day implants. These implants have prefabricated shapes that extend well beyond the obvious area of augmentation into the surrounding areas. Such implants are referred to as "anatomic" or "extended" implants and are commercially available in a variety of materials and dimensions. Placement of an extended implant results in augmentation of the target area with smooth contour transition into the surrounding areas. This technique results in dramatic aesthetic results that are natural and subtle. Almost any area of the face is amenable to augmentation for aesthetic or reconstructive purposes (Figure 12–2).

The most common commercially available implant materials are silicone and

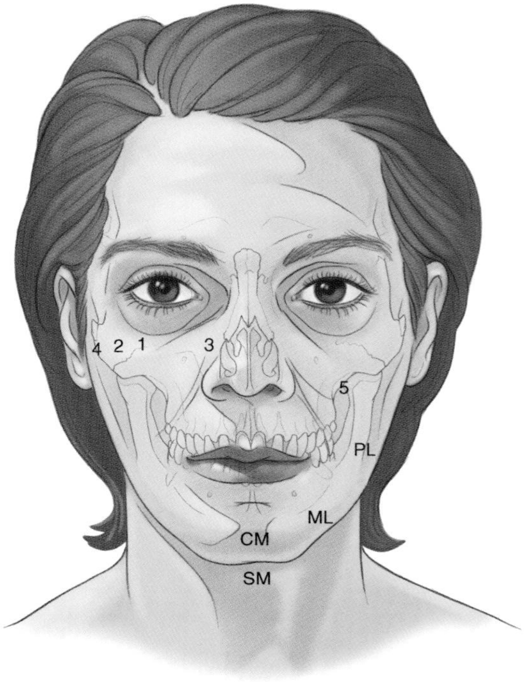

Figure 12–1. Terino's zonal anatomy of the face. The cheek is divided into five zones: 1, infraorbital foramen to the medial third of the zygomatic arch; 2, middle third of the zygomatic arch; 3, paranasal region; 4, lateral third of the zygomatic arch; 5, submalar zone—the site of age-related soft tissue atrophy and descent as well as lipodystrophy of other etiologies. Zones 1 and 2 comprise the malar region. The chin is divided into four zones: CM, central mentum zone; ML, midlateral zone; PL, posterolateral zone; SM, submandibular zone.

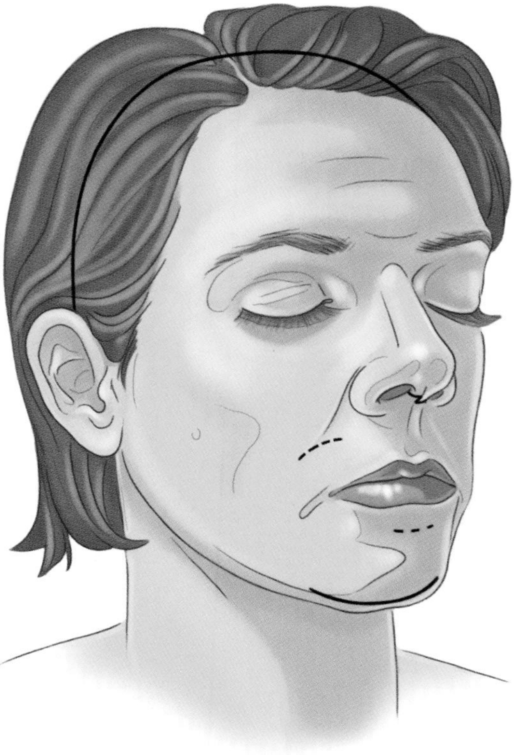

Figure 12–2. Diagram shows the incisions frequently used to access the areas of the facial skeleton that can be corrected with alloplastic implant augmentation. Solid lines = cutaneous incisions; dotted lines = mucosal incisions.

polyethylene. Silicone implants are smooth, allowing easy insertion and removal. However, smooth implants are associated with a greater likelihood of implant migration, thicker capsule formation with increased likelihood of contracture, and underlying bone resorption. Polyethylene implants are porous and promote local tissue ingrowth. Porous implants are less likely than smooth implants to migrate once in place and less likely to stimulate formation of thick scar capsules or underlying bone resorption. However, porous implants are more difficult to insert, require wider tissue dissections for placement, and are difficult to remove. Porous implant materials may be associated with a higher risk of infection; however, they may also have lower rates of extrusion compared to silicone due to tissue ingrowth and incorporation.

Both smooth and porous implants are available in pre-made shapes and sizes that can be trimmed to individual fit intraoperatively. Both types of implant materials can be fixed in place with screws, wires, or sutures according to surgeon preference, or situated in a well-designed tissue pocket without fixation.

Facial implants are also available as custom-made molds. Custom-made implants can be cast directly from impressions of the defect area made from commercially available soft molding materials or indirectly from computerized reconstructions (such as three-dimensional computerized tomography), permitting calculation and subsequent custom manufacture of individualized implant shapes and sizes.

The recommended tissue plane of placement for facial implants is the subperiosteal plane. This plane offers an easily identifiable level of dissection, is relatively bloodless, and minimizes the risk of nerve injuries. Expected soft tissue augmentation with facial implants can be estimated at a 0.66:1 ratio of soft tissue augmentation to implant height.

ANATOMY

The aesthetic appearance of the face is governed by geometric principles. These include symmetry, balance, and overall harmony of outward appearance with respect to age, ethnicity, and culture. However, the concept of aesthetics by definition contains a subjective element. Precise numeric relationships of facial features have been studied and described by numerous authors, but there is no one technique for facial aesthetic analysis that is universally accepted or applicable to all patients. The aesthetic surgeon should be familiar with and able to apply various techniques for facial analysis, while at the same time using aesthetic judgment when it comes to the individual patient.

The face has three primary and two secondary areas of anatomic prominence that define its overall appearance and balance. The primary areas are the nose, the malar-zygomatic eminence of the cheek, and the jawline. The secondary areas are the forehead and the paranasal regions.

As a principle, aesthetically pleasing outward appearances of the face are related to smooth contours and balanced soft tissue fullness. Deficient or excessive projection in primary areas of prominence, such as the cheek and the chin, disrupt the perception of continuity and diminish the outwardly pleasing aspects of facial appearance. For instance, malar fullness and prominence result in a youthful, healthy outward appearance, while malar-submalar deficiency results in a drawn, harsh, aged appearance.

The general proportions of the face can be assessed using geometric relationships based on the traditional division of the face into thirds (Figure 12–3). The upper third of the face is the most variable in terms of numeric measures due to variability in hairline position among individuals and is the least important aesthetic third. The lower and middle thirds of the face should be of nearly equal heights, although in some patients the lower third of the face may be smaller in both the horizontal and vertical dimensions and still remain aesthetically pleasing. The lower third of the face is further subdivided into an upper one-third and lower two-thirds by a line drawn through the oral commissures and stomion. This analysis becomes significant in evaluating the chin.

Changes in the dimensions of one of the thirds of the face can affect the overall perception of the shape of another third. For instance, augmentation of the cheeks resulting in a horizontal widening of the middle third of the face can decrease the impression of an overly long narrow face and has been described by Terino.

The width of the face is divided into equal fifths by lines drawn at the lateralmost projections of the face (bizygomatic distance), the lateral canthi, and the medial canthi (Figure 12–4). Each vertical fifth is approximately the width

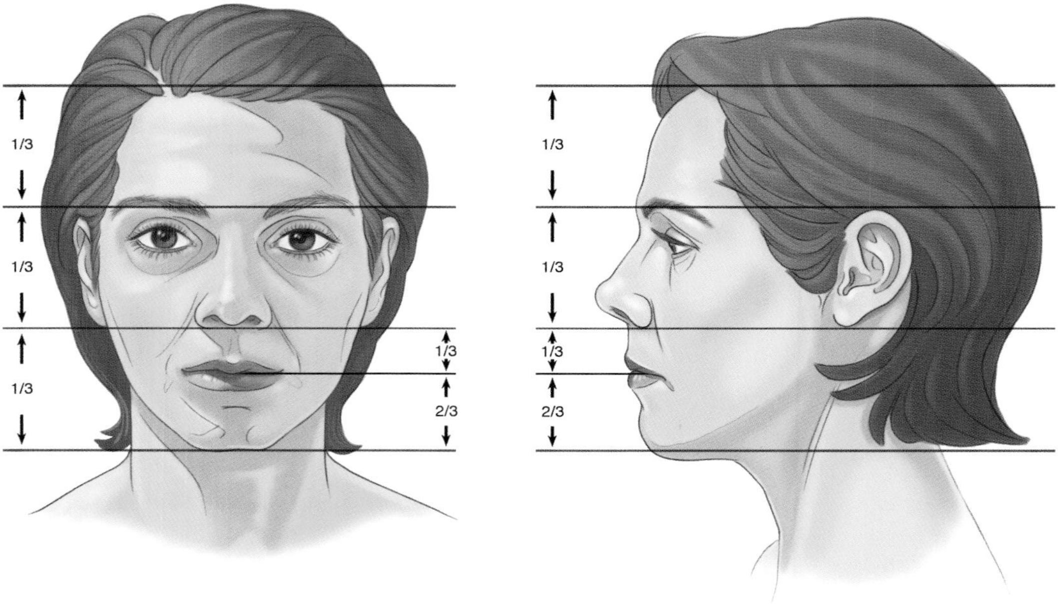

Figure 12–3. The face is divided into thirds drawn at the hairline, brows, the alar base, and the menton. The height of the lower third of the face is approximately the height of the middle third of the face and is further divided into an upper one-third and a lower two-thirds by a line drawn through the stomion. On profile view, the horizontal thirds of the face can be approximated by lines at the hairline, glabella, alar base, and menton. The lower third of the face can be further subdivided into an upper third and a lower two-thirds by a line drawn through the oral commissures and stomion.

of the eye. The distance between the medial canthi is approximated by the width of one eye. The widest portion of the face on frontal view lies at the level of the zygomatic arches and averages up to 20% greater than the bitemporal distance in men, and about 15% in women. The bigonial distance averages 10% less than the bitemporal distance in men and 15% less in women (Figure 12–5).

The balanced profile is characterized by a convex outline described by Legan and Burstone and is defined by the anterior projections of the forehead (glabella), nose, and chin (pogonion) (Figure 12–6).

The anatomy underlying the facial appearance has two distinct elements: bone and soft tissue. Accurate evaluation of the aesthetic area in question must identify and distinguish between defects related to skeletal structure and those related to soft tissue deficiencies.

Soft tissue deficiencies are congenital or acquired. In the aesthetic setting, soft tissue deficiency is often acquired and secondary to aging (Figure 12–7). Skin drooping and volumetric loss are the visible result. Facial implants can provide effective correction of mild to moderate age-related soft tissue changes in the malar-submalar and jowl regions. Implant augmentation of soft tissue changes should be limited to implant heights that will not result in an abnormal-appearing underlying contour. In addition, implants do not address the

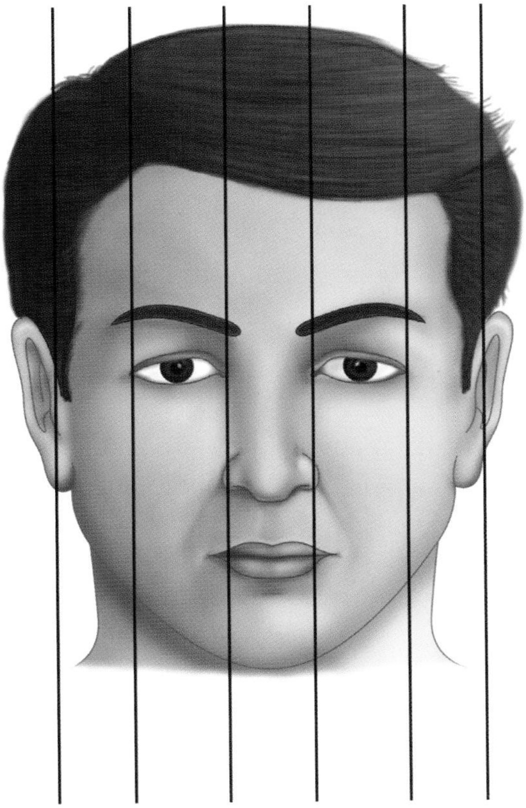

Figure 12–4. The face can be divided into vertical fifths measuring the width of an eye.

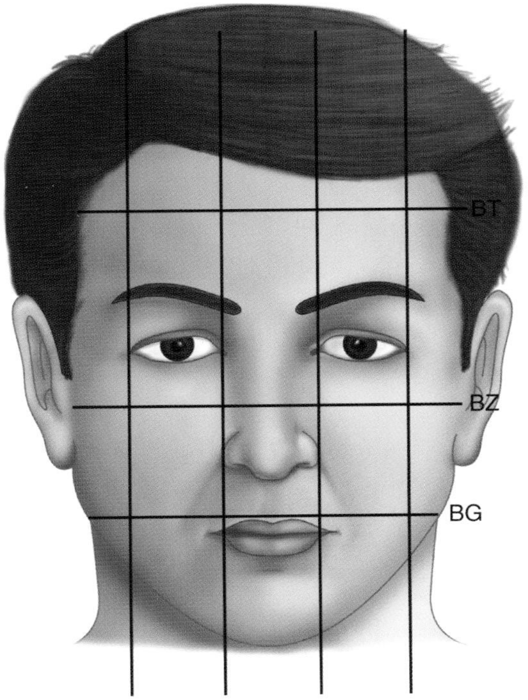

Figure 12–5. The bitemporal (BT) distance is the width across the forehead from frontotemporal to frontotemporal junction. The bizygomatic (BZ) distance is the widest portion of the face on the frontal view, measured from zygion to zygion, the lateralmost point of the zygomatic arch; this distance averages 10%–20% greater than the BT distance. The bigonial (BG) distance measures the distance between the lateralmost aspect of the gonia on frontal view; it averages 10%–15% less than the BT distance. Note that the gonion by definition is identified on lateral view and can then be translated to the frontal view. Accurate identification on frontal view is difficult without locating the level of the gonion on lateral view first.

underlying biologic mechanisms of age-related changes in soft tissue. Implant augmentation for soft tissue aging fills an increasingly lax and atrophied skin envelope that results from progressive soft tissue descent related to gravity and tissue compositional change with age. More severe degrees of soft tissue atrophy and sagging may be indications for other surgical procedures, such as rhytidectomy.

Skeletal deficiencies present an underlying structural defect upon which the soft tissue elements rest. Skeletal deformities can also be congenital or acquired. Skeletal deficiencies suitable to implant correction are mild to moderate in severity and typically fall in the range of 5–10 mm deficiencies in the cheek and chin areas, and up to 5 mm in deficiency over the nasal dorsum. The absolute perpendicular

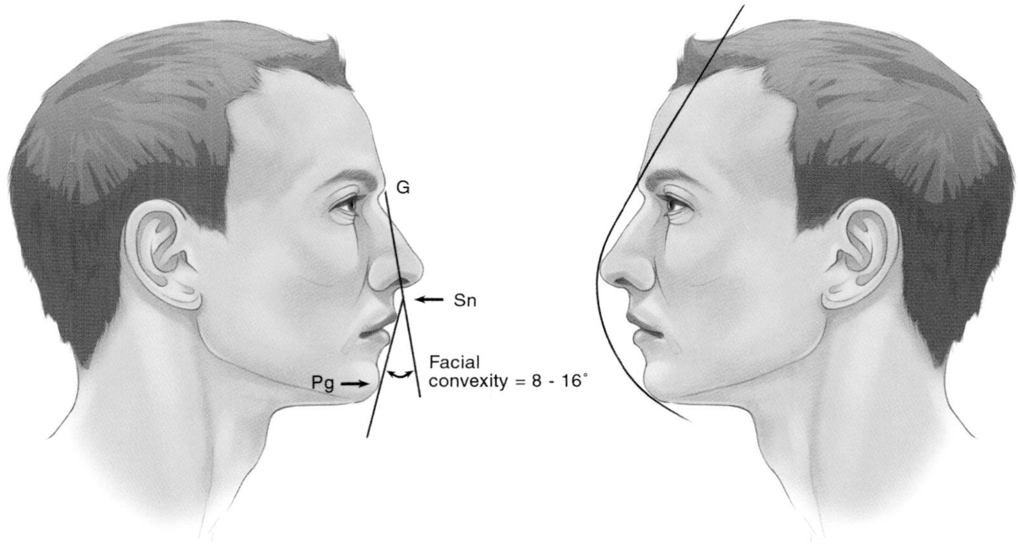

Figure 12–6. Legan and Burstone's facial convexity. G, glabella; Sn, subnasal point; Pg, pogonion.

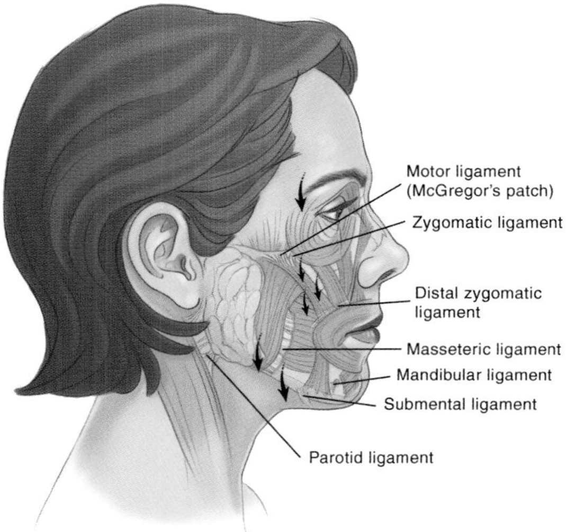

Figure 12–7. Skin drooping and volumetric loss are the visible soft tissue results of aging.

height of any implant augmentation should take into account the overlying skin quality and tension.

Skeletal or soft tissue deformities of more severe degrees may be indications for orthognathic or craniomaxillofacial surgeries. These deformities include congenital phenotypes, such as severe midface retrusion or hypoplasia, vertical maxillary excess, micrognathia greater than 10 mm in sagittal deficiency, micrognathia with associated vertical mandibular excess, any condition involving significant malocclusion and craniofacial syndromes.

Ideal facial proportions and relationships serve as guidelines to the identification of physical deformity, the assessment of the objective severity of the deformity, and the planning of operative intervention. Such criteria are not definitive in every case. Numeric quantifications of "ideal" anatomic relationships by definition do not represent the full range of normals. It is also important to remember that many of the numeric analyses of facial relationships are primarily based on the study of white features, and therefore may not apply to all ethnic groups. Recognition of normal variations in outward appearance due to age, gender, ethnicity, and overall facial balance is important in developing sound aesthetic judgment. The principles of symmetry and balance can help guide aesthetic assessment across all groups.

PATIENT PREPARATION

Initial consultation should determine the patient's specific concerns. Satisfactory outcome depends on accurate identification of the patient's aesthetic goals. After initial consultation, it may be useful to schedule a subsequent follow-up office visit about 4 weeks later to give the patient time to think about surgery, ask additional questions, and make an informed decision.

A thorough past medical and surgical history is obtained, with special attention to prior related surgical procedures. Functional deficits related to the area of concern are assessed and if identified, should be addressed prior to aesthetic interventions. Focused radiographic examination is necessary only if there is a specific anatomic question or a need for clarification of prior surgical interventions.

Photodocumentation of preoperative and postoperative findings should be standard for all cases. The operative plan, recovery course, expected outcomes, and potential complications should be reviewed in detail with the patient and are part of the informed consent (see Chapter 1).

Medications that predispose to increased risk of surgical bleeding, including aspirin and vitamin E, should be discontinued 1 week or more prior to surgery. Medical conditions that predispose to coagulopathy or thromboembolic disease or that represent significant cardiovascular disease or general anesthetic risk should be carefully evaluated and may represent contraindications to elective aesthetic surgery.

Facial implant augmentation is performed on an outpatient basis unless it is scheduled in combination with another procedure that may require hospitalization. Implant augmentation may be done under local or general anesthesia. General anesthesia offers control of a secure airway and the possibility of more complete patient comfort and cooperation. Implant augmentation may also be performed under intravenous sedation without general anesthesia, but this does not decrease the risk of associated perioperative anesthetic morbidity or monitoring requirements compared with general anesthesia.

A local field block is performed in all implant procedures using 0.5–1% lidocaine with dilute epinephrine at 1:100,000–400,000. Local anesthetic infiltration aids in dissection and provides hemostasis; if a longer-acting anesthetic is used, it can confer some postoperative pain control. Prophylactic antibiotics are given perioperatively.

► CHIN IMPLANT

ANATOMY

In the setting of normal occlusion and mild to moderate microgenia, the aesthetically pleasing chin profile can be evaluated using varying soft tissue landmarks and relationships. It is useful to be familiar with several described relationships, since no one relationship has been identified that can be routinely applied to all patients. Quantitative measurement tools can be classified into two categories: one category of tools is used to help determine the anterior-most projection of the chin in profile. The other category describes the relative relationships of the structures of the lower third of the face.

On profile view, the anterior projection of the chin can be assessed using the soft tissue landmarks of the nose-lip-chin plane. The nose-lip-chin plane extends from a point one-half the distance of the nasal length through the upper and lower lip vermilion. This plane should form a 2–4 degree posterior angle with a plumb line dropped vertically from the glabella and a 10 degree posterior angle with a line running from the nasion through the subnasale.

The anteriormost projection of the chin can also be identified by a vertical plumb line dropped from the anteriormost projection of the white roll of the lower lip or, alternatively, by a vertical plumb line dropped from the labial surface of the lower central incisors.

The relationship between the structures of the profile of the lower third of the face to each other can be demonstrated by a lower lip lying slightly posterior to the upper lip by up to 2 mm (Figure 12–8), and the anteriormost projection of the chin lying up to 2 mm posterior to the lower lip. Alternatively, the relative position of the lips and chin can be assessed by a line drawn from the nasal tip to the pogonion. The lips should lie posterior to this line, with the anteriormost projection of each lip a similar distance posterior to the line so that again, the lower lip lies slightly posterior to the upper lip.

Strong anterior projection of the chin confers a masculine appearance. There is less aesthetic tolerance for a masculinized anterior chin in a female face than there is for a neutral or slightly posteriorly placed chin in a male face. Aesthetic judgment plays a role in the management of anterior chin projection in the individual patient.

In anterior view, the width of the mandible is approximated by bigonial distance and is equal to the bitemporal distance. A narrower mandibular width and more obtuse curvature of the mandibular angle is more aesthetically accepted in women than in men.

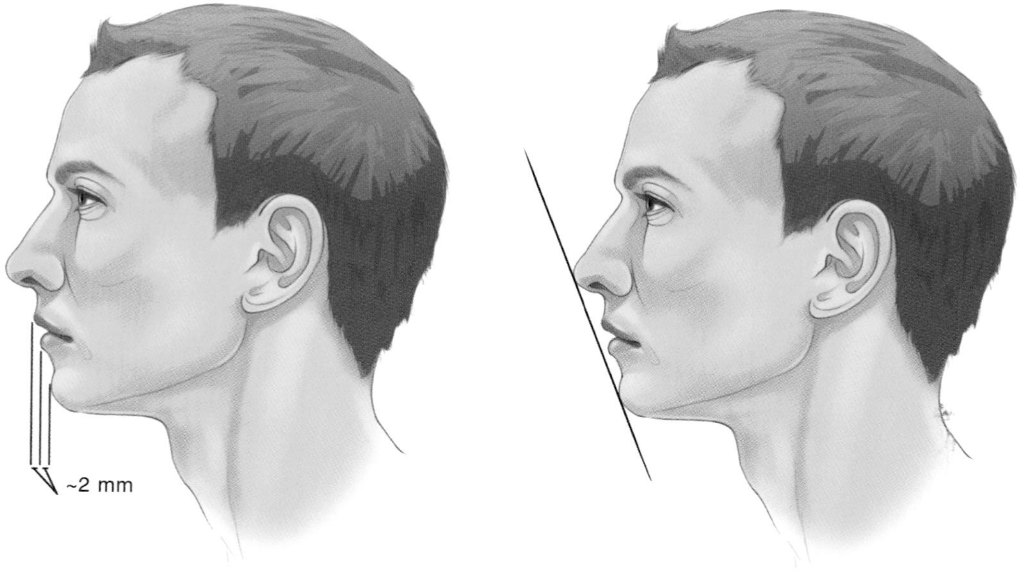

Figure 12–8. Relationship of chin to lips. The lower lip lies up to 2 mm posterior to the upper lip; the chin lies up to 2 mm posterior to the lower lip. The upper lip lies up to twice as far posterior as the lower lip relative to a line drawn from the nasal tip to the anterior chin.

being addressed. Soft-tissue atrophy related to facial aging or malar lipodystrophy should include augmentation of the submalar region (Figure 12–1, Zone 5), with or without inclusion of the malar areas, for effective restoration of volume. Defects that are skeletal in nature are addressed with augmentation to the area of bony deformity.

Identifying the infraorbital nerve may help protect the nerve from injury but is not routine. The infraorbital nerve exits the maxilla through the infraorbital foramen, which is typically located on the maxilla just medial to the forward-gazing pupil and about 10 mm inferior to the orbital rim. Applying digital pressure externally over the infraorbital foramen during subperiosteal elevation can help prevent dissection in the vicinity of the nerve.

Trimming of commercially available implants and suture or screw fixation is performed based on surgeon preference. If the tissue pocket is well-sized to the desired implant position, fixation may not be necessary. Handling of implant materials should be kept to the minimum possible.

As in chin implant placement, the wound should be closed in layers with meticulous approximation of tissues and without tension.

COMPLICATIONS

Complication rates for malar implants are higher than those seen with chin implants. Infection rates average 2%. Displacement rates average 2% for malar implants compared to < 0.5% for chin implants. As in chin implants, major nerve injury is rare. Infraorbital nerve paresthesia usually represents edema and traction injury that is self-limited and resolves with observation. Complete numbness should prompt consideration of nerve impingement or possible transection injury and should be surgically explored if symptoms do not resolve within 2 weeks.

▶ NASAL IMPLANT

ANATOMY

Traditional aesthetic analysis of the nose is often based on the nasal anatomy seen in whites and uses both relative and absolute measurements. Ethnic nasal phenotypes may vary significantly from the white phenotype (Figure 12–10). Absolute measurements can become difficult to apply across races; relative proportions and harmony tend to remain useful indicators of overall aesthetic outcome in all cases.

Facial analysis of the nose for implant augmentation examines three key components: the dorsum, the tip/columella, and the nostrils.

The dorsum is assessed by comparing it to a straight line drawn from the radix to the tip. The amount of deficiency present under this line is evaluated and may be considered significant, or a low-lying dorsum. The presence of negative "scooped" curvature to the dorsum and the distal extent of the deficiency is noted. Nasal implants require apposition to the full length of the dorsum to avoid visible step-offs mid-dorsum, and this may necessitate lowering dorsal height distally.

The tip is evaluated for projection, definition, and cartilaginous resilience. The columella is evaluated for bowing or retraction. Nostrils are evaluated for shape, width, and alar flare. Skin quality along the entire dorsum and tip of the nose is noted. Finally, assessment should be made of the nasolabial angle and the presence or absence of premaxillary retrusion and paranasal midface hypoplasia.

If the tip projection is inadequate, techniques for increasing tip projection are similar to those used in traditional rhinoplasty and can be combined with dorsal implant augmentation. Likewise, the approach to other deficiencies of the nose that are identified during examination and aesthetic analysis for dorsal nasal implant augmentation, including

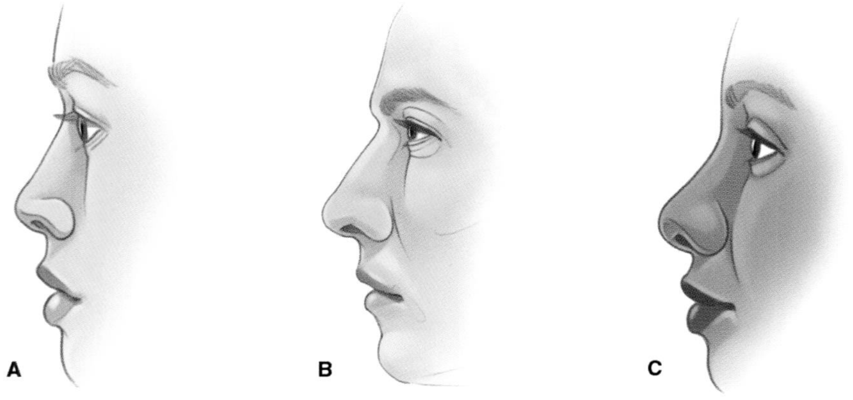

Figure 12–10. Ethnic variations in idealized aesthetic balance of the nose in profile. A) Asian. B) White. C) Black.

alar flare, wide alar base, excessive columellar show, and hanging or boxy tips, can be addressed with proper planning using open rhinoplasty techniques at the same time as implant augmentation.

Like chin and malar/submalar implants, nasal implants are commercially available in several shapes, sizes, and materials and can be trimmed to individual needs intraoperatively.

PATIENT EVALUATION & SELECTION

The use of nasal implants is indicated in the aesthetic and reconstructive treatment of the low-lying nasal dorsum. In reconstructive cases, autogenous tissues are preferable, but when the availability of autogenous tissue is inadequate, synthetic implant materials can be a useful resource.

For aesthetic purposes, nasal implants offer a simple technique for correction of the low-lying dorsum. In settings in which there is no plan to perform other major surgical interventions, the placement of a nasal implant is a minimally invasive procedure.

The low-lying nasal dorsum is an anatomic feature that carries ethnic distribution. The low-lying dorsum is characteristic of East Asian and Southeast Asian populations as well as some black and Hispanic populations. Aesthetic surgery aimed at altering ethnic features should be approached with sensitivity. Results that remain consistent with the patient's overall outward appearance are desireable. Screening and counseling of patient expectations to this end will help promote satisfactory outcomes.

Any history of prior surgical or nonsurgical enhancements of the nose, including procedures involving injection or placement of permanent or nonpermanent moldable or free-form injectable liquid materials, should be obtained.

TECHNIQUE

Nasal implant augmentation is easiest performed with an open technique. Access to the nasal dorsum is achieved with a stair-step incision in the columella. This incision may be extended into the nostrils on either side with a marginal incision. The skin and soft tissue of the tip are then carefully dissected free from the lower lateral cartilages, taking care not to inadvertently cut the cartilages. A subperiosteal pocket is created over the dorsum of the nose. The dorsum is resected as needed to permit the implant to lie flat and to extend along the full length of the dorsum to the tip. Care should be taken to preserve vascularized intact periosteal tissues around the pocket and to create a pocket that does not put any implant pressure on the soft tissues of the tip. The pocket is irrigated with antibiotic solution when completed, and the implant is inserted with minimal handling and avoidance of contact with nasal mucosa. The wound is closed in layers.

COMPLICATIONS

Compared with implant augmentation of other areas of the face, nasal implants have a high rate of complications (Table 12–1, Terino and Flowers; Rubin). The relatively sparse overlying soft tissue coverage available at the nasal dorsum and the increased likelihood for soft tissue tension contribute to higher rates of implant exposure and extrusion. Attention to sterile technique, avoidance of contact with contaminated nasal mucosa, use of preoperative and postoperative antibiotics, minimal tissue handling and dissection, and avoidance of tension in the overlying tissues is of particular importance in placement of the nasal implant compared to other implant augmentation sites of the face.

▶ TABLE 12–1. COMPLICATION RATES OF IMPLANTS BY LOCATION

Location	Overall Infection Rate	Extrusion Rate
Chin	1.4%	<0.5%
Malar	2.4%	<0.5%
Nasal	2.4%	5.2%

REFERENCES

Guyuron B et al. A critical comparison of osteoplastic and alloplastic augmentation genioplasty. *Aesthetic Plast Surg.* 1990 Summer;14(3):199–206. [PMID: 2399851]

Legan HL, Burstone CJ. Soft tissue cephalometric analysis for orthognathic surgery. *Journal of Oral Surgery.* 1980;38:744–751.

Rubin JP et al. Complications and toxicities of implantable biomaterials used in facial reconstructive and aesthetic surgery: a comprehensive review of the literature. *Plast Reconstr Surg.* 1997 Oct;100(5):1336–53. [PMID: 9326803]

Talmor M, Hoffman LA, LaTrenta GS. Facial atrophy in HIV-related fat redistribution syndrome: anatomic evaluation and surgical reconstruction. *Ann Plast Surg.* 2002 Jul;49(1):11-7; discussion 117-8.

Terino EO, Flowers RS, eds. *The Art of Alloplastic Facial Contouring.* St. Louis: Mosby; 2000.

Warren SM et al. Chin surgery V: treatment of the long, non-projecting chin. *Plast Reconstr Surg.* 2007 Sep;120(3):760–8. [PMID: 17700129]

Yaremchuk MJ. Facial skeletal reconstruction using porous polyethylene implants. *Plast Reconstr Surg.* 2003 May;111(6):1818–27. [PMID: 12711941]

Yaremchuk MJ. Improving aesthetic outcomes after alloplastic chin augmentation. *Plast Reconstr Surg.* 2003 Oct;112(5):1422–32. [PMID: 14504528]

Yaremchuk MJ. Mandibular augmentation. *Plast Reconstr Surg.* 2000 Sep;106(3):697-706. [PMID: 10987481]

Zide BM et al. Chin surgery I: Augmentation—the allures and the alerts. *Plast Reconstr Surg.* 1999 Nov;104(6):1843–53. [PMID: 10541191]

CHAPTER 13

Breast Augmentation

Nicholas Vendemia, MD, Tal T. Roudner, MD, Brian D. Cohen, MD, & Lloyd A. Hoffman, MD

Congenital or acquired micromastia is a commonly encountered clinical condition. The association between a feminine appearing breast and a positive self-image is strong. According to the American Society for Aesthetic Plastic Surgery (ASAPS), 307,230 breast augmentation procedures were performed in 2008. With both the publicity and the relative success of breast augmentation, plastic surgeons must make an effort to be educated in the arenas of patient selection, technique selection, perioperative surgical management, complications, and patient counseling relative to breast augmentation.

ANATOMY

The breast is made up of both fatty and glandular tissues. The ratio of the fatty to glandular tissue varies with age and among individuals. Younger women have a higher proportion of the dense glandular tissue composing their breasts, while older women have a higher fatty component. As estrogen production decreases during menopause, glandular breast tissue atrophies, and the fatty tissue predominates in proportion.

The suspensory ligaments of Cooper run throughout the breast parenchyma from the deep pectoralis fascia to the dermis of the skin and provide a support structure for the soft tissues of the breast. With age and the long-standing effects of gravity, these ligaments relax and result in breast ptosis.

The female breast extends from approximately the second rib superiorly to the fifth rib inferiorly. The superior portion overlies the pectoralis major muscle, the serratus anterior muscle inferiorly, and the axillary fascia laterally. The pectoralis major is extremely important in providing muscle coverage for the breast implant in the subpectorally augmented breast. The serratus anterior muscle may also be elevated during breast reconstruction to obtain a sufficient muscle layer laterally to provide complete muscle coverage for an expander or implant. The rectus fascia often must be elevated to place the implant or expander in an inferior position when lowering the inframammary fold (IMF).

The blood supply to the breast is derived from the perforating branches of the internal mammary artery, the thoracodorsal artery, the lateral thoracic artery, the thoracoacromial artery and the lateral intercostal perforators.

The blood from these arteries supports the glandular tissues, soft tissue, while the breast skin relies on the subdermal capillary plexus for vascular support.

Sensory innervation of the breast is mainly derived from the anterolateral and anteromedial branches of thoracic intercostal nerves T3–T5. Supraclavicular nerves from the lower fibers of the cervical plexus (C3–C4) also provide innervation to the upper and lateral portions of the breast. Sensation to the nipple is mainly derived from the lateral cutaneous branch of T4, which enters the nipple areola complex (NAC) inferolaterally.

PATIENT EVALUATION & SELECTION

Most breast augmentation procedures are performed to correct glandular hypoplasia, breast asymmetry, or a combination of both. It is important to identify patients with unrealistic expectations for the operation, and those who expect their newfound self-esteem to resolve problems in their personal lives. Such patients will invariably be dissatisfied with their results, and their surgeon, and should not be considered for undergoing elective surgery. Asking the patient to bring photographs that depict how she would like her breasts to appear clothed and unclothed may help the surgeon gauge expectations. In addition to discussing the patients' expectations for the operation, time should be reserved during the consultation to talk about the objective benefits, risks, and potential complications of the planned procedure. Ensuring that the patient is well informed and that her expectations are realistic are keys to a successful encounter. Attempts to provide an augmentation that appears as natural as possible and that meets the patient's expectations within the limits of safety concerns should be the surgeon's goal.

A. History

It is of critical importance to obtain a full history before scheduling any elective surgical procedure. Preexisting medical and surgical history must be carefully outlined, with special attention to any first-degree family history of breast cancer, anticipated pregnancy, recent weight changes, and any previous breast surgery. The results of the patient's last mammogram, if applicable, should be recorded, as should the patient's current and desired bra size.

B. Physical Examination

A full physical examination with a comprehensive breast examination should always be performed with particular attention to masses; scars; and nipple size, color, and position. Natural asymmetry between the breasts and NACs is common and should be discussed with the patient preoperatively. The patient may not be aware of such subtle differences and may view postoperative asymmetry as a complication of the operation rather than an expected result due to the asymmetric presentation prior to the procedure. The surgeon must also pay close attention to the preoperative IMFs, as asymmetric IMFs must be addressed with caution. Plans to readjust the IMF, including possible complications, must be made clear to the patient during the preoperative evaluation.

The breast parenchyma should be examined with documentation of the amount, quality, and distribution of the parenchyma. Striae of the skin represent poor elasticity and must be taken into account when deciding on the appropriate procedure. Two centimeters of soft tissue pinch in the superior pole of the breast indicates adequate tissue for coverage of a subglandular implant. A superior pinch test result of less than 2 cm is an indication for submuscular placement of the implant in order to decrease the chance of rippling, visibility, and palpability of the implants. Precise measurements must be taken, including

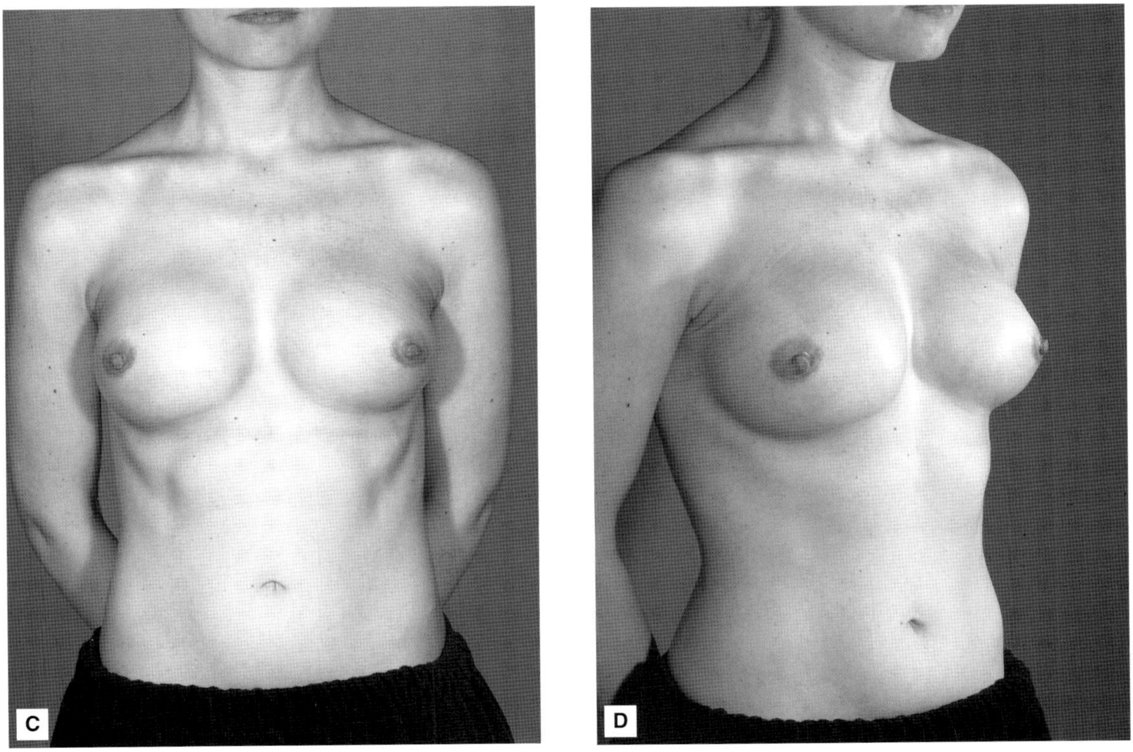

Figure 13–1. (Continued)

on the volume and position of the sizer, the permanent implant is placed after a thorough inspection for hemostasis and copious antibiotic irrigation.

The myotomy (if performed) and the deep soft tissues are closed with a 2-0 absorbable suture. The dermis is closed with a 3-0 absorbable suture, and the skin is closed with a 4-0 absorbable suture in a running subcuticular fashion. Sterile dressings and a surgical bra are applied at the conclusion of the procedure. Figure 13–1 shows the preoperative and postoperative photographs of a woman who received silicone implants through a periareolar incision.

B. Inframammary Breast Augmentation

The patient is marked preoperatively in the standing position with the arms relaxed at the sides and shoulders level. Marking begins with the IMF, chest midline, breast meridian, and the anterior axillary line. The superior border of the pocket to be dissected is marked. The incision is marked along the proposed post-augmentation IMF crease with the most medial point at the level of the nipple, extending laterally for 4.5 cm. If the incision is made above the anticipated IMF, it will show on the breast mound. If the incision is made below

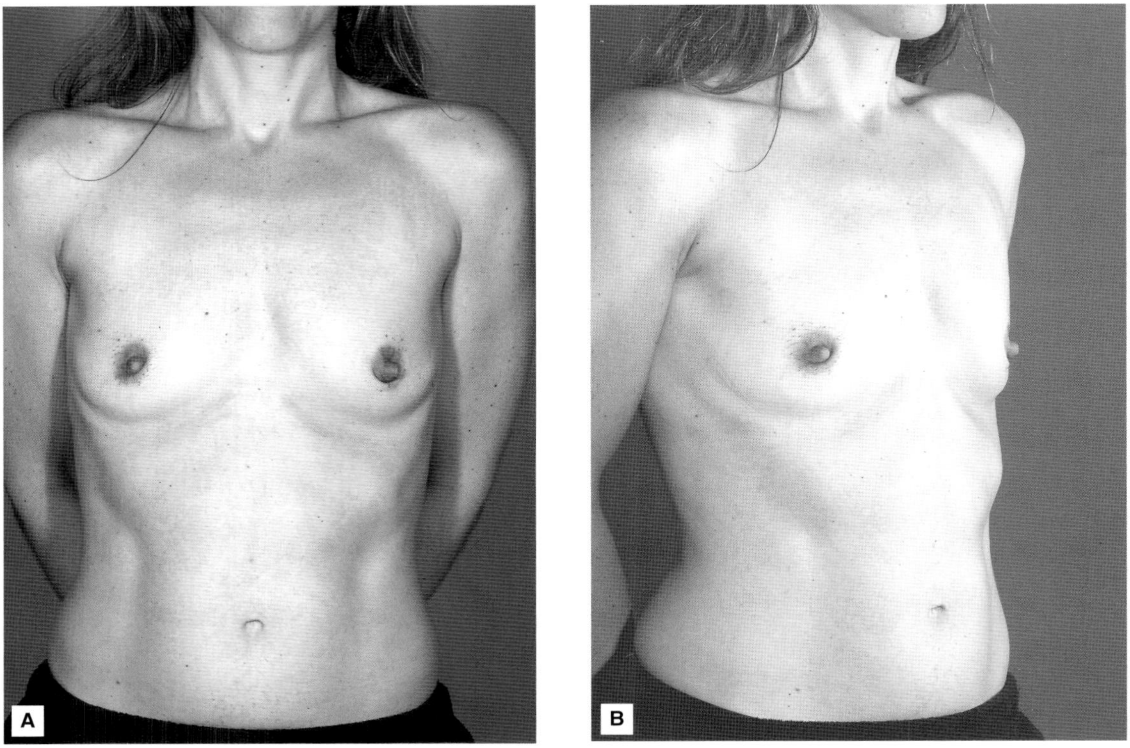

Figure 13–2. **A, B:** Preoperative photos of a 28-year-old woman with "A cup" breasts. **C, D:** Postoperative photos after placement of submuscular 194 mL silicone implants through a periareolar incision.

the anticipated IMF, it may appear on the chest wall. The IMF is marked from the point that lies on a vertical line passing through the medial border of the NAC, to a point 3–6 cm lateral to that along the fold.

After the skin incision, the skin edges are retracted with skin hooks, and a combination of electrocautery and blunt dissection is used to expose the lateral border of the pectoralis major muscle and its investing fascia. With the surgeon and assistant carefully elevating the pectoralis major with tooth forceps, a myotomy is created using the using the electrocautery instrument, ultimately exposing the undersurface of the muscle and allowing entry into the loose areolar plane between the pectoralis major and the chest wall. A combination of gentle finger dissection and electrocautery is then used to elevate the pectoralis muscle away from the chest wall thereby creating the submuscular pocket. Constant assessment of the advancement of the dissection in relation to the external anatomy and skin markings is of crucial importance to avoid crossing the chest midline or violating the IMF. Once the submuscular pocket correlates with the preoperative markings, hemostasis must be obtained using the electrocautery and insulated forceps.

An implant sizer is then placed and positioned in the pocket, and the incision is stapled temporarily. The patient is placed in the sitting position on the operating table, and any

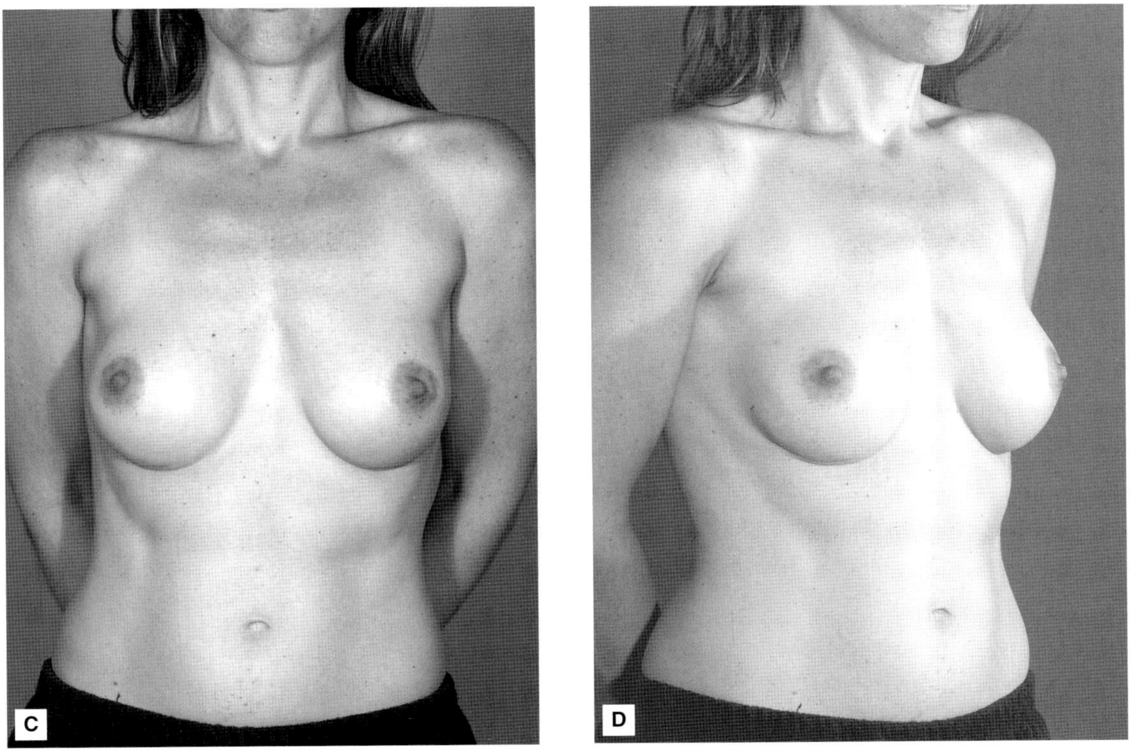

Figure 13–2. (Continued)

necessary adjustments in size or position are noted. Of note, surgical staples are *only* used in the presence of an implant sizer and *never* when final adjustments are being made with the permanent implant. The sizer is removed and replaced as many times as necessary to confirm proper implant placement relative to the pocket and preoperative markings. Once no further adjustments are necessary based on the volume and position of the sizer, the permanent implant is placed after a thorough inspection for hemostasis and copious antibiotic irrigation. The myotomy and the deep soft tissues are closed with a 2-0 absorbable suture. The dermis is closed with a 3-0 absorbable suture, and the skin is closed with a 4-0 absorbable suture in a running subcuticular fashion. Sterile dressings and a surgical bra are applied at the conclusion of the procedure. Figure 13–2 shows the preoperative and postoperative photographs of a woman who received saline implants through an inframammary incision.

C. Endoscopic Transaxillary Breast Augmentation

The patient is marked preoperatively in the standing position with the arms relaxed at the sides and shoulders level. Marking begins with the IMF, chest midline, breast meridian, and the anterior axillary line. The superior border of the pocket to be dissected is marked. The markings of the axillary incision are made with the patient's arms in 90 degrees of abduction. The surgeon then identifies the highest axillary crease above the hairline previously marked. An incision ranging from 3.0 cm to 5.0 cm is marked at the axillary crease described above. When using silicone gel implants, the incision should be large enough to enable insertion of the implant without traumatizing the tissues.

After the skin incision, the skin edges are retracted with skin hooks, and a combination of electrocautery and blunt dissection is used to expose the lateral border of the pectoralis major muscle and its investing fascia. The dissection should be limited to the anterior axillary line to avoid injury to the intercostobrachial nerve and the axillary contents (eg, brachial plexus, axillary artery, vein). The loose areolar plane between the pectoralis major and minor muscles is entered using the electrocautery instrument exposing the undersurface of the muscle. The right angle retractor and the 10-mm 30-degree endoscope are inserted under the muscle and a submuscular pocket is created under direct vision using the insulated electrocautery instrument. A low continuous suction should be applied to the endoscope to help clear the smoke and improve visualization. Constant assessment of the advancement of the dissection in relation to the external anatomy and skin markings is of crucial importance to avoid crossing the chest midline or violating the IMF. Percutaneous placement of 20-gauge needles along the IMF can facilitate its identification internally during dissection of the pocket. Once the submuscular pocket correlates with the preoperative markings, hemostasis must be obtained using the electrocautery and insulated forceps.

An implant sizer is then placed and positioned in the pocket, and the incision is stapled temporarily. The patient is placed in the sitting position on the operating table, and any necessary adjustments in size or position are noted. Of note, surgical staples are *only* used in the presence of an implant sizer and *never* when final adjustments are being made with the permanent implant. The sizer is removed and replaced as many times as necessary to confirm proper implant placement relative to the pocket and preoperative markings. Once no further adjustments are necessary based on the volume and position of the sizer, the permanent implant is placed after a thorough inspection for hemostasis and copious antibiotic irrigation.

The deep soft tissues are closed with a 2-0 absorbable suture. The dermis is closed with a 3-0 absorbable suture, and the skin is closed with a 4-0 absorbable suture in a running subcuticular fashion. Sterile dressings and a surgical bra are applied at the conclusion of the procedure.

D. Transumbilical Breast Augmentation

The patient is marked preoperatively in the standing position with the arms relaxed at the sides and shoulders level. Marking begins with the IMF, chest midline, breast meridian, and the anterior axillary line. The superior border of the pocket to be dissected is marked. The proposed incision is marked at an inconspicuous point on the superior portion of the umbilicus. Since a tunnel between the umbilical incision and the breast pockets must be created, it may be helpful to mark the skin overlying the proposed location of these subcutaneous tunnels.

After the skin incision, the soft tissues are bluntly dissected with the index finger and a blunt clamp to expose the rectus fascia. The endotube and the blunt obturator are guided in the plane just above the rectus fascia to create a subcutaneous tunnel connecting the umbilicus to each breast pocket. External palpation of the obturator with the opposite hand during advancement allows for a safe dissection. When approaching the costal margin, the obturator is carefully advanced above the lower ribs into the breast pocket.

If a subglandular augmentation is desired, the obturator is guided above the pectoralis muscle at the level of the IMF and directed cranially in the plane just above the pectoralis muscle fascia. Once the obturator has reached the level of the nipple, it is removed and the endoscope is used to confirm proper hemostasis. Next, a tissue expanding device similar to an implant sizer is inserted into the pocket, and is inflated to a volume that is approximately 1.5 times the volume of the intended permanent implant. The inflation of this device is responsible for bluntly dissecting the subglandular pocket that will house the permanent prosthesis. The permanent implant is then placed in a similar manner to the expander device. Finally, the endotube and the endoscope are guided back into the pocket under careful guidance and the pocket is inspected for proper placement, adequate hemostasis, and proper position of the implant valve.

The dermis is closed with a 3-0 absorbable suture, and the skin is closed with a 4-0 absorbable suture in a running subcuticular fashion. Sterile dressings, a surgical bra, and an abdominal binder are applied at the conclusion of the procedure.

COMPLICATIONS

As in any surgical procedure, a discussion of the potential complications with the patient is imperative. Although breast augmentation is a relatively safe procedure with a high satisfaction rate, complications do arise. The potential for bleeding, seroma formation, infection, extrusion, changes in nipple sensation, hypertrophic scars, inability to breast feed, capsular contracture, implant deflation, implant displacement, asymmetry, synmastia, implant visibility, implant rippling, galactorrhea, and superficial thrombophlebitis must all be discussed preoperatively with the patient, and the procedure should not be scheduled without clear documentation of informed consent.

Capsular contracture is the most common complication of breast augmentation. Contracture rates up to 30% have been reported. Spear et al described a clinical classification system that grades the severity of the contracture:

Grade I: The capsule is not palpable or visible, and the breast feels soft.
Grade II: The capsule is palpable but not visible.
Grade III: The capsule is palpable and visible.
Grade IV: The breast is hard, painful, and distorted.

The etiology of the capsular contracture remains elusive. Two common theories describe formation of the capsule in relation to hypertrophic scarring and subclinical infection. Stimulation of myofibroblasts is believed to occur as a reaction to a hematoma, seroma, or possible silicone bleed. The myofibroblast activation leads to scarring and formation of a capsule. Other foreign materials such as powder or lint may induce a similar reaction. Thus, all members of the operating room team must wear powder free gloves.

Subclinical infection by normal skin flora has been implicated as another possible cause of capsular contracture. The infectious process suggests that a biofilm formed on the implant surface contains the infective organism. Use of antibiotic irrigation prior to insertion of the implant may decrease this subclinical colonization.

Hematoma formation is one of the most common surgical complications (2%–3%) and is a concern until approximately 2 weeks postoperatively. The patient may complain of sudden breast swelling and pain that is usually asymmetric. This may happen spontaneously but is more common after trauma to the breast or intense physical activity that transiently increases blood pressure. Hematoma formation increases the rate of infection and subsequent capsular contracture. Hematomas should be treated as surgical emergencies, and patients should undergo exploratory surgery as soon as possible. Every attempt to identify the source of the bleed should be made, and after confirmation of hemostasis, the implant may be reinserted after copious antibiotic irrigation of the pocket.

The rate of seroma formation after augmentation is approximately 1%. Large seromas may be drained under ultrasound guidance if necessary, but the risk of infection as a result of this procedure should be carefully weighed against the potential benefits.

The rate of infection after breast augmentation is relatively low at 0.5%–2% but carries significant morbidity when it occurs. Infections can range from a mild cellulitis to deep abscesses resulting in subsequent implant extrusion. Infections usually present with symptoms of swelling, erythema, tenderness, and fever. The most common microorganism is *Staphylococcus aureus*; but *Staphylococcus epidermidis*, *Propionibacterium acnes*, and *Serratia* species, may also be causative. In an effort to prevent postoperative implant infection, standard preoperative antibiotic prophylaxis should be the norm. Every patient should receive an intravenous dose of a first- or second-generation cephalosporin 30 minutes prior to the skin incision. Clindamycin or vancomycin may be used for patients with penicillin allergies. In addition to routine antibiotic prophylaxis, careful preoperative antiseptic skin preparation, and the use of antibiotic irrigation intraoperatively are additional preventive measures that should be instituted in every case.

Changes in nipple sensation may occur in up to 10% of patients undergoing breast augmentation. The periareolar approach carries the highest risk of sensation changes, while the TUBA approach has the lowest risk. Minimizing dissection at the level of the pectoralis fascia inferomedially and inferolaterally to the NAC affords the lowest risk of trauma to the nipple's nerve supply.

Galactorrhea, an uncommon complication of augmentation mammaplasty, appears to result from injury to or irritation of the thoracic nerves. Treatment includes use of bromocriptine or intercostal blocks.

Superficial thrombophlebitis (Mondor disease) may occur in up to 2% of patients. It usually presents as a thrombosis of veins on the inferior aspect of the breast resulting in a hard cord that is tender and palpable. The condition is temporary and usually resolves over a course of several weeks with warm compresses and NSAID therapy.

Breast asymmetry due to implant displacement is always a possibility, especially when smooth, nontextured implants are used. When seen early in the postoperative period, maneuvers to correct the asymmetry, such as taping the breasts or wrapping the chest with an elastic cloth bandage, may be all that is necessary to correct the problem. However, when postoperative malpositioning is refractory to nonoperative measures, the patients should be expeditiously brought back to the operating room for formal repositioning of the implants.

For the patient with asymmetric IMFs, it is likely that one fold will need to be lowered. In lowering the IMF, it is essential that the incisions are at the same level and that the original fold is scored to provide ample room for the implant to fill the pocket. If the old IMF is not scored, the patient may be left with a double-bubble deformity.

Visible or tactile rippling of the implants is most commonly seen in subglandular augmentations where the soft tissue coverage is minimal and when larger implants are used. Slightly overfilling saline implants, using silicone implants, or using a submuscular approach may avoid this complication, especially in patients with low body fat percentages.

Deflation of saline implants has been reported to be as high as 5.5%. Underfilling the implant, chest trauma, spontaneous deflation, manufacturer defects, implant age, and the addition of antibiotics or corticosteroids to the intraluminal filler, have been implicated as possible causes.

The risk of silicone implant rupture increases with the aging of the implant. The rate of rupture is different between different types of implants and is more difficult to detect when silicone is used. The presence of rupture may by asymptomatic and undiagnosed for years. When a patient with a silicone implant notes pain, or a change in the size of the breast, an MRI should be obtained to rule out a rupture. In most cases, the rupture is intracapsular, but when left untreated, an intracapsular rupture may become extracapsular and lead to extravasation of the silicone gel. When the rupture is contained within the capsule, it may be treated by simple capsulectomy and implant removal. With extracapsular extravasation of the silicone gel, a significant granulomatous reaction may develop, which makes the implant exchange much more challenging.

OUTCOMES ASSESSMENT

A. Primary Augmentation Patients

In the Allergan Core study for primary augmentation patients, 396 (87%) of the original 455 patients had a breast measurement within 18 months of surgery. Of these 396 patients, 41% increased by one cup size; 45% increased by two cup sizes; 8% increased by more than two cup sizes; and 6% had no increase or decrease. Of the original 455 patients, 364 (80%) provided a satisfaction rating at 4 years after implantation, with 346 (95%) of these patients indicating that they were satisfied with their breast implants. For primary augmentation patients, the SF-36, which measures mental and physical health, showed a slight improvement after 4 years.

In the Mentor Core study for primary augmentation patients, 370 (67%) of the original 551 patients were included in the analysis of cup size at 3 years. Of these 370 patients, 359 (97%) experienced at least one cup size increase; the average increase in circumferential chest size was 2.8 inches. At 3 years, 456 (83%) of the 551 patients enrolled completed the patient satisfaction questionnaire. Of these 456 patients, 445 (98%) stated to their surgeon that they would have the breast implant surgery again.

B. Revision-Augmentation Patients

In the Allergan Core study, 87% of 111 revision-augmentation patients who responded to the satisfaction survey indicated that they were satisfied with their breast implants. For revision-augmentation patients, the SF-36, which measures mental and physical health, showed no significant changes in these scales after 4 years. Patient responses to questions on the Tennessee Self Concept Scale, Rosenberg Self Esteem Scale, and Body Esteem Scale regarding overall self-concept/self-esteem and body image showed no changes 4 years after receiving implants.

In the Mentor Core study for revision-augmentation patients, 116 (79%) of the original 146 patients were included in the analysis at 3 years. For these 116 patients, the average increase in circumferential chest size was 2.4 inches. At 3 years, 118 (81%) of the 146 patients enrolled answered the patient satisfaction questionnaire. Of these 118 patients, 111 (94%) stated to their surgeon that they would have the breast implant surgery again.

REFERENCES

Adams Jr WP et al. Enhancing patient outcomes in aesthetic and reconstructive breast surgery using triple antibiotic breast irrigation: six-year prospective clinical study. *Plast Reconstr Surg.* 2006 Jan;117(1):30–6. [PMID: 16404244]

Collins N et al. Ten-year review of a prospective randomized controlled trial of textured versus smooth subglandular silicone gel breast implants. *Plast Reconstr Surg.* 2000 Sep;106(4):786–91. [PMID: 11007389]

Cunningham BL et al. Saline-filled breast implant safety and efficacy: a multicenter

retrospective review. *Plast Reconstr Surg.* 2000 May;105(6):2143–9. [PMID: 10839417]
Lesavoy MA. Breast Augmentation Techniques. In: Mathes SJ, ed. *Plastic Surgery, 2nd ed. Volume VI: Trunk and Lower Extremity.* Philadelphia: Saunders; 2006:35–46.

Slavin SA, Greene AK. Augmentation Mammoplasty and Its Complications. In: Thorne CH, ed. *Grabb and Smith's Plastic Surgery, 6th ed.* Philadelphia: Lippincott Williams & Wilkins; 2007:575–84.

Spear SL et al. Classification of capsular contracture after prosthetic breast reconstruction. *Plast Reconstr Surg.* 1995 Oct;96(5):1119–23. [PMID: 7568488]

Tebbetts JB et al. Five critical decisions in breast augmentation using five measurements in 5 minutes: the high five decision support process. *Plast Reconstr Surg.* 2006 Dec;118(7 Suppl):35S–45S. [PMID: 17099482]

CHAPTER 14

Breast Reduction in Women

Peter Korn, MD, Lloyd Gayle, MD, Nicholas Vendemia, MD, & Christine Rohde, MD

According to the American Society of Aesthetic Plastic Surgeons, 153,087 women underwent breast reduction procedures in 2007, making breast reduction the fifth most common surgical procedure performed by plastic surgeons. This number reflects the high prevalence of macromastia with its associated symptoms, as well as the efficacy of breast reduction surgery to alleviate symptoms and improve physical appearance.

The etiology of macromastia is thought to be related to increased sensitivity to circulating estrogens at the level of the end-organ. Women ranging in age from puberty to old age seek consultation for breast reduction surgery. The presence of macromastia often leads to unfavorable aesthetic appearance, difficulty with clothing, social embarrassment, and decreased self-esteem. Furthermore, it is often associated with multiple somatic symptoms, such as pain and fatigue in the cervical and thoracic spine, poor posture, grooving of the skin and underlying soft tissues of the shoulders, and intertriginous rashes at the inframammary fold (IMF). It has been shown that macromastia exerts a significant impact on the patient's overall health and quality of life. Medical management focuses on weight loss, adequate support using properly fitted bras with wide straps, nonsteroidal anti-inflammatory drugs, and physical therapy. However, these measures are ineffective in satisfactorily relieving symptoms in most patients. Attempted weight loss was reported to be completely inefficient in more than half and offered partial relief in only 10% of surgical candidates. Furthermore, the presence of macromastia makes it difficult for most patients to participate in exercise programs. Breast reduction surgery has been shown to be an effective means of alleviating symptoms associated with macromastia and in improving the patient's quality of life. These benefits as well as the improvement in aesthetic appearance make breast reduction both a reconstructive and aesthetic surgical procedure.

ANATOMY

Important anatomic considerations include the blood supply, innervation, the lactiferous system as well as the aesthetic considerations regarding breast size and contour.

The breast has a rich blood supply from multiple sources, including perforating branches of the internal mammary artery, the lateral thoracic artery, the thoracodorsal artery, intercostal artery perforators, and the thoracoacromial artery. The blood supply to the nipple-areola complex (NAC) is carried through the glandular breast tissue but also receives contributions from the subdermal plexus of the breast skin. While the early, mostly dermal pedicle, designs relied on the subdermal plexus as the source for NAC perfusion, glandular contribution is now generally considered to be more robust.

The innervation of the breast is based on the underlying dermatomes. The sensation of the NAC (erogenous as well as tactile) is provided for the most part by the anterolateral and anteromedial branches of the fourth intercostal nerve with additional innervation contributed by adjacent dermatomes. Anatomic studies have shown that the fourth intercostal nerve divides into a superficial as well as a deep branch, the latter being situated on top of the pectoralis fascia and reaching the NAC through the breast parenchyma. This explains why nipple sensation can be preserved with a variety of pedicle designs.

The lactiferous ducts of the breast parenchyma consist of 15–25 ducts that converge from the periphery toward the nipple. Thus, any undermining of the NAC is associated with significant disruption of the lactiferous system and reduced ability to breastfeed.

The ideal breast size and contour has been a matter of debate. While the patient's individual body habitus and desire regarding breast size needs to be taken into account, some general guidelines are well established. Most studies on breast aesthetics focus on ideal position of the nipple-areola. Penn quantitatively defined the position in "aesthetically perfect" breasts using an equilateral triangle with 21 cm-long limbs between the suprasternal notch and nipples as well as between the nipples; the average nipple-to-IMF distance was 6.9 cm. While these measurements are generally used as a good starting point, adjustments need to be made based on individual patient and the technique of breast reduction used. For instance the nipple-to-IMF distance often needs to be longer than 7 cm to accommodate a more projecting breast, such as in a vertical breast reduction.

PATIENT EVALUATION & SELECTION

Evaluation of the patient focuses on the degree of macromastia (the patient's cup size), its effect on appearance, as well as its associated symptoms and their effect on the patient's quality of life. The signs and symptoms associated with macromastia need to be confirmed, correlated with the degree of macromastia, and well documented. Confounding comorbidities, such as cervical radiculopathy, need to be excluded. Other important aspects with respect to breast procedures include an obstetric history, lactation and nursing history, future pregnancy and nursing plans, breast size over the last several years, any family or personal history of breast cancer, as well as breast cancer screening history. The general history focuses on risk factors for an elective surgical procedure, such as advanced age, obesity, medical comorbidities, or a smoking history.

The degree of macromastia is assessed, and the weight to be reduced on each side is estimated. The breast size as well as the desired amount of reduction is commonly expressed in cup sizes. However, it needs to be taken into account that cup sizes are poorly standardized, and that many women wear bras that are poorly matched to their breast size. As a general guideline, it has been estimated that in an average sized woman (chest girth 36–38 inches) 200 g of tissue resected corresponds to a reduction by one cup size. This estimate varies, however, proportional to the patient's chest girth.

The degree of ptosis is documented according to Regnault. Standard preoperative measurements of the breasts are obtained with the patient in the upright position. The distances from the suprasternal notch to nipple as well as nipple to IMF are crucially important as a guide in selecting the appropriate technique. While the presence of mild to moderate elongation in these distances allows the use of a vertical resection pattern, a more extensive elongation usually suggests the addition of a horizontal skin resection component. If the nipple position is well below the level of the IMF, consideration should be given to use a purely horizontal skin resection pattern.

The skin quality is assessed with focus on skin elasticity, the presence of stretch marks as well as the presence of intertrigo. The integrity of nipple sensation needs to be assessed, since it is commonly reduced in patients with marked macromastia and ptosis. The presence of shoulder bra strap grooving is assessed and documented. Furthermore, the presence of any breast masses and scars from previous breast surgery needs to be evaluated. Standardized multiple view preoperative photographs are obtained for insurance approval and documentation.

PATIENT PREPARATION

Preoperative counseling should cover the following points: the expected scar appearance and the possibility of unfavorable scarring; the expected breast shape and any temporary postoperative irregularities; the possibility of reduced or lost postoperative lactation potential or nipple sensation, as well as the chance of partial or complete nipple loss. Especially with vertical scar breast reductions, the patient should be prepared for an unnatural appearance during the early postoperative period that may require some time to resolve. Representative early and late postoperative photographs are helpful to ensure the patient's understanding. Presurgical markings on the patient, performed at the time of consultation, are often useful to facilitate patient understanding of planned surgical incisions and the resulting scars. The preoperative discussion of the operative goals and expectations needs to demonstrate a reasonable consensus between the surgeon and patient.

Standard preoperative laboratory studies are obtained as indicated for patient age and comorbidities. A preoperative mammogram obtained within 1 year of the anticipated date of surgery is mandatory for patients aged 35 years and older. Any patient with first-degree relatives with breast cancer should be asked about the age at which their relatives were diagnosed with breast cancer, and appropriate early screening mammograms should be performed.

On the day of surgery, the skin markings are done with the patient in the standing position. The standard markings include the midline of the anterior chest, the IMFs, the breast meridians, and the desired position of the NAC. The breast meridians are marked along a line crossing the clavicles at 6–8 cm lateral to the suprasternal notch and going through the center of the breast mound as well as through the IMF. In most patients, this line transverses the nipple; however, care must be taken not to use the nipple as a guideline in patients with abnormally deviated nipple positions. The new desired nipple position is then marked along the breast meridian, most commonly at the level of the anterior projection of the IMF (Pitanguy's point) or slightly above. In most patients, the point is at about 21 cm from the suprasternal notch. In patients with heavy ptotic breasts, this point should be marked 1–3 cm lower to compensate for the anticipated upward movement once the skin is relieved from the excess weight. In patients with good upper-pole fullness, the new nipple position can be placed slightly higher; however, in patients with a convex upper pole with little fullness, care must be taken not to place the nipple too high on the anticipated new breast mound.

The markings of the skin resection pattern can be done either freehanded or using a template and will be discussed with the individual techniques. Skin resection is most commonly performed in a Wise pattern or a vertical excision. The areolar opening can either be marked in a keyhole pattern as part of the initial markings (Wise pattern), or marked at the end of the procedure after closure of the vertical and horizontal skin excisions (modified Wise pattern). A purely horizontal resection resulting in a scar along the IMF can be done if the NAC is situated well below the IMF due to ptosis of the breast.

The patient is positioned supine on the operating table with the arms extended and secured on arm-boards. Care is taken to assure symmetric positioning. The procedure is usually performed under general anesthesia. A dose of an intravenous antibiotic (commonly a first-generation cephalosporin) should be administered 30 minutes prior to the surgical incision.

TECHNIQUE

The following general principles and operative steps apply to all techniques of breast reductions. Xylocaine 0.5% with epinephrine 1:200,000 may be infiltrated along the incisions and planed dissection. If a significant amount of suction-assisted lipectomy is anticipated, 1 L of tumescent fluid is infiltrated (500 mL per side), with most of the fluid infiltrated laterally on the chest wall.

The skin is incised along the preoperative markings. The use of a commercially available breast tourniquet or a rolled gauze designed tourniquet may assist the following steps. The NAC is marked and incised in a circular fashion using a 42–45 mm diameter with the skin under minimal stretch. Next, the dermoglandular pedicle is deepithelialized using a blade, scissor, electrocautery, or laser. The parenchymal dissection is commonly done using the electrocautery. Care is taken not to undermine the pedicle. The skin and parenchymal resection is performed next. Exposure of the pectoralis fascia and underlying muscle should be avoided so that the risks of compromising nipple sensation and creating postoperative pain control issues are minimized. The volume of breast tissue resected is weighed to assist in achieving a symmetric result. Furthermore, the final weight provides data to the insurance companies. Suction-assisted lipectomy may be used to improve the final contour, especially to address any residual fullness over the lateral chest wall. After hemostasis is obtained and the wounds are irrigated, the incisions are temporarily closed to ensure an adequate volume, shape, and symmetry. For the inspection of the preliminary result, the patient is often placed in a sitting position. When placing stitches into the breast parenchyma, it is important to take small bites of fibrous tissue that can be tied down loosely to avoid tissue necrosis. The skin is closed with buried deep dermal sutures and then a subcuticular suture. Placing closed suction drains is always an option, but no statistically significant advantage has been demonstrated. Incisions are dressed with steri-strips, and a surgical brassiere is commonly used for patient comfort. After confirming the viability of the NAC postoperatively, most patients are discharged the day of or morning after surgery. Patients are instructed to shower starting the day after surgery and carefully pat the tape dry. Patients are advised to use the surgical brassiere or a sports bra continuously for 6 weeks.

A. Choosing the Pedicle Design and Skin Resection Pattern

A variety of breast reduction techniques have been used historically and are still in use based on the surgeon's preferences and individual patient's anatomic considerations. The key elements that define each procedure are the skin-resection pattern, the pedicle design, and

TABLE 14–1. POTENTIAL PATTERNS OF SKIN RESECTION BASED ON THE CHOSEN TISSUE PEDICLE

Tissue Pedicle	Possible Skin Resection Patterns
Inferior pedicle	Wise pattern/Horizontal scar only
Medial pedicle	Wise pattern/Vertical scar only
Superior pedicle	Wise pattern/Vertical scar only
Superomedial pedicle	Wise pattern/Vertical scar only/Horizontal scar only
Superolateral pedicle	Wise pattern/Vertical scar only/Horizontal scar only
Central mound	Wise pattern/Vertical scar only/Horizontal scar only
Liposuction reduction	No skin excised

the parenchymal-resection pattern. To tailor the technique of breast reduction to the individual patient's needs, it is best to consider the pedicle design/parenchymal-resection pattern as well as the skin-resection pattern as separate components. While some pedicle designs and parenchymal-resection patterns suggest a specific skin resection pattern, a wide spectrum of possible combinations can be used to accommodate individual preoperative findings (Table 14–1).

The appropriate skin resection pattern is determined by the amount of preoperative skin excess. Patients with significant ptosis and excessive breast skin in the vertical and horizontal dimension are best approached with the Wise pattern (Figures 14–1 through 14–4). In patients with less pronounced skin excess, the length of the horizontal limb can be limited to spare the medial and lateral pole of the IMF. A vertical scar technique (Figures 14–5 through 14–8) is best suited for patients with mild to moderate ptosis and decent skin elasticity. In this case, the remaining vertical skin redundancy can be addressed by gathering the skin during closure of the vertical scar, raising the IMF, allowing for more projection, and excising a slightly larger areolar opening. Even though many surgeons use vertical scar techniques preferentially in patients requiring mild to moderate reductions, there is no true limitation in terms of weight reduction.

A horizontal scar technique can be used in patients with significant vertical skin excess/ptosis. In order to use this technique, the projected new nipple position must be at least 7 cm above the superior border of the areola, so that the inferior border of the skin flap remains above the pigmented areola skin. The remaining horizontal redundancy is addressed during closure of the inframammary incision by gathering the superior flap skin, especially in the area of breast meridian. Some pleating of the redundant skin typically resolves early postoperatively. More extensive horizontal skin excess, however, is better addressed using the Wise pattern.

Suction-assisted lipectomy is commonly used as an adjunct to excisional techniques for final contouring. This is especially useful to reduce any excess subcutaneous fat lateral to the breast. The use of liposuction alone without an excisional procedure has been used successfully for reduction mammaplasty in selected patients with mostly fatty breast hypertrophy. Appropriate candidates include patients with mild to moderate breast hypertrophy in the absence of significant skin excess and ptosis, including adolescent patients with developmental unilateral breast hypertrophy. Even though the volume reduction may accentuate breast ptosis, this is usually compensated for by liposuction-induced scarring and skin tightening as well as by the

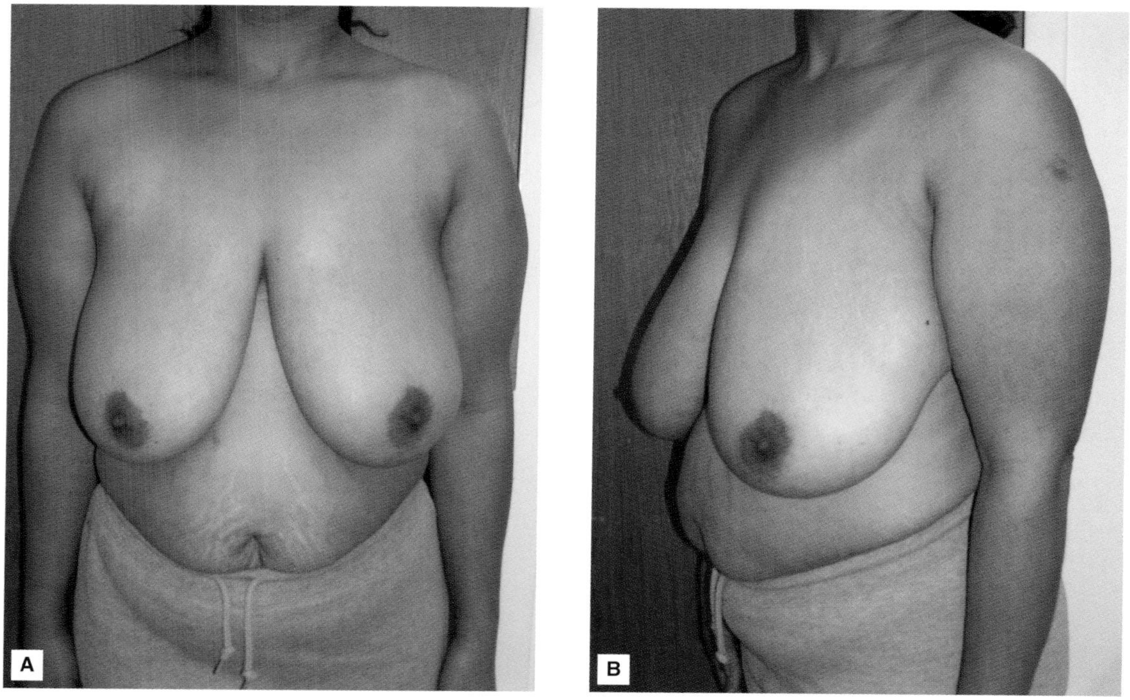

Figure 14–1. Patient is a candidate for Wise pattern skin resection due to the moderate ptosis with skin excess in both the horizontal and vertical dimensions. **A:** Anterior view. **B:** Lateral view.

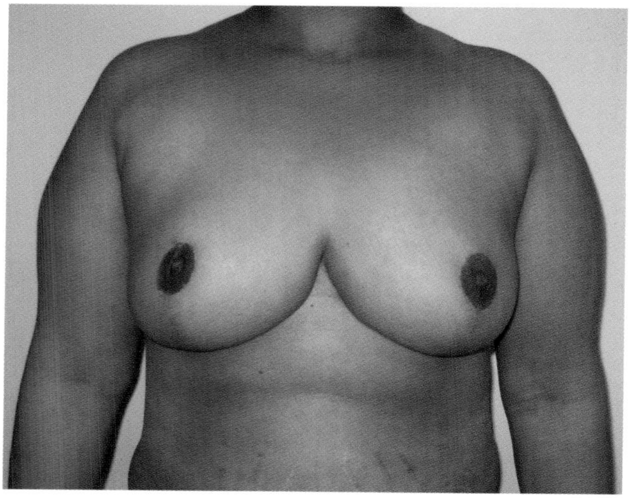

Figure 14–2. Postoperative view after Wise pattern skin resection, inferior pedicle reduction (1175 g resected from the left breast, 1120 g from the right breast). Note that the skin excess has been corrected in both the vertical and horizontal dimensions compared with the preoperative pictures shown in Figure 14–1.

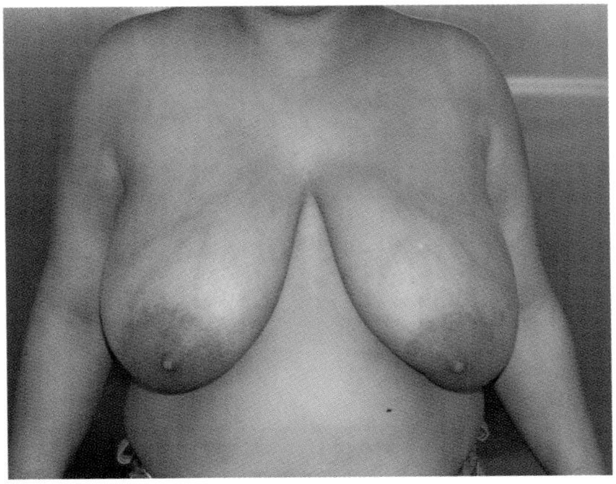

Figure 14–3. Patient is a candidate for the Wise pattern skin resection due to moderate to severe degree of ptosis, and poor skin elasticity with skin excess in both horizontal and vertical dimensions.

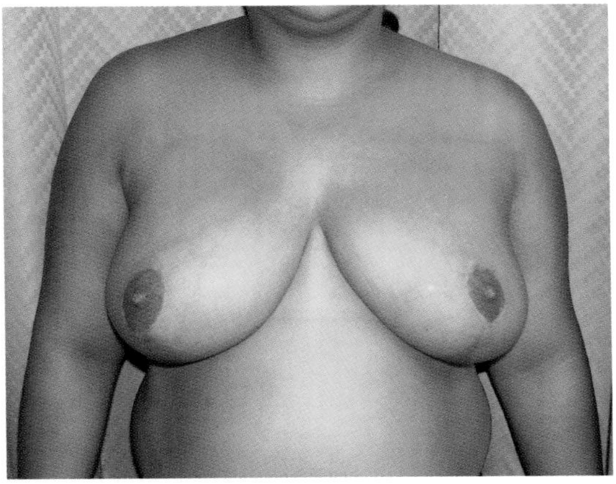

Figure 14–4. Postoperative view after Wise pattern skin resection, inferior pedicle reduction (645 g resected from the left breast, 540 g from the right breast).

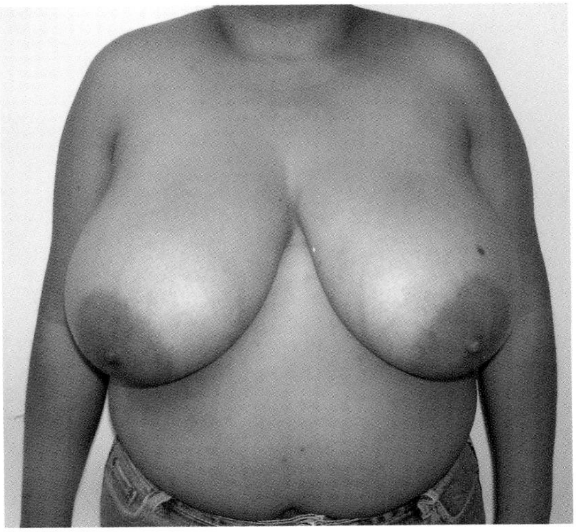

Figure 14–5. Patient is a candidate for vertical pattern skin resection due to moderate ptosis with good skin elasticity and skin excess mainly in the horizontal dimension. Excess skin in the vertical dimension can be addressed by gathering during wound closure.

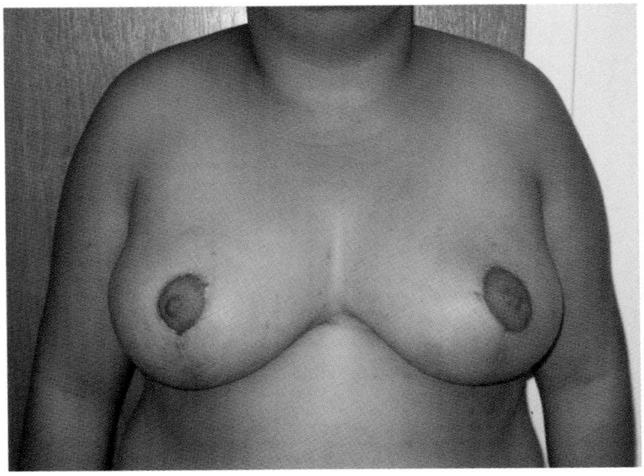

Figure 14–6. Postoperative view after vertical pattern skin resection, medial pedicle reduction (1000 g resected from left breast, 1015 g from the right breast). The majority of the skin resection has taken place in the horizontal dimension of the breast, and the vertical skin excess was gathered during wound closure.

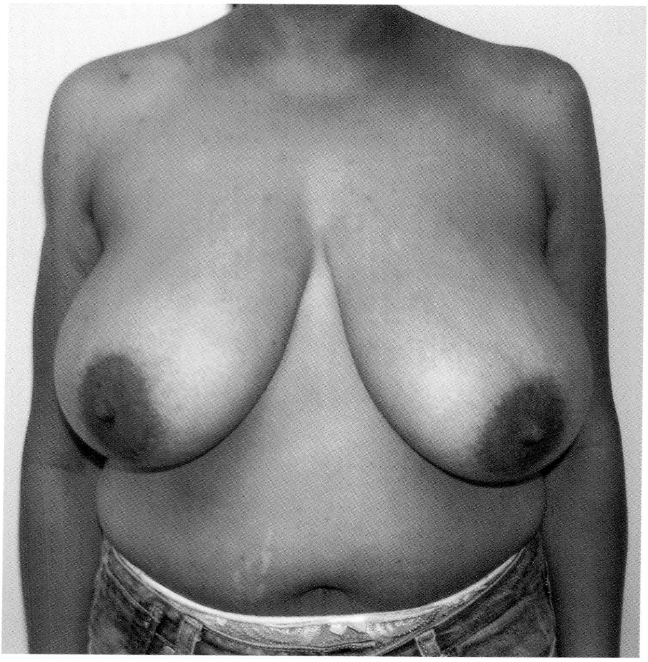

Figure 14–7. Patient is a candidate for vertical pattern skin resection. Note the moderate degree of ptosis with relatively good skin elasticity.

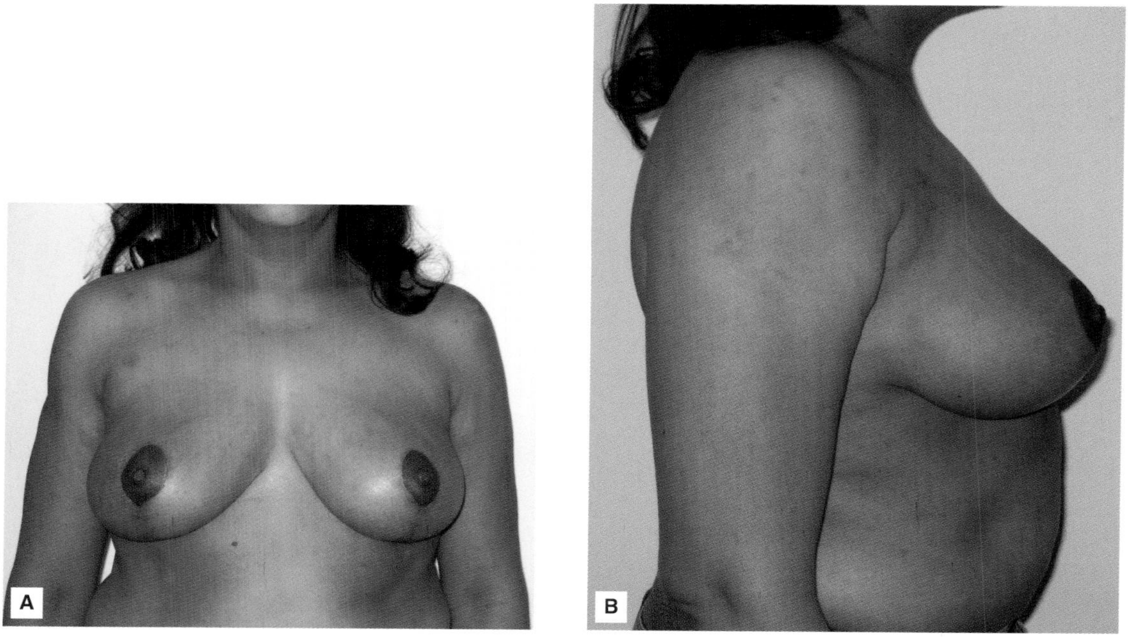

Figure 14–8. A: Postoperative anterior view after vertical pattern skin resection, medial pedicle reduction (480 g resected from left breast, 410 g from the right breast). **B:** Postoperative lateral view after vertical pattern skin resection, medial pedicle reduction.

decrease in breast weight, limiting the gravitational pull on the breast, thereby elevating the NAC. Furthermore, in patients with significant comorbidities and potential wound healing problems, a minimally invasive reduction of excess breast weight using liposuction may be preferable to an excisional procedure. This may offer particular advantages in the patient with a known tendency to keloid scarring, which would preclude a satisfactory aesthetic outcome with traditional skin incisions.

B. Inferior Pedicle/Wise Pattern Technique

The inferior pedicle technique has been proven to be safe and easily reproducible in a wide variety of breast sizes, and remains the most frequently used technique. The skin resection is typically based on a Wise pattern, resulting in an inverted T closure. The vertical limb is kept short (4.5–6.5 cm) to minimize the development of postoperative pseudoptosis. The combined length of the horizontal limb on the upper skin flaps should be equal to or greater than the incision along the IMF to allow for closure around the volume of the breast tissue. The NAC is carried on an inferiorly based dermoglandular pedicle, the base of which is 8–10 cm wide and centered around the meridian.

Circumscribing the NAC using a 42–45 mm diameter cookie cutter under moderate skin stretch commences the procedure. Next, the outline of the inferior pedicle is incised and the skin overlying the pedicle is deepithelialized. The dermoglandular wedge-shaped pedicle is then created by carrying medial and lateral incisions down toward the chest wall taking care not to undermine the pedicle. The incisions of the Wise-pattern are then completed. The excess skin and breast tissue medially, laterally, and superiorly is then excised. Most of the volume should be reduced laterally in order to maintain an aesthetically pleasing shape with medial and upper pole fullness.

C. Medial or Superomedial Pedicle/Vertical Scar Technique

The vertical scar technique as described by Lejour and Hall-Findley has gained increasing popularity. It refers to a skin and parenchymal resection pattern based on a vertical ellipse. Closure is achieved by approximating medial and lateral parenchymal pillars that support the breast shape and minimize the tension on the skin closure. The medial (or superomedial) pedicle is the pedicle of choice, as it rotates easily into position and facilitates adequate lateral breast resection; furthermore, it has a reliable blood supply and postoperative nipple sensation has been described to be as good as other pedicle designs.

The initial skin markings are similar to the Wise pattern, excluding the medial and lateral horizontal lines. The nipple should be placed at the anterior projection of the IMF, oftentimes higher than with a Wise pattern because there is less "bottoming out" expected over time. The areolar opening is marked more in a mosque-dome shape rather than circular. The medial and lateral vertical lines are then marked as a continuation of the breast meridian while the breast is manually displaced laterally and medially, respectively. The lines are joined together, staying 2–4 cm above the level of the IMF, which is commonly raised 1–2 cm after the reduction.

The medial pedicle is designed to originate from the areolar opening with its upper half and from the medial vertical margin with its lower half. This allows easy rotation of the pedicle into the areolar opening. The width of the pedicle base measures 6–10 cm, depending on the size of the reduction and the pedicle length.

The procedure is commenced circumscribing the areola and deepithelializing the pedicle, which is then dissected toward the chest wall with minimal undermining. Even a full thickness medial pedicle is mobile and easily rotates into position. The skin resection follows the preoperatively marked vertical ellipse. Since the remaining breast parenchyma, rather than the skin, holds the shape, it is important not to take too much skin and thus to avoid horizontal skin tension that impedes projection. The areolar opening can either be excised initially along with the elliptical skin excision, or alternatively can be marked and excised after the completion of the reduction and closure of the vertical excision.

The parenchymal resection is carried out by beveling outward, especially laterally and inferiorly. Visualizing the Wise pattern during the parenchymal resection is a good guide for mentally outlining the tissue that must be resected. The vertical incision length corresponds to the vertical pillar height. For an average C cup, it is important to leave behind a lateral pillar of parenchyma that measures about 7 cm. The inferior border of the medial pedicle becomes the medial pillar. The flap at the margins should be at least 1 cm thick, and beveling is performed as needed to resect the necessary breast tissue. Thinning out the flap just superior to the IMF allows the fold to rise and minimizes puckering of redundant skin in this area. However, care must be taken not to make the skin flap too thin, which may result in a scar contracted to the chest wall. The medial and lateral pillars of breast tissue are then sutured together with a few interrupted 2-0 or 3-0 absorbable sutures. This shaping causes coning of the breast tissue, and increases projection as desired. Suction-assisted lipectomy can be used after a preliminary closure to improve the contour of the IMF. Any remaining fullness or asymmetry can also be addressed this way especially along the lateral chest wall and the preaxillary areas as needed.

During skin closure, the discrepancy between the redundant length of the vertical skin edges and the desired areola to IMF distance needs to be addressed. Skin gathering is avoided superiorly, and only a minimal amount of skin is gathered inferiorly. If the skin is of poor quality or substantially redundant, it can be removed as a short inverted T. For more significant vertical skin excess a full (modified) Wise pattern skin excision can be used. Such a combination of a medial pedicle technique together with the Wise pattern skin excision has gained increasing popularity as an alternative for the inferior pedicle technique for larger breast reductions (Figure 14–9).

D. Central Mound Technique

The central mound technique popularized by Balch and Hester refers to a technique that bases the NAC on the underlying parenchyma rather than on a dermal or dermoglandular pedicle. The parenchymal reduction is then achieved by tangential resection of the more superficial

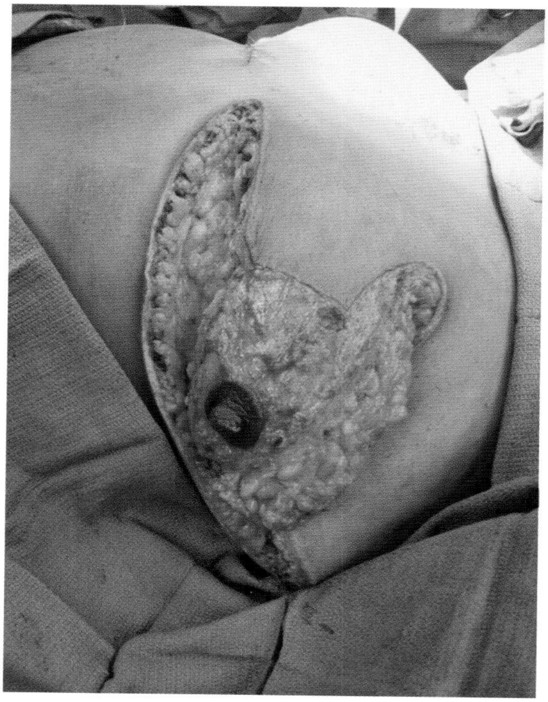

Figure 14–9. Intraoperative view of a Wise pattern medial tissue pedicle breast reduction.

layers of the breast mound. The skin resection is most commonly based on a Wise pattern; however, since the nipple transposition and parenchymal reduction is totally independent from the overlying skin flap, any design of skin resection is technically possible. This allows addressing a wide variety of breast sizes and shapes, making the central mound technique the "breast reduction for all seasons."

The areola is circumscribed and a rim of surrounding dermis is deepithelialized. Leaving deepithelialized dermis on the entire lower pole of the central mound is optional but is often done unless a large volume reduction is performed. The medial and lateral skin flaps are then raised at 1–1.5 cm thickness and the plane carried superiorly to the level of the clavicle. Care must be taken to proceed with the dissection in a smooth plane between the subcutaneous tissue and breast parenchyma. Eventually, the entire breast mound is freed from the overlying skin envelope. Next, the breast mound is reduced and shaped by resecting excess breast tissue in a circumferential tangential fashion using the electrocautery. For accurate shaping, it is critical to maintain the NAC in its desired position at all times. After the desired volume is achieved, the shape of the mound is stabilized with several absorbable parenchymal stitches. In general, several stitches are placed into the peripheral breast tissue with a medial and superior vector to support the tissue against gravity without distorting the desired shape. Once a well-shaped central mound is obtained, skin closure is achieved in standard fashion. The areolar opening is excised using a small diameter (eg, 38 mm) and the NAC inset.

E. Free Nipple Graft

The classic free micrograph breast reduction uses a straightforward amputation of the ptotic inferior breast tissue, usually combined with a Wise pattern skin closure. The NAC is transferred to its desired position as a full thickness skin graft. The major drawback of this technique relates to the universally observed loss of pigment, loss of projection, and loss of sensation in the NAC. However, a free nipple graft may be the primary technique of choice in patients with massive macromastia and ptosis, when the benefits of minimizing the amount of dissection, decreasing operating time and achieving predictable nipple take outweigh the disadvantages associated with a nipple graft. Furthermore, a free nipple graft as a secondary procedure can be used to salvage the NAC compromised by an ischemic pedicle.

The NAC is harvested at the beginning of the procedure and thinned by trimming any excess subdermal and deep dermal tissue. The parenchymal reduction is done by amputation of the lower breast tissue and excess skin is resected using the Wise pattern or horizontal resection pattern. The incisions are then closed and the areola graft bed prepared at the desired location by deepithelialization. After the NAC is grafted, a bolster dressing is applied to optimize take.

F. Liposuction Reduction Mammaplasty

Liposuction reduction mammaplasty in the female breast should be done using traditional liposuction technique. Ultrasound-assisted liposuction should be undertaken with caution in the female breast because of concerns regarding the unknown long-term sequelae associated with ultrasound-induced parenchymal injury and scarring with subsequent mammographic changes.

A stab incision is made just above the lateral aspect of the IMF with an optional second incision above the medial aspect of the IMF. Generally the incisions and aspiration should be designed to preserve the option of a pedicle reduction in case of inadequate results after the liposuction. Standard tumescent solution is infiltrated using 500–1500 mL of infiltrate per side. Ten minutes should be allowed for appropriate vasoconstriction before starting the procedure. Blunt-tipped 3–4 mm multihole cannulas are then used for pretunneling as well as for lipoaspiration proceeding with fan-shaped movements from the deep plane to more superficial levels. Terminate the suction when the target volume of aspirate is reached or an unacceptably bloody aspirate is obtained. The addition of superficial undermining of the skin in the superiomedial and lateral areas using a blunt 3-mm cannula not on suction may help stimulate skin retraction to correct ptosis. No wound closure is performed to allow some egress of fluid, and the breasts are then molded and dressed using elastic foam tape.

COMPLICATIONS

Analysis of the BRAVO study showed an overall complication rate of 43% (77 of 179 patients), most of which were minor. The most common complication was delayed wound healing (21.6%). Other complications included spitting sutures, hematoma, nipple necrosis, hypertrophic scars, fat necrosis, seroma, and infection. Increased resection weight correlated with increased risk. However, the presence of complications had no negative impact on the beneficial effects on preoperative symptoms.

Wound dehiscence and delayed healing typically affect the point where the vertical and horizontal suture lines meet. This can be prevented by leaving an additional margin of deepithelialized skin along the margin of the flaps. Furthermore, during closure of the horizontal suture line, the flaps should be advanced toward the vertical suture line to eliminate any tension.

The risk of nipple loss is a concern when long pedicles are designed in patients with large volume reduction (eg, an inferior pedicle greater than 20 cm). In such patients, consideration should be given to using a central mound technique, which theoretically optimizes nipple blood supply, or to use a free nipple graft. If a compromised nipple is encountered intraoperatively or postoperatively, the procedure should be converted to a free nipple graft.

Loss of nipple sensation occurs in about 10%–15% of patients of the breast reduction as a result of disrupting the continuity of the fourth and adjacent intercostals nerves to the nipple. Limiting the depth of resection to leave some breast tissue over the pectoralis fascia and limiting undermining of the pedicle may help protect nipple innervations. Likewise, using the central mound technique adheres to these principles and minimizes the incidence of loss of sensation.

Studies comparing common dermoglandular pedicle designs showed limited impact of the pedicle origin on nipple sensation. More than 85% of patients after vertical reduction with medial pedicle recover sensation close to preoperative levels.

The ability to breastfeed may be affected by breast reduction surgery, but it is difficult to determine the validity of such conclusions. The patient's choice and ability to breastfeed is influenced by multiple physical as well as psychological factors. Women who had breast reduction surgery commonly chose not to breastfeed independent of their physiologic ability to do so, making it more difficult to assess the physiologic impact of the procedure. One study compared breastfeeding success in women who had undergone breast reduction surgery with women in a control group; results showed that 21% and 4% of women in the breast reduction surgery group were successful at 1 and 4 months respectively, compared with 70% and 22% of women in the control group.

OUTCOME ASSESSMENT

Assessing the outcome after breast reduction must include aesthetic considerations and quality of life aspects. The latter were evaluated prospectively in the BRAVO study. In this study, symptoms related to macromastia (such as pain and decreased overall health status) were substantially improved by breast reduction. Likewise, quality of life scores and the ability to engage in physical activity were significantly improved. An important finding is that the benefits from breast reduction were not associated with body weight, bra cup size, or weight of resection, with essentially all patients benefiting from surgery.

Aesthetic considerations focus on the breast shape, projection, as well as scarring. As the Wise pattern addresses both vertical and horizontal skin redundancy it allows for the greatest flexibility in shaping and redraping the skin envelope. Compared with the vertical scar or horizontal scar techniques, it provides a more predictable and instantaneous contour at the expense of a larger scar. Conversely, the benefit of omitting the horizontal or vertical scar is associated with increased puckering and irregularities of redundant skin along the suture line, especially in patients with significant skin excess. These irregularities typically resolve over 3 weeks to 6 months postoperatively. However, a secondary procedure to address more significant redundancy that does not result postoperatively is needed in 10%–20% of patients after purely vertical breast reduction.

The amount and quality of scars on the breasts is a major concern in patients undergoing reduction mammaplasty. In general, the scars heal well around the NAC. The vertical scar rarely hypertrophies, but it is the most visible and least accepted scar according to patient surveys. The inframammary incision not uncommonly shows some thickening of the scar, particularly in the medial portion.

The shape after breast reduction is highly dependent on the technique. In general, the inferior pedicle breast reduction tends to result in a boxier shaped breast, whereas the vertical scar technique often results in a temporarily unnatural appearing cone-shaped breast with exaggerated projection. A major long-term issue of the breast reduction is the development of pseudoptosis or "bottoming out." This is a significant problem seen, in particular, after inferior pedicle reductions, where the shape of the inferior pole relies on the strength of the skin supporting the weight of pedicle. Longer term results of vertical breast reductions, however, demonstrated improved shape and decreased incidence of pseudoptosis compared with inferior pedicle reductions. Improved projection occurs because the parenchyma resection is performed through a vertical ellipse; approximating the lateral and medial parenchymal pillars with parenchymal stitches cones the breast and supports the shape. The central mound technique also adheres to the principal to provide parenchymal support for the breast shape, rather than relying on the skin envelope. The intraoperative shaping of the central mound provides the surgeon with maximal control and flexibility over the immediate postoperative breast shape. Ultimately, the choice of technique is determined largely by the surgeon's preference and experience, with most surgeons using one or two techniques with good outcomes and high patient satisfaction in most patients. However, including a greater variety of techniques allows the surgeon to account for the large heterogeneity in breast sizes and shapes and to tailor the breast reduction to the individual patient.

REFERENCES

American Society of Aesthetic Plastic Surgeons. http://www.cosmeticplasticsurgerystatistics.com/statistics.html#2007-NEWS. Accessed July 29, 2009.

Balch CR. The central mound technique for reduction mammaplasty. *Plast Reconstr Surg.* 1981 Mar;67(3):305–11. [PMID: 7232563]

Collins ED et al. The effectiveness of surgical and nonsurgical interventions in relieving the symptoms of macromastia. *Plast Reconstr Surg.* 2002 Apr 15;109(5):1556–66. [PMID: 11932597]

Courtiss EH et al. Reduction mammaplasty by the inferior pedicle technique. An alternative to free nipple and areola grafting for severe macromastia or extreme ptosis. *Plast Reconstr Surg.* 1977 Apr;59(4):500–7. [PMID: 847026]

Cunningham BL et al. Analysis of breast reduction complications derived from the BRAVO study. *Plast Reconstr Surg.* 2005 May;115(6):1597–604. [PMID: 15861063]

Gonzalez F et al. Reduction mammaplasty improves symptoms of macromastia. *Plast Reconstr Surg.* 1993 Jun;91(7):1270–6. [PMID: 8497527]

Hall-Findlay EJ. Vertical breast reduction. In: Shenaq SM, Spear SL, Davison SP, eds. New Trends in Reduction and Mastopexy, Seminars in Plastic Surgery. 2004;18:211–24.

Hester TR Jr et al. Breast reduction utilizing the maximally vascularized central breast pedicle. *Plast Reconstr Surg.* 1985 Dec;76(6):890–900. [PMID: 4070458]

Lejour M. *Vertical Mammaplasty and Liposuction.* St. Louis, MO: Quality Medical Publishing; 1994.

Penn J. Breast reduction. *Br J Plast Surg.* 1955 Jan;7(4):357–71. [PMID: 13230442]

Regnault P. Breast ptosis. Definition and treatment. *Clin Plast Surg.* 1976 Apr;3(2):193–203. [PMID: 1261176]

Reus WF et al. Preservation of projection after reduction mammaplasty: long-term follow-up of the inferior pedicle technique. *Plast Reconstr Surg.* 1988 Oct;82(4):644–52. [PMID: 3420186]

Robbins TH. A reduction mammaplasty with the areola-nipple based on an inferior dermal pedicle. *Plast Reconstr Surg.* 1977 Jan;59(1):64–7. [PMID: 831241]

Wise RJ. A preliminary report on a method of planning the mammaplasty. *Plast Reconstr Surg.* 1956 May;17(5):367–75. [PMID: 13335513]

Yousif NJ et al. Elimination of the vertical scar in reduction mammaplasty. *Plast Reconstr Surg.* 1992 Mar;89(3):459–67. [PMID: 1741469]

CHAPTER 15

Breast Lift

Katherine Heiden, MD, Tal T. Roudner, MD, & Jason A. Spector, MD

Mastopexy is a cosmetic surgical procedure designed to improve the appearance of ptotic, or "sagging" breasts. Although a wide variety of techniques are available, the choice of which one to use depends primarily on the severity of ptosis. In essence, a mastopexy is a reduction of the excessive breast skin envelope without significant parenchymal resection. As such, approaches to mastopexy have often mirrored those of reduction mammoplasty. Similar to breast reduction, current approaches to mastopexy emphasize smaller incisions that result in less scarring.

In properly selected patients, mastopexy can produce aesthetically excellent results with a high degree of patient satisfaction.

ANATOMY

The female breast lies along the anterior chest wall extending from the second through the seventh ribs and from the sternal edge to the mid axillary line. It derives its blood supply from multiple sources: internal mammary artery perforators, the lateral thoracic artery (originating from the axillary artery), the thoracodorsal and thoracoacromial arteries, as well as perforators from the third through fifth intercostal arteries. These arteries form a rich collateral circulation that supplies the breast parenchyma, overlying skin, and the nipple areola complex (NAC). Venous drainage follows the arterial supply, namely via the axillary vein, internal mammary vein, and the intercostal veins. Lymphatic drainage of the breast is mainly via an extensive axillary lymph node basin and, to a lesser extent, via the internal mammary lymph nodes located along the course of the internal mammary vessels.

Sensory innervation to the breast comes from the second through the seventh intercostal nerves as well as the cervical plexus. The medial breast and overlying skin is supplied by the anterior cutaneous branches of the second through the seventh intercostal nerves, while the lateral breast and overlying skin receives innervation from the lateral cutaneous branches of the second through the seventh intercostal nerves. Innervation of the nipple is thought to be largely via the lateral cutaneous branch of the fourth intercostal nerve, with lesser contributions from proximate intercostals branches.

Within an individual's lifetime, the size, shape, and contour of the breast changes with age, weight gain or loss, and after pregnancy. In the middle of the last century, Penn attempted to define the dimensions of the "aesthetically perfect" breast by recording measurements of 150 women. Penn found that the sternal notch to nipple distance averaged 21 cm, while the average nipple to inframammary fold (IMF) distance was 6.9 cm. This study, however, suffered from an extremely limited and homogenous sample size. Although often cited, this study is mostly of historic interest, since the breast metrics described in that study are not commonly seen in the contemporary population. Ultimately, the 'desired' size of the breast depends on an individual's size and body habitus. Most plastic surgeons agree that a NAC diameter of 4 cm is aesthetically pleasing while the appropriately positioned nipple lies anterior to the level of the IMF.

PATIENT EVALUATION & SELECTION

The universal complaint among women seeking a mastopexy is sagging or deflated breasts. Most women seeking mastopexy have a relative deficiency of breast tissue in relationship to their breast skin envelope. In large-breasted women, the ptosis is exacerbated by excessive, heavy breasts. This latter group of women will require resection of both skin and glandular tissue (reduction mammoplasty) in order to correct their deformity.

Originally published by Regnault in 1976, the most commonly utilized and clinically relevant grading system for breast ptosis describes the relationship of the NAC to the IMF (Table 15–1). Although it is useful and serves as a general guideline to describe different degrees of ptosis, the utility of this classification system is limited in that there may be vast differences in the severity of ptosis within the most severe grade. Pseudoptosis, a distinct entity from true ptosis (see below), is caused by deflationary descent of the breast parenchyma with normal location of the nipple. This is seen in a number of clinical scenarios, including, but not limited to, postpartum involution of breast tissue, excess skin following extensive weight loss, and following explantation of a breast implant.

All mastopexy procedures are described based on two major variables: (1) the pattern of skin incisions (and resultant scars), and (2) the parenchymal pedicle utilized to provide blood supply to the (transposed) NAC. In general, the type of skin incision and the nipple pedicle are independent of each other, and various combinations of the two are possible. For the remainder of the chapter, the procedures

TABLE 15–1. DEFINITIONS OF PTOSIS SEVERITY

Degree of Ptosis Severity	Description
First-degree (mild)	Nipple is within 1 cm of the level of the IMF and above the lower contour of the gland and skin envelope.
Second-degree (moderate)	Nipple is 1–3 cm below the level of the IMF but above the lower contour of the gland and skin envelope.
Third-degree (severe)	Nipple is more than 3 cm below the level of the IMF and below the lower contour of the breast and skin envelope.
Pseudoptosis	Glandular ptosis with nipple at or above the IMF.

IMF, inframammary fold.

will be categorized and described according to the three general types of skin incisions used: periareolar, vertical, and inverted T. Any of these operations may be combined with an augmentation or reduction according to the clinical scenario.

The severity of ptosis dictates the appropriate operation; in general, mild ptosis can be corrected with smaller incisions, while more severe ptosis requires more extensive skin resections and consequently larger scars. Mild (first-degree) ptosis may usually be treated using a circumareolar incision. Moderate (second-degree) ptosis may often be corrected with a vertical technique, and severe (third-degree) ptosis is typically corrected with an inverted T or "Wise"-pattern incision.

For patients with minimal ptosis, breast augmentation alone may provide the necessary volume to elevate the NAC (see Chapter 13). This is often the case in the setting of postpartum glandular involution. When the ptosis is more than several centimeters, excision of skin will be necessary with the specific pattern chosen depending on the severity of the ptosis. Conversely, when a large excess of breast parenchyma is the cause of the patient's ptosis, a formal reduction mammaplasty (see Chapter 14) in combination with a generous skin resection may be required to achieve the optimal lift with the best durability.

Although these recommendations represent general guidelines, the most appropriate surgical approach must be determined on an individual basis, taking into consideration not only technical issues, but also surgeon comfort with different techniques as well as patient expectations (eg, scar, durability of repair). Of great importance, the patient must decide the degree of scarring she is willing to accept. Some women will accept a suboptimal result to avoid excess scarring, while others are less concerned about scarring.

Recurrence of some degree of ptosis will be the rule, and it is imperative to discuss this with patients in the preoperative setting so that patients may have realistic goals and expectations before proceeding with surgery. In addition, the patient must be informed of the attendant risks of decreased nipple sensation and the extremely small, but finite, possibility of partial or complete necrosis of the NAC. The likelihood of nipple necrosis is increased in cases of severe ptosis where the NAC is transposed over a long distance.

PATIENT PREPARATION

Before undergoing mastopexy, all patients age 35 years and older should undergo a preoperative mammogram to rule out occult malignancy. A second mammogram should be obtained approximately 6 months postoperatively to serve as a new baseline followed by yearly mammograms thereafter. Patients should be informed that nipple sensation will likely be decreased in the early postoperative period regardless of the approach used. Although there are few mastopexy-specific studies to document it, data from the reduction mammoplasty literature demonstrate that most patients will experience a return to their baseline nipple sensation within 1 year of surgery. Patients also need to be counseled regarding the possibility that mastopexy may impact their ability to breastfeed successfully. Despite the paucity of peer-reviewed studies regarding the impact of mastopexy on breastfeeding, several studies on (more invasive) reduction mammoplasty have shown that the percentage of women who are able to successfully breastfeed after breast reduction is equivalent to those who had not had previous breast surgery.

PREOPERATIVE MARKINGS

Before starting any type of mastopexy procedure, standard preoperative skin markings are used to mark important anatomic landmarks

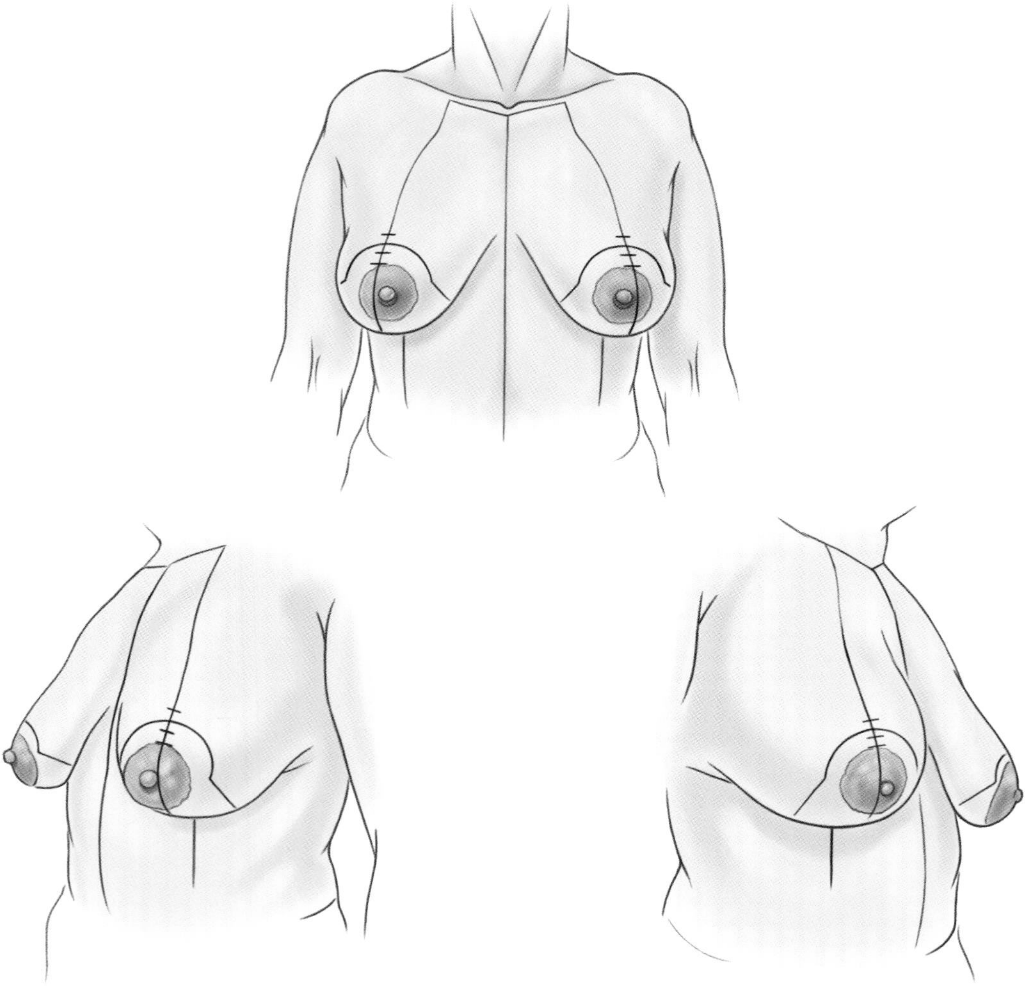

Figure 15–1. Preoperative markings. A line is drawn along the breast meridian from the clavicle to the inframammary fold (IMF). Next, the IMF is marked from the lateral breast margin to the sternum. The nipple areola complex (NAC) is then marked in its planned position using a 4 cm circle. If using an inverted-T type of incision, a keyhole pattern is also drawn.

(Figure 15–1). These include a line along the breast meridian originating from the clavicle and extending to the IMF on both breasts. The IMF is marked along its length from the lateral breast margin to the sternum. The "new" NAC is marked in its planned position using a diameter of approximately 4 cm. (This may be done with a cookie cutter.) If using an inverted-T type of incision, a keyhole pattern of skin excisions is also marked.

Proper preoperative markings are essential for proper intraoperative placement of vital landmarks such as the new nipple position. However, it is not uncommon to make intraoperative revisions of the amount of skin resected, the effects of which can be best envisioned using tailor-tacking techniques. Changing the location of the nipple intraoperatively should be done with extreme caution.

Because of inevitable bottoming out of the breast over time (no matter which technique is used), the preferred new nipple position location is approximately 1 cm below the IMF. It is better to place the nipple position too low than too high, as the former problem can be easily remedied, whereas an inappropriately high nipple can be an intractable problem.

TECHNIQUES

A. Periareolar

The Benelli periareolar, or "donut," mastopexy is indicated in cases of mild ptosis. While it usually results in a well-camouflaged periareolar scar, major shortcomings include a tendency toward flattening out of the breast over time, widening of the NAC, and high recurrence rates. In a mastopexy procedure without glandular excision, the blood supply to the nipple is largely uninterrupted, therefore obviating the need for a designated vascular pedicle.

The procedure is begun by marking two concentric skin incisions around the circumference of the NAC, leaving an inner NAC with an approximate diameter of 4 cm (most commonly 38 mm or 42 mm) (Figure 15–2). Best results are achieved if the diameter of the outer circle does not exceed three times the diameter of the inner circle, in order to minimize tension and wrinkling around the NAC. Further variations exist that use concentric ovals rather than circles.

Next, the intervening skin "donut" is circumferentially de-epithelialized. At this point in the operation, a decision is made regarding reshaping of the glandular tissue. This may be accomplished in a number of different ways, such as plicating the inferior glandular tissue to the chest wall or by incising the inferior breast parenchyma vertically and reapproximating it to increase projection.

At this point, a nonabsorbable purse-string suture (eg, Gore-Tex) is placed in the dermis around the limits of the outer skin incision. This suture is tightened, pulling the dermis of the outer concentric circle to the level of the inner circle, and effectively lifting the NAC. The periareolar incision is then closed with interrupted deep dermal sutures (taking care not to lacerate the Gore-Tex purse-string suture), followed by a running subcuticular stitch. Rippling of the skin around the nipple is expected at the conclusion of the operation and should disappear by 6 months.

B. Vertical Scar

The vertical scar technique combines the periareolar procedure described above with a vertical incision of varying length from the NAC downward toward the IMF. This technique is ideal for cases of moderate ptosis. Like the periareolar technique, it may be combined with either a reduction or augmentation to optimize the result. It results in a longer scar than the periareolar technique; however, the vertical component reduces tension on the suture line around the NAC and lowers the incidence of NAC widening (Figure 15–3).

The markings are very similar to the vertical reduction mammoplasty, although the length and width of the inferior limb of the incision will vary significantly depending on the amount of skin that requires excision. The choice of pedicle used to transpose the NAC will also depend on the individual requirements but in general a medial or superior pedicle technique (or some combination thereof) will often allow for better parenchymal shaping as well as leave maximal fullness in the aesthetically important superomedial portion of the breast.

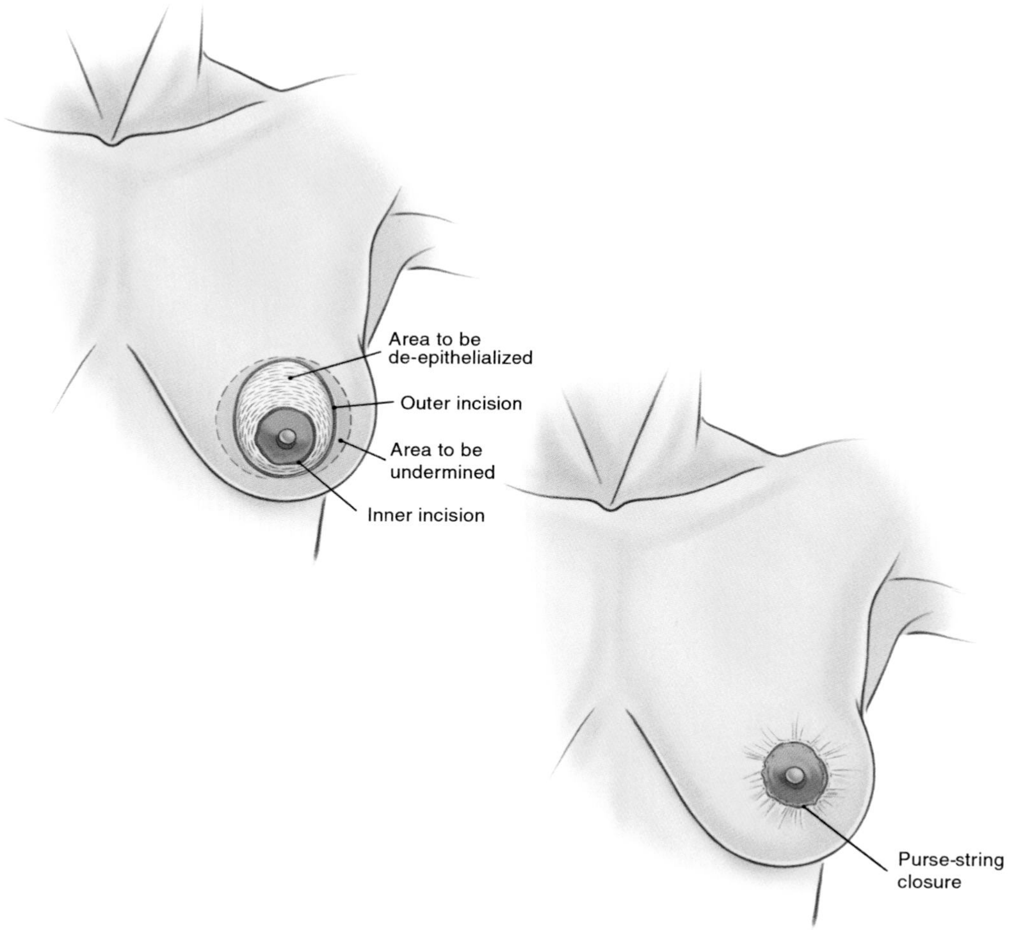

Figure 15–2. Diagram of mastopexy using the periareolar technique.

Several techniques for parenchymal redistribution to improve projection and fullness have been described. Many of these techniques rely on tucking the inferior portion of the gland under the more superior portion of the breast. Although this will increase projection, in the immediate postoperative period the breast takes on an unaesthetic tubular or "snoopy" like appearance (Figure 15–4). Patients need to be informed of this preoperatively and reassured that as the parenchyma bottoms out over the next few months the breast assumes a more natural and pleasing shape. Often, there is insufficient breast tissue remaining to provide adequate projection in which case placement of an implant will provide optimal results.

C. Inverted T (Wise Pattern)

The inverted T technique uses periareolar, vertical, and horizontal incisions in the shape

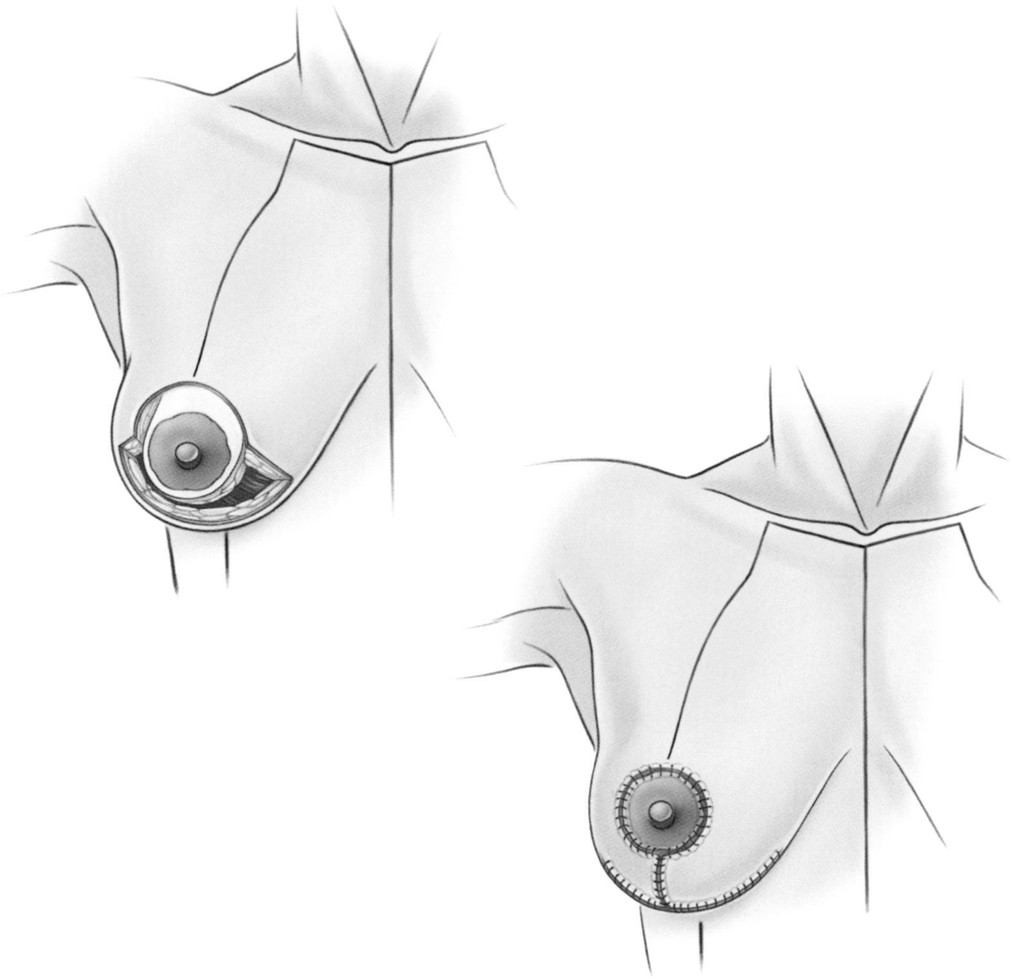

Figure 15–3. Diagram of mastopexy using vertical technique.

of an inverted T with the horizontal incision along the IMF. The preoperative skin markings and incisions are identical to those used for Wise-pattern reduction mammaplasty (see Chapter 14). This procedure is ideal for cases of third-degree (severe) ptosis. While this does result in more extensive scarring, significant amounts of vertically and horizontally excessive skin may be resected safely. The results are both reliable and reproducible. This pattern, originally described by Wise in 1956, is widely used for breast reduction and has been described in various forms by many authors. Again, the pedicle used to transpose the NAC depends on the distance to be moved, with care taken to provide adequate width for long pedicles. Often in cases of significant ptosis, the blood supply to the NAC can be tenuous

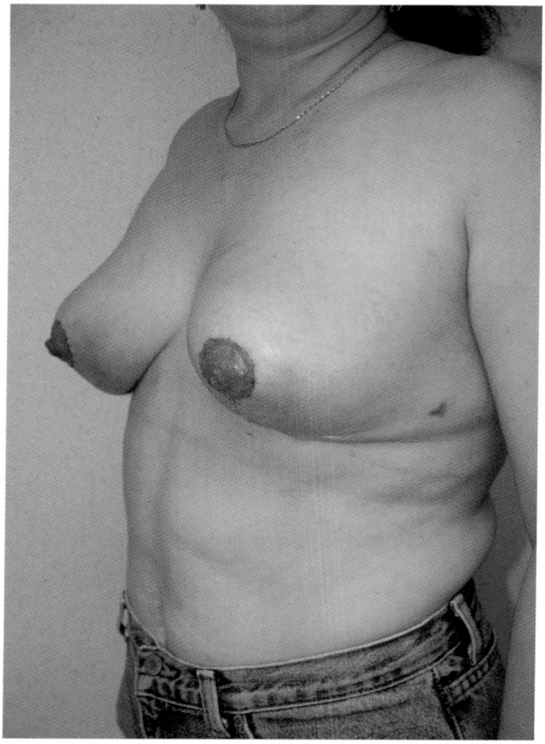

Figure 15–4. The so-called "snoopy" appearance of the breast following vertical scar mastopexy can be expected to resolve within several months following the procedure.

and use of a free nipple graft should be duly considered.

A recently published survey of American Society for Aesthetic Plastic Surgery (ASAPS) members addressed current physician preferences and satisfaction using different mastopexy techniques. The results demonstrated that the most popular technique remains the inverted-T incision (45%), with a trend toward popularization of the vertical scar technique in the last 5 years (overall 18%). Satisfaction was greatest using the vertical scar technique. The periareolar technique resulted in the lowest physician satisfaction and led to the greatest number of surgical revisions (50%).

COMPLICATIONS

The overall complication rate for mastopexy is low (~8%); however, most data in the literature come from single-institution case series. Although scarring is an expected outcome of mastopexy (rather than a complication), poorly healed incisions often lead to patient dissatisfaction and surgical revision. A recent review of the literature reported the expected morbidities according to the mastopexy technique performed (periareolar, vertical, inverted T, or L scar). The morbidities described ranged from hematoma, seroma, and fat necrosis to poor scarring, decreased nipple sensation, and skin or nipple necrosis.

Another recent retrospective review analyzed 150 patients (298 breasts) who underwent mastopexy. During the 36-month follow-up period, there were no major complications. Fifteen percent of patients experienced a minor complication, the most common being poor scarring (6%), seroma (2.7%), hematoma (2%), and minor infection (1.3%). There were no cases of flap loss or nipple necrosis. Thirteen of the 150 patients (8.6%) had revisions, most commonly for poor scarring (75%). Complication rates may vary depending on the surgeon's experience with breast surgery.

Another important question that was recently addressed is whether breast reconstruction with tissue expanders/implants can be safely performed in patients who have previously undergone mastopexy or reduction, or both. The authors analyzed the success rate, complication rate, and cosmetic outcome following tissue expander/implant placement in patients who had previously undergone breast reduction or mastopexy (or both) using inverted T incisions. Based on the results, the authors concluded that previous mammoplasty or mastopexy surgery does not increase the complication rate or compromise aesthetic outcomes, and that breast reconstruction with tissue expanders/implants is safe and effective in patients who have previously undergone mammoplasty with inverted T scars.

OUTCOMES ASSESSMENT

Objective patient satisfaction data following mastopexy are limited, and the studies that are available are retrospective. In a recently published retrospective analysis of patients undergoing combined augmentation/mastopexy, the authors included an objective aesthetic analysis of their results in addition to a patient satisfaction survey. Of 34 patients undergoing a single-stage augmentation/mastopexy, the overall complication rate was 8.8%, the majority of which were due to capsular contracture (6%). The aesthetic ratings were highest for postoperative ptosis and asymmetry correction and lowest for postoperative NAC size. The authors found that while patients were generally satisfied with the result, more than half (54%) of patients desired further surgery to improve their appearance, most commonly to increase the degree of breast lift.

REFERENCES

Benelli L. A new periareolar mammaplasty: the "round block" technique. *Aesthetic Plast Surg.* 1990 Spring;14(2):93–100. [PMID: 2185619]

Cruz NI et al. Lactational performance after breast reduction with different pedicles. *Plast Reconstr Surg.* 2007 Jul;120(1):35–40. [PMID: 17572542]

Graf R et al. Reduction mammaplasty and mastopexy using the vertical scar and thoracic wall flap technique. *Aesthetic Plast Surg.* 2003 Jan–Feb;27(1):6–12. [PMID: 12687296]

Hall-Findlay EJ. A Simplified Vertical Reduction Mammaplasty: Shortening the Learning Curve. *Plast Reconstr Surg.* 1999 Sep;104(3):748–59.

Kilgo MS et al. Tissue expansion after inverted-T mammaplasty: can it be performed successfully? *Ann Plast Surg.* 2003 Jun;50(6):588–93. [PMID: 12783005]

Lassus C. A 30-year experience with vertical mammaplasty. *Plast Reconstr Surg.* 1996 Feb;97(2):373–80. [PMID: 8559820]

Lejour M. Vertical mammaplasty: early complications after 250 personal consecutive cases. *Plast Reconstr Surg.* 1999 Sep;104(3):764–70. [PMID: 10456529]

Nahabedian MY et al. Viability and sensation of the nipple-areolar complex after reduction mammaplasty. *Ann Plast Surg.* 2002;49(1):24–31. [PMID: 12142591]

Penn J. Breast reduction. *Br J Plast Surg.* 1955 Jan;7(4):357–71. [PMID: 13230442]

Regnault P. Breast ptosis. Definition and treatment. *Clin Plast Surg.* 1976 Apr;3(2):193–203. [PMID: 1261176]

Ritz M et al. Fascial suspension mastopexy. *Plast Reconstr Surg.* 2006 Jan;117(1):86–94. [PMID: 16404254]

Rohrich RJ et al. Mastopexy preferences: a survey of board-certified plastic surgeons. *Plast Reconstr Surg.* 2006 Dec;118(7):1631–8. [PMID: 17102738]

Rohrich RJ et al. The limited scar mastopexy: current concepts and approaches to correct breast ptosis. *Plast Reconstr Surg.* 2004 Nov;114(6):1622–30. [PMID: 15509961]

Spear SL et al. Concentric mastopexy revisited. *Plast Reconstr Surg.* 2001 Apr 15;107(5):1294–9. [PMID: 11373576]

Spear SL et al. One-stage augmentation combined with mastopexy: aesthetic results and patient satisfaction. *Aesthetic Plast Surg.* 2004 Sep–Oct; 28(5):259–67. [PMID: 15529204]

Stevens WG et al. Mastopexy revisited: A review of 150 consecutive cases for complication and revision rates. *Aesthet Surg J.* 2007 Mar–Apr; 27(2):150–4. [PMID: 19341640]

Wise RJ. A preliminary report on a method of planning the mammaplasty. *Plast Reconstr Surg.* 1956 May;17(5):367–75. [PMID: 13335513]

CHAPTER 16

Abdominoplasty & Abdominal Contouring Procedures

Mark Schwartz, MD & Sophie Bartsich, MD

Abdominal contouring is one of the most commonly performed cosmetic procedures today. In 2008, 121,653 abdominoplasties were performed in the United States. The standard abdominoplasty continues to be the mainstay of midline reshaping for patients with an obvious skin deformity; however, recent advances in liposuction and surgical technique allow for a re-adaptation of the procedure to suit individual needs. Through careful evaluation of skin, fat, and muscle quality, patients can be stratified into different treatment groups, each with a customized surgical plan.

Factors that play important roles in determining body shape and contour include aging, genetics, gender, and parity. Lifestyle and medication regimens may also contribute to varying degrees to changes in abdominal girth and firmness. While there are behavioral modifications that can significantly improve the appearance of the abdomen, surgical intervention is often warranted to achieve the desired result.

Even for patients who are not overweight, inherent weight distribution patterns may preclude a desired waistline, despite efforts with diet and exercise. Female patients in particular will often experience permanent changes in their abdominal profile after childbearing, with varying degrees of secondary skin and muscle laxity or deformity. Patients who have undergone abdominal surgery may have disfiguring scars, corresponding soft tissue folds, or resultant diastasis. Finally, some patients with minimal contour irregularities may seek less invasive methods of improvement. After careful evaluation and counseling, the appropriate surgical intervention can achieve highly satisfying results.

▶ ANATOMY

The anterior abdominal wall is composed of several distinct layers of soft tissue. Beneath the skin and subcutaneous fat lie Camper fascia and the more membranous Scarpa fascia. In the center of the abdomen, the next layer of tissue is the rectus abdominus muscle, bounded by the anterior and posterior rectus sheaths above the arcuate line. Beneath the arcuate line, the rectus has only an anterior sheath, making that layer weaker posteriorly.

The lateral aspects of the abdominal wall are composed of four layers: the external oblique, the internal oblique, the transversus abdominus, and the transversalis fascia. While all of the above muscles contribute to the shape and contour of the abdomen, it is the rectus abdominus that is chiefly responsible for the outline of the mid abdomen.

In performing an abdominoplasty, the skin and subcutaneous fat is dissected off of the anterior rectus sheath and the external oblique muscles. Identification of the relevant tissue planes is critical to a proper dissection, especially in the event of prior surgery (ie, cesarean section) or abdominal hernias. It is also important to distinguish between the different muscle groups, their fascia, and their orientation when performing the tissue plication.

If the muscle layers or their fascia appear particularly weak, mesh may be used to ensure the strength of the abdominal wall. Variations in intra-abdominal pressure, postoperative changes in the distribution of tension lines, and long incisions will promote the formation of tissue bulges or hernias over time. The long-term result of abdominal contouring depends on the integrity of the structural components of the abdominal wall, and any reconstruction of this area must preserve or restore their stability.

The anterior abdominal wall can be divided into three main zones based on blood supply (Figure 16–1). Zone I is the superomedial portion of the abdominal wall. Blood supply to zone I is provided by the superior epigastric artery, a continuation of the internal mammary artery. While the inferior blood supply to the abdominal wall is of greater magnitude, most tissue flaps based on the abdominal wall and muscles rely primarily on the superior epigastric blood supply.

The inferior portion of the abdominal wall is supplied by the deep and superficial inferior epigastric vessels, and is known as zone II. The deep inferior epigastric artery is a branch of the external iliac artery, and the superficial inferior epigastric artery is a branch of the femoral artery. Low transverse abdominal incisions interrupt this blood supply and render the lower abdominal region largely compromised, since the blood supply from the superior vessels originates too proximally to compensate well. As a result, the majority of the vascular supply to the lower abdomen after an abdominoplasty must originate laterally.

Zone III represents the lateral aspects of the anterior abdominal wall. It is supplied by the circumflex iliac artery (a branch of the external iliac vessel) and perforating branches of the intercostal arteries. While this blood supply is the weakest of the three zones, it becomes critically important for survival of the abdominoplasty flap and proper healing of the incision. Many surgeons choose to limit the lateral dissection in order to maximize perfusion to the medial portion of the flap.

▶ PATIENT EVALUATION & SELECTION

There are no exact guidelines for patient selection; therefore, clinical judgment and experience play significant roles. The overall criteria by which to evaluate a patient for abdominal contouring involve assessments of skin, muscle, and fat superficial to the peritoneum. Skin must be examined for laxity, compliance, and elasticity. Skin redundancy must also be addressed as well as folds and the presence of a pannus (Figure 16–2). The rectus muscle must be evaluated for conditioning and the presence of a diastasis. The amount of subcutaneous fat should be estimated as well as its pattern of distribution. Finally, a good analysis of the aesthetic abdominal wall must establish the above characteristics of the tissue both superior and inferior to the umbilicus, including a general estimation of the supraumbilical tissue reaching the inferior incision line if stretched.

Changes in body shape are generally due to soft tissue phenomena; however, there are cases in which bony irregularities are the cause. Therefore, the evaluation of a patient

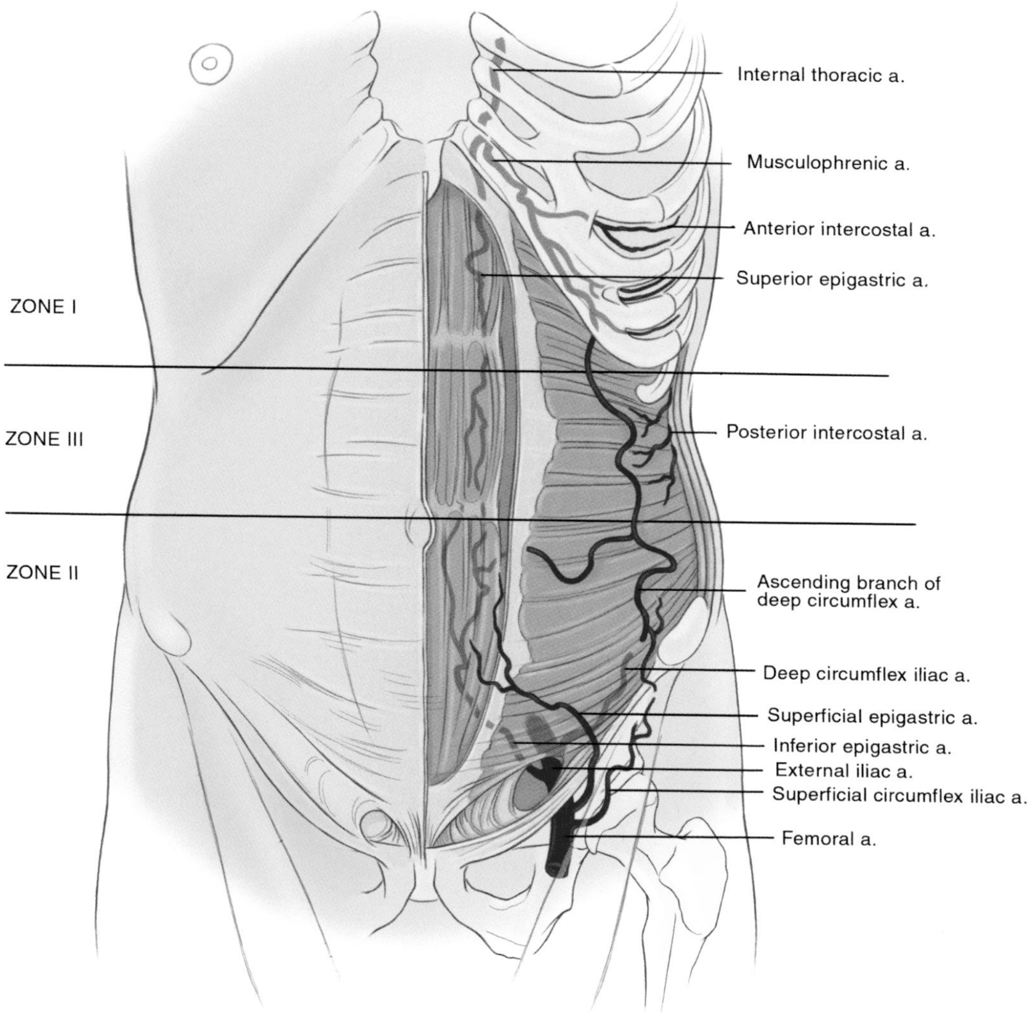

Figure 16–1. Blood supply to the anterior abdominal wall.

who is considering abdominal contouring must include a thorough assessment of their general body type and structure as well as their skeletal silhouette.

A. Physical Examination

In order to establish eligibility for abdominal contouring, all patients require a thorough history of physical examination. The patient's weight on initial evaluation should be documented.

Patients who are obese are advised to lose a certain amount of weight before undergoing surgery because the weight loss may change their evaluation and because the operative course could be dramatically improved. Ideally, a patient's weight should be consistent for 6 months before abdominal contouring surgery.

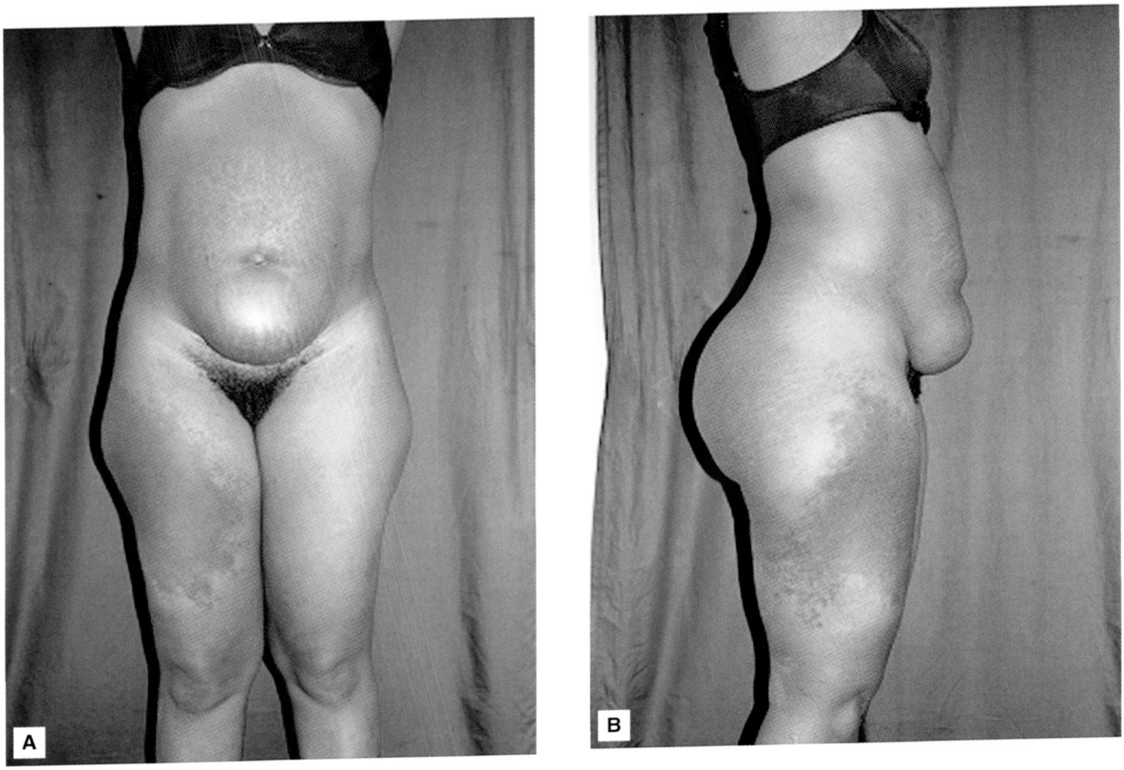

Figure 16–2. **A, B:** Preoperative abdominoplasty candidate, with significant pannus and muscle laxity. **C, D:** Postoperative result after pannus excision and imbrication of the abdominal wall.

While some patients have a tapered waistline despite being overweight, others have a straighter shape. For the latter, creating the desired hourglass silhouette may be more difficult and may involve more advanced surgical techniques for reducing the diameter of the mid-abdomen. Some patients who are dissatisfied with their abdominal shape may also have a significant amount of intra-abdominal adipose tissue. Patients should be advised that intra-abdominal adipose tissue is not amenable to aesthetic surgical treatment.

The physical examination should be conducted with the patient in a variety of positions. The patient should be evaluated both standing upright and leaning forward. The arms should be straight down while upright, and folded behind the waist while leaning forward. The patient's silhouette should be examined from both frontal and lateral views in order to fully appreciate positional variation in apparent laxity.

The physical examination begins with an evaluation of the skin overlying the abdomen. Obvious deformities or laxity should be noted. The surgeon should pinch the skin and assess its general turgor, stretching it to determine compliance and elasticity. Skin that demonstrates good compliance is more amenable to stretching, whereas skin that has more elastance is more likely to resume its original shape and size after less invasive fat-reducing procedures.

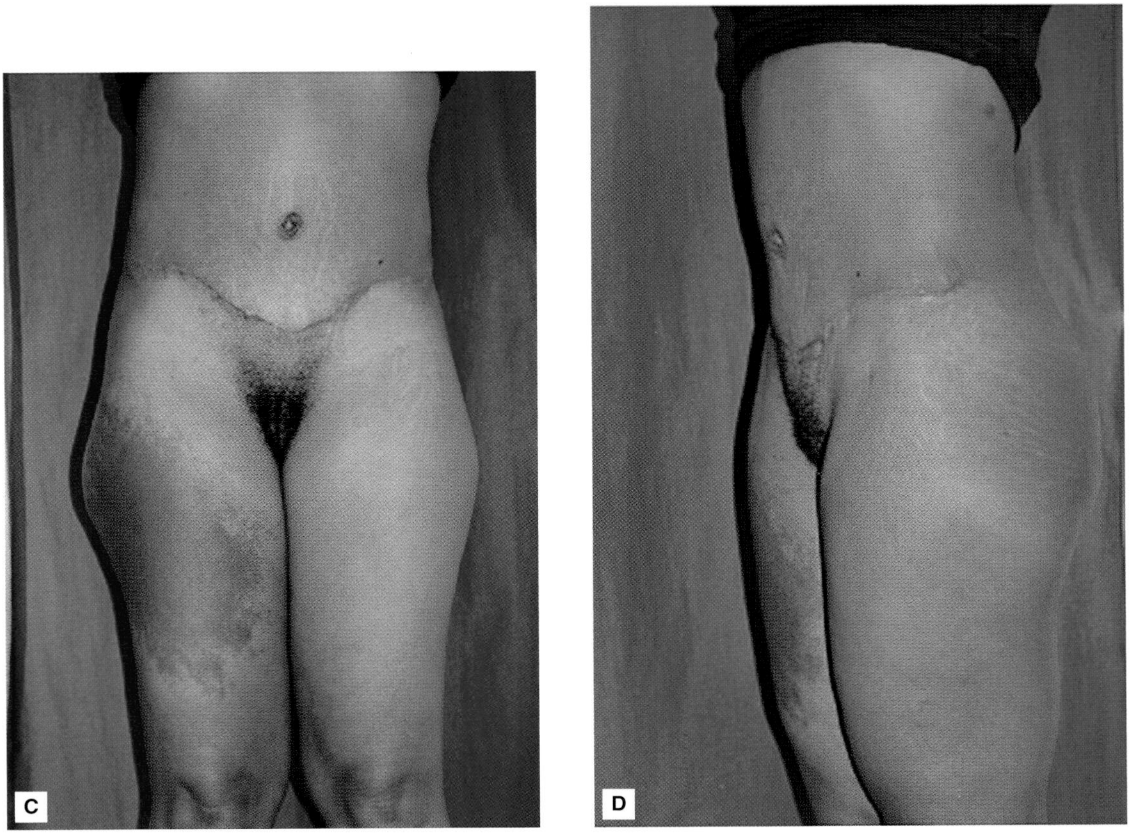

Figure 16–2. (Continued)

The main muscle group of the mid-abdomen is the rectus abdominus. It consists of two vertical strips of muscle, separated by a thin line. Surgery, pregnancy, obesity, and many other factors may compromise the integrity of the linea alba. A careful examination should note any weakness in the rectus abdominus, as well as the presence of any degree of diastasis between the two muscles. The patient should also be evaluated for the presence of an abdominal hernia. If the patient has a current indication for another surgical procedure of the abdomen, the two interventions may be performed concurrently.

The patient should be evaluated for fat distribution patterns. Adipose tissue is omnipresent in the abdomen. A significant amount of it can be removed with liposuction, but it must be extraperitoneal. For patients with notable adipose tissue on the flanks, liposuction may be a recommended adjunct to abdominoplasty.

The patient should also be evaluated in the supine position. While lying flat, the abdomen should be assessed for shape (scaphoid vs concave). A scaphoid abdomen while supine is indicative of intra-abdominal girth. If a significant amount of the abdominal diameter is due to intra-abdominal fat as opposed to subcutaneous fat, a good result from extra-abdominal body contouring is less likely.

Finally, the abdomen must be carefully examined for the presence of scars, and a thorough history of prior surgery must be taken. Scar tissue may create significant adhesions, making the aesthetic procedure more difficult and potentially more complicated. For patients with strategically placed abdominal scars, the pattern of blood supply to the abdomen may be altered significantly enough to influence the feasibility of a given procedure. Considering that one of the greatest concerns in the survival of any tissue flap is adequate perfusion, this element of patient evaluation cannot be overestimated. One particularly important scar to be aware of is that from an open cholecystectomy because it risks devascularizing the large zone between the costal margin and the superior portion of the abdominoplasty incision.

B. Choosing the Proper Technique

Some patients are amenable to any of the various surgical interventions, and the decision becomes a matter of patient preference. In other situations, the surgeon may recognize limitations to performing certain procedures, and care should be taken to avoid undergoing less appropriate interventions due to patient request.

The scarring that results from abdominal contouring is often a major concern among patients. While the overall aesthetic improvement usually merits the resultant scar, it is important to stress the nature of the long-term deformity associated with this procedure. The goal is an aesthetically pleasing result with minimized scar formation. While the standard abdominoplasty incision is a transverse arch on the lower aspect of the abdomen, there are options for incision placement. Consultation with the patient should involve a discussion regarding clothing fit and dress habits. Ideally, the incision line should be covered by underwear and bathing suits (Figure 16–3).

Similarly, some patients may opt to not undergo an abdominoplasty because of the scar, but excision of redundant skin may be the only available method for producing the desired effect. Patient preference should be an integral part of the decision-making process with regard to choice of abdominal contouring procedures, but it should only come into play once the reasonable options have been delineated.

▶ PROCEDURES

According to the Matarasso classification system, patients can be categorized into one of four groups for abdominal reshaping. Categories are based on degree of skin laxity, excess subcutaneous fat, and muscle flaccidity. Category I includes those patients with no skin excess of muscle deficits; the treatment is liposuction alone. Category II includes patients with some skin excess of muscle laxity and fat; these patients can have mini-abdominoplasty. Patients with considerable skin and muscle issues who need full abdominoplasty are classified in category III and those patients with these same issues who require abdominoplasty with liposuction are classified in category IV. The basis of this system recognizes that each of these issues must be approached individually.

Redundant skin can only be remedied with excision (Figure 16–4). Only patients with taut, elastic skin and lipodystrophy are good candidates for liposuction alone. Both the degree and location of excess skin should be noted, and for patients in whom this is limited to the infra-umbilical area, a standard abdominoplasty is often unnecessary for the desired result. In patients with significant fat deposition, liposuction is often an adjunct to abdominoplasty, and using it in conjunction

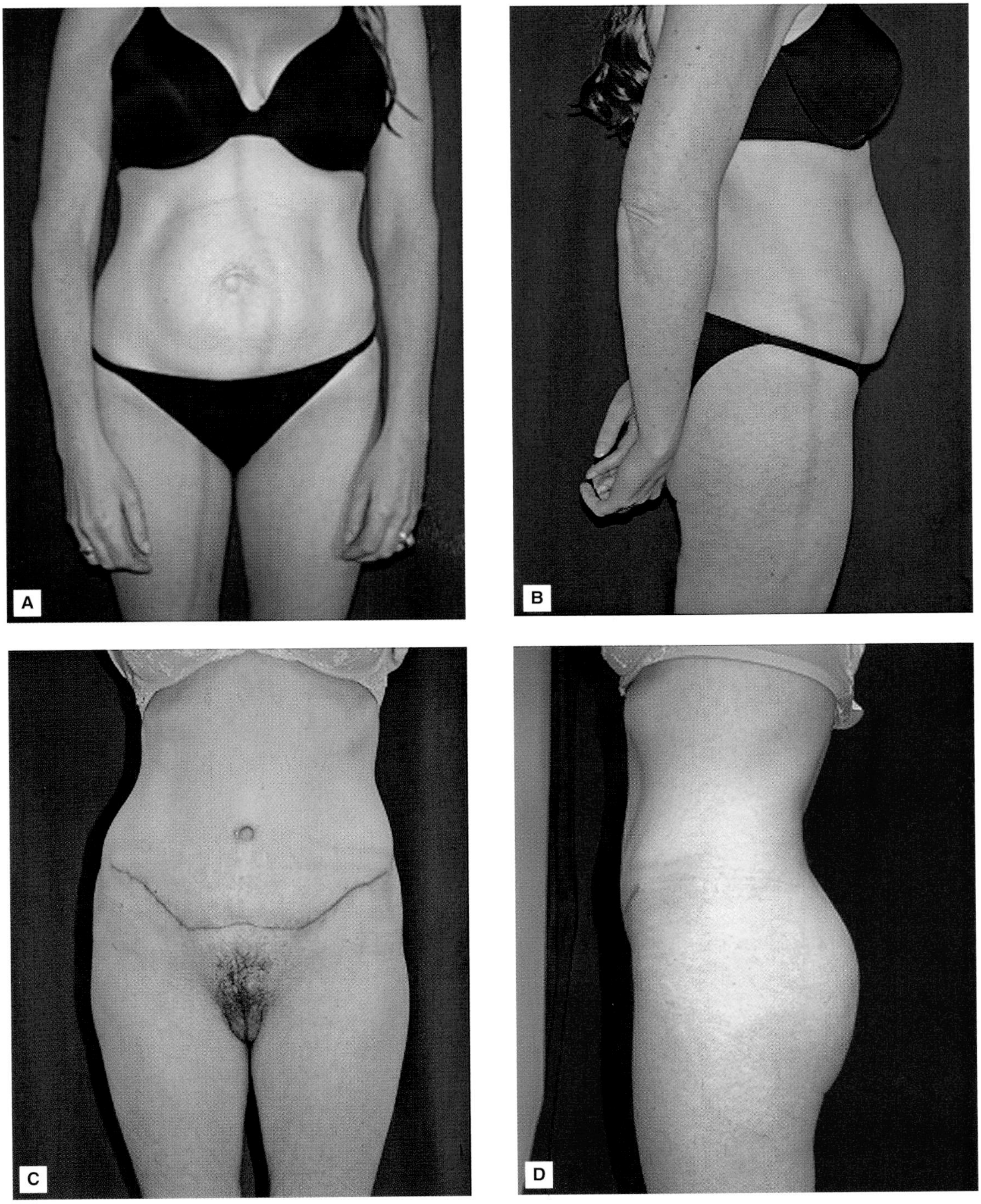

Figure 16–3. **A, B:** Preoperative abdominoplasty candidate with significant abdominal wall laxity. **C, D:** Postoperative result, using a low abdominal incision, easily hidden by a bathing suit.

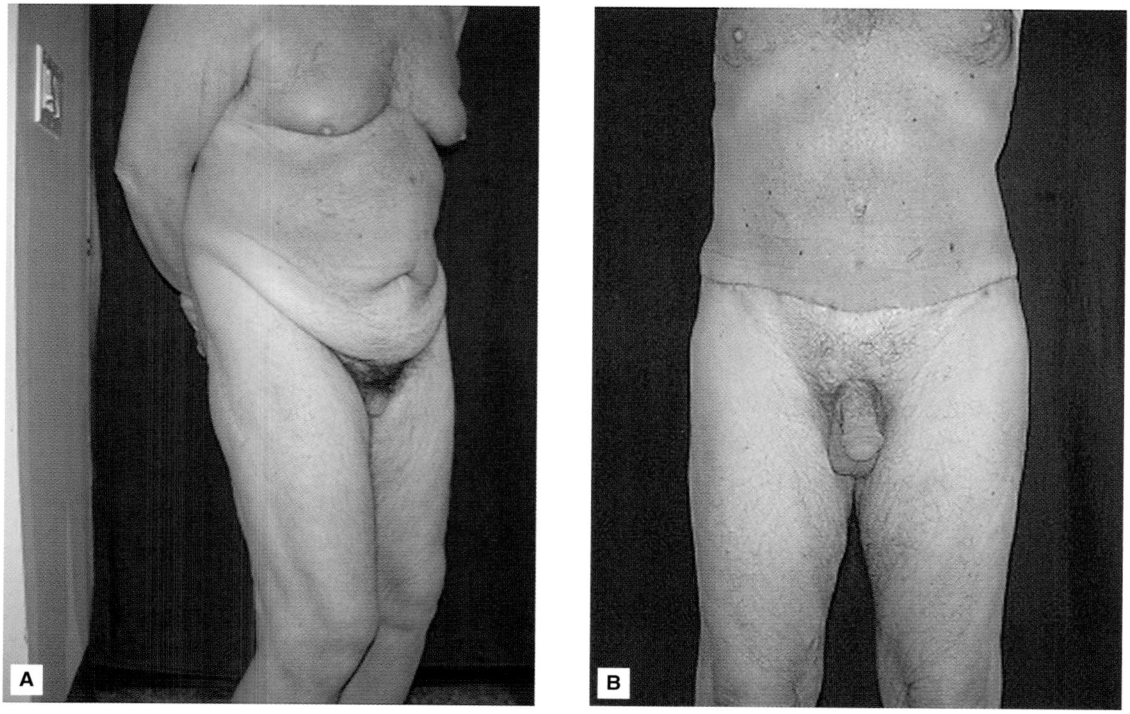

Figure 16–4. **A:** Preoperative abdominoplasty candidate with significant skin redundancy. **B:** Postoperative result, with repositioning of the umbilicus.

with the latter can allow for treating a larger area than with abdominoplasty alone. In cases of muscle laxity, the muscular abdominal wall must be tightened in order to decrease the girth of the midsection.

Using these guidelines for abdominal reshaping, various forms of abdominoplasty can be combined with liposuction to achieve the desired result. Overall, most patients undergoing abdominal contouring surgery will undergo liposuction alone.

LIPOSUCTION ALONE

For many patients desiring abdominal body contouring, the target area is subcutaneous fat. This is particularly true for women, for whom sex-specific fat deposition patterns tend to create pockets superficial to the abdominal musculature. By virtue of its location, this fat is readily accessible by liposuction alone.

Liposuction is the aspiration of subcutaneous fat with the use of specifically designed cannulas inserted into the subcutaneous space through several small incisions. With the use of different cannulas, fat extraction can be tailored to the different areas of the body, as well as to the variability of fat textures and densities. The result is a reduction in fatty tissue and an improvement in body contour with minimal invasiveness and scarring.

Because liposuction does not involve the removal of excess skin, it is not an effective body contouring procedure for all patients. A thorough evaluation of skin quality and turgor is necessary prior to any recommendation of liposuction alone as a cosmetic procedure. In patients with significant subcutaneous fat and limited skin elastance, liposuction may result in appropriate fat reduction but significant skin deformity. For these patients, a more invasive procedure such as abdominoplasty is recommended to produce a better result.

A. Patient Evaluation

Prospective liposuction patients must undergo a thorough physical examination. Visual examination includes assessing the mid-section from anterior, posterior, and lateral views. The patient should be examined while standing straight and while leaning forward. All skin redundancy should be noted, as well as any deformity resulting from position changes. The abdominal skin itself should be pinched and assessed for turgor and elasticity. If a significant volume reduction is planned, the enveloping skin must be able to compensate for the decrease in girth by appropriately shrinking to match the new contour. Skin that has already been stretched (ie, in women who have borne children) and does not demonstrate good recoil will require excision in order to achieve the desired form. The abdomen should also be evaluated for existing scars, as their presence may determine port site location.

When counseling a patient regarding potential liposuction, it is of paramount importance to explain that the procedure is strictly intended for body contouring, and not weight reduction. The ideal liposuction candidate is generally fit, with good skin elasticity, and stable weight. For such a patient, the procedure seeks to target defined pockets of fat that fail to respond to diet and exercise. Resolution of these problem areas leads to an improved appearance and body contour, maximizing results. Finally, it is important to recognize that liposuction will not alter the quality of the overlying skin, and as such it is not effective for the treatment of cellulite.

B. Patient Preparation

As with most plastic surgery procedures, preoperative marking is of great importance. Extensive markings should be made before any skin preparation. With the patient standing, target areas should be topographically outlined. It is imperative to mark the patient while standing because the soft tissues will shift and flatten once the patient is lying flat on the table. Target areas are identified, and concentric circles are used to describe areas with increasing fat density.

In patients undergoing liposuction of the abdomen, there are usually several target areas. Many of these patients are also undergoing liposuction of the flanks, hips, or thighs. Because of this, it is often most convenient to prepare the entire torso, hips, and thighs prior to beginning the procedure. Furthermore, the patient will likely require turning or, at the very least, extensive repositioning throughout the course of the process. In order to facilitate this, the patient should be prepared circumferentially while standing and should then be positioned on the surgical table lying on top of sterile drapes. The patient can then be easily repositioned and manipulated during the procedure without the need for further preparing nor concern for contamination of the field.

C. Technique

A series of small incisions are made surrounding the target areas. Entry ports must be large enough to accommodate the cannulas that will be used but should be small enough to minimize scarring. They should be strategically positioned to allow access to a significant portion of the target area and to be hidden as eventual scars. Lower body skin folds and groin creases are generally good locations for this purpose.

Once the entry points are established, areas to be treated are extensively infiltrated with tumescent fluid. Tumescent fluid is generally composed of a mixture of lidocaine, epinephrine, and Ringer lactate solution. Using a specialized cannula, the target fat is penetrated in long horizontal strokes, creating pathways for future suction, and allowing dissipation of the tumescent fluid. Once the tissues have been thoroughly infiltrated, they become turgid, often taking on a "cobblestone" appearance. This "pre-tunneling" provides a guide for the suction cannulas, and the expanded volume of the target area aids in maneuverability. The total lidocaine dose in this procedure should not exceed 30 mg/kg.

The combination of lidocaine and epinephrine provides extensive local anesthesia as well as significant vascular constriction. This limits blood loss and also decreases the need for general anesthesia. Many liposuction procedures are amenable to sedation, given the degree of local pain control. It is important to note that a significant portion of the large amount of solution that is injected during tissue tumescence is absorbed by these tissues, and with it a significant amount of lidocaine. However, with appropriate dilution, and effective vasoconstriction in the setting of epinephrine use, lidocaine toxicity during liposuction remains extremely rare.

Once appropriate tumescence has been achieved in the target areas, aspiration may begin. Using the existing tracts, fat is aspirated using long horizontal strokes. Care must be taken to fan out over the target are so as to avoid localized depressions. The tissues should be intermittently pinched to assess thickness and degree of infiltrate remaining. Bleeding should be minimal, and the aspirate should have a milky yellow appearance throughout the majority of the case. At the conclusion of the procedure, the patient should demonstrate the desired contour in the target areas.

The liposuction aspirate is collected into vacuum containers and disposed of after the procedure is concluded. In the event that the suctioned fat is intended for further use (ie, reinjection at another anatomic site), it must be collected using a sterile syringe. It can then be used as a fat graft for augmentation.

D. Complications

The most common complication after liposuction of the abdomen is contour deformity. This is usually due to technique and excess suctioning from particular areas (depressions). In order to avoid this, a variety of suction cannula sizes should be used to maximize the overall smoothness of the result. Experienced surgeons will often alternate between cannulas, using larger caliber ones at first and then downsizing during the procedure. Strokes should be parallel to the plane of the body, and should be distributed evenly over the target area.

One of the most morbid potential complications of the procedure remains puncture. Superficial punctures with suction cannulas can damage the skin, creating disfiguring scars. Deep punctures can penetrate the abdominal musculature, or more critically, can enter the abdomen and puncture a viscus. While by far the most concerning of potential complications, the incidence of a hollow-viscus injury is extremely low in liposuction. The incidence of such morbidity is usually attributable to alterations in superficial anatomy, as caused by prior surgical procedures and their resulting scars.

Blood loss is generally not significant during liposuction limited to the abdomen. Estimates range from 8% to 10% of the total aspirate. The color and quality of the aspirate is noted during the procedure; it will invariably become more sanguinous toward the end of the process as the amount of fat is reduced and the tumescent fluid has been largely evacuated. While small blood vessels may be broken during aspiration, larger caliber vessels are generally encased in fibrous tissue that remains undisrupted by the cannula tracks. As a result, bleeding is usually minimal, and blood supply to the overlying skin is not interrupted despite the significant undermining involved in the procedure.

As with any operative procedure, there is the possibility of infection. Wound complications are very rare with liposuction, likely owing to the use of proper sterile technique as well as copious irrigation. Entry points are often left open after the procedure, allowing fluids to express themselves and avoiding stasis of fluid collections.

E. Postoperative Care

While the majority of the tumescent fluid is aspirated, a significant portion is absorbed into the surrounding tissues. As a result, it will egress in the postoperative phase, usually within the first 48 hours. Patients should be counseled to expect drainage from the incision sites for the first few days after surgery. This may be uncomfortable, particularly if they are continuously wearing a cloth undergarment for support. Soilage of linens and clothing may continue for days, and the use of protective disposable pads is recommended.

Use of a compression garment is often recommended for abdominal liposuction. Patients are advised to wear these garments continuously for 3 weeks after surgery. This will generally prevent excessive swelling, and provide support for the new body contour. Pain is usually minimal, and the patient may resume normal activities within 3–4 weeks.

Surgeons should explain that the final result will not be apparent until the patient is completely healed. In the initial postoperative phase, significant tissue swelling occurs, particularly if the patient is not using a compression garment, and they may initially feel larger than they were prior to the procedure. Once the excess fluid has been expressed and the inflammation and bruising have abated, the results can be evaluated. This process usually takes 3–6 months.

F. Other Techniques

Ultrasound-assisted liposuction has become an adjunct to conventional liposuction. Using this technique, ultrasound waves are emitted into the fat prior to its aspiration in an effort to melt it without significant mechanical force. Vibration of the ultrasound probe also promotes channel formation in the subcutaneous tissues with less effort than is required with manual tunneling. Ultrasound probes used in this technique have been adapted to include suction tips, allowing for simultaneous fat breakdown and aspiration.

There are several issues of concern with regard to ultrasound-assisted liposuction. Because the ultrasound cannulas are usually of wider bore than conventional suction cannulas, entry points must be made larger to accommodate them. This results in more prominent scarring. Once in use, the ultrasound probe heats over its entire length, increasing the risk of burning surrounding tissues. Vibration of the device has also been implicated in nerve damage for the practicing surgeon.

While the use of ultrasound-assisted liposuction is widely practiced, it remains a subject of much debate. In areas with great fat density, such as the back, ultrasound-assisted liposuction can be helpful for dissolving thick fat pockets and facilitating aspiration of the tissue. For many other areas, such as the abdomen, conventional liposuction has been reported to be equally effective. Overall, there has been significant criticism of ultrasound-assisted liposuction, with the prevailing argument being that both techniques achieve similar results.

STANDARD ABDOMINOPLASTY

Despite some technical innovations, the basic procedure for an abdominoplasty has remained the same; however, the setting in which these procedures are performed has changed. Many body contouring procedures are now performed in ambulatory surgical facilities, and patients are discharged the same day. Some surgeons are choosing to perform some of these procedures under conscious sedation, limiting the risks and complications of general anesthesia. Liberal use of local anesthetic can compensate for the lack of general anesthesia and may even help prolong the pain-free period postoperatively with the use of long-acting analgesics. The use of conscious sedation has not been demonstrated to produce increased morbidity. Local blocks can further facilitate effective outpatient management by minimizing postoperative pain through the principle of preemptive anesthesia.

One of the main concerns with abdominoplasty is the pressure that is placed on the suture line. Because the skin is stretched, it is usually closed under tension. The point of greatest tension is in the medial aspect of the wound, therefore the dissection of the abdominal flap must reach its most superior point in the median plane of the body.

While the central portion of the abdominoplasty wound is the most tenuous, it is the lateral aspects of the wound that remain the most challenging in terms of the aesthetic outcome. The tension on the lateral aspect of the wound is usually far less than in the central position, due to the elliptical nature of the incision. Often, there is even a certain amount of skin redundancy at the lateral borders of the suture line. This, coupled with differential wound lengths on the superior and inferior portions of the ellipse, may often cause "dog ears." Several methods have been suggested to minimize on lateral bulging of the wound, and these will be discussed later.

A. Patient Selection

Patients who are good candidates for abdominoplasty generally have moderate to marked skin laxity, variable subcutaneous fat, and some muscular weakness. For these patients, it is not possible to achieve a smooth midline contour without excising the redundant tissues. Compliant skin is not only favorable but required for the success of the operation.

The abdominoplasty involves extensive incisions, making scarring a critical topic in counseling patients regarding the procedure. While a successful operation does lead to a smooth, flattened, aesthetically pleasing midline, scarring is significant. Although efforts are made to strategically place future scars and minimize their visibility, the incision involved in this procedure extends the entire width of the abdomen. While most swimwear can cover the scar, there is still the risk of abnormal scarring. It is important to establish that these patients are willing to accept the resultant blemish and its implicit aesthetic limitations in exchange for the body contouring result.

Because a large ellipse of tissue will be removed from the abdomen, it is of paramount importance that the resultant defect be amenable to closure. If the skin on the upper portion of the abdomen does not have the required "give" to later reach the inferior margin of the resected skin paddle, the wound will not close, and the results can be severely disfiguring. It is therefore important to assess skin compliance in these patients, to stretch the skin superior to the umbilicus, and anticipate its likelihood of meeting the suprapubic region once undermined.

Because most abdominoplasty patients are women, a careful evaluation must include any plans for future pregnancy. While this is not an absolute contraindication to performing the procedure, it should be taken into consideration. For patients who have demonstrated decreased skin elasticity, it should be noted that a pregnancy is likely to affect the final result of the contouring procedure. Patients who are concerned about this are well advised to delay planning the operation until they have completed childbearing.

B. Patient Preparation

Preoperative marking is performed with the patient standing. The midline is described, from the xiphoid process to the anterior vulvar commissure. This will provide a constant gauge of symmetry and will be an eventual guide for reapproximation of the edges of the resected skin paddle. The umbilicus is circumscribed, and the iliac crests are marked. The superior wound margin must lie superior to the umbilicus, extending laterally toward the iliac crests.

The inferior incision line will become the new "bikini line," and should be low enough to be concealed by clothing. At the midline, the inferior wound edge should be approximately 5–7 cm from the anterior vulvar commissure. This positioning should represent the new pubic hairline. The lateral extensions of the inferior wound margin should curve superiorly in order to be concealed by clothing cut high on the hips.

In the event that the patient has scars from prior abdominal surgery, all efforts should be made to incorporate those wounds into the resected tissue paddle. Ideally, the inferior wound margin should extend 1 cm beyond Pfannenstiel incisions to provide a fresh wound margin for healing. This may make the procedure more technically difficult if it extends the necessary surgical area. Careful consideration should be given to a history of any prior abdominal operations in these patients.

The patient is placed supine on the operating table and the entire abdomen is prepared from above the xiphoid process to the mid-thigh area. While the patient will be lying flat for the majority of the procedure, setup must allow for flexing of the surgical table at the patient's waist at the time of wound closure. If liposuction is planned in conjunction with the abdominoplasty, patient preparation must take this into consideration as well.

C. Technique

Some surgeons elect to infiltrate the surgical area prior to performing an abdominoplasty. Similar to the tumescence performed with liposuction, the subcutaneous tissues are imbued with a dilute solution of lidocaine and epinephrine. This provides anesthesia, vasoconstriction, and prepares the field for liposuction if it is planned. In combined liposuction/abdominoplasty procedures, liposuction is performed first.

The first step in an abdominoplasty is the circumscription of the umbilicus (Figure 16–5). The umbilicus is retracted from the abdominal wall and incised at the established markings and the stalk is exposed. The inferior incision is then made, and dissection of the flap begins. Dissection preserves the fascia overlying the abdominal musculature, and it extends superiorly to the xiphoid process. The lateral margins of the flap do not need to reach as superiorly because it will require a far greater amount of movement at the midline compared with the sides. Furthermore, because a significant portion of the blood supply to the flap relies on circulation from zone III, extensive lateral dissection should be avoided, since it may compromise perfusion and wound healing.

Once the flap has been raised, the umbilicus remains intact on its stalk. Using a nonabsorbable suture, the remaining musculofascial layer is imbricated superior and inferior to the umbilicus, in order to tighten it and narrow the abdomen. Strategic imbrication can be used to create a specific shape at the waist and accentuate the midline silhouette. The fascia may then be infiltrated with long-acting local anesthetic to provide greater pain control in the postoperative period.

Prior to excising the skin paddle, the proposed markings are checked with the operating table positioned like a beach chair to provide flexion at the midline while relaxing the knees. The inferior portion of the paddle is transected at the midline, beneath the umbilical site defect. The excess skin is then pulled down so that its superior edge may meet the inferior margin of the wound. While the superior margin is already marked, it can be adjusted at this time to accommodate the effective elasticity of the flap, as well as any unforeseen asymmetries. It can also be extended superiorly in cases where the degree of stretch had been underestimated. In the event that it does not have enough give to meet the other edge of the wound, the superior margin cannot be readjusted inferiorly without creating

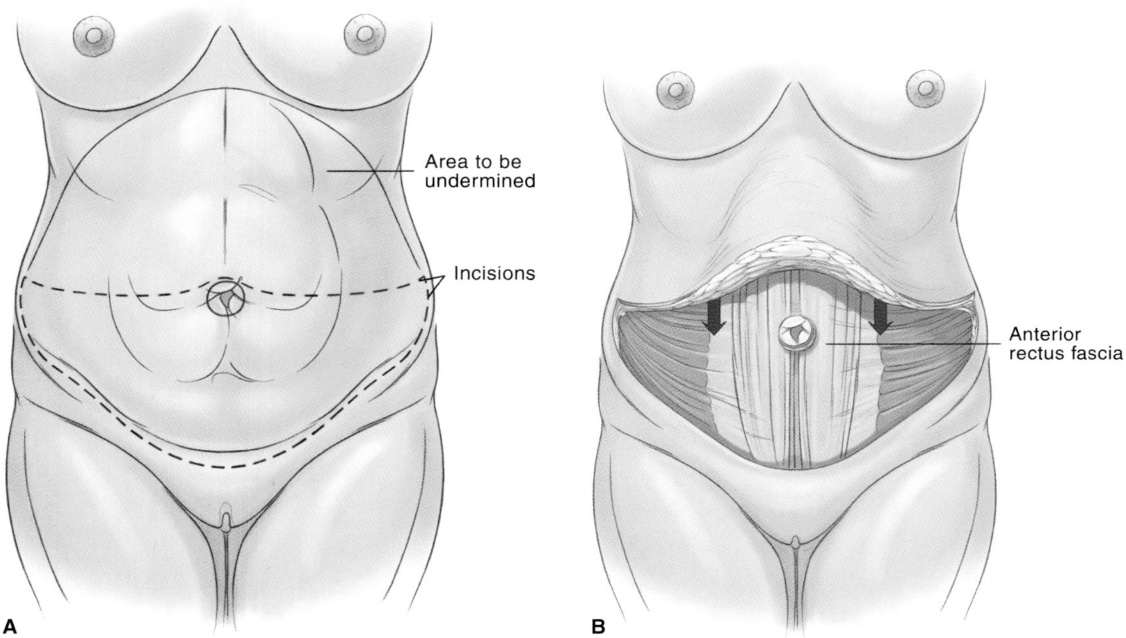

Figure 16–5. Steps in standard abdominoplasty. **A:** The incision lines to be made and the area to be undermined are shown. The area to be undermined is under the fasciocutaneous flap and above the rectus fascia, extending up to the breast bone. **B:** The resultant opening with the flap flipped up is shown. The umbilicus is circumscribed and left in place. **C:** The flap is pulled down to the inferior incision and split down the middle. The flaps are then excised at an angle to prevent a dog-ear. **D:** A hole is made in the pulled-down flap at the natural position of the umbilicus. The circumscribed umbilicus is then pulled through this opening.

additional scarring around the umbilicus. If the skin paddle is excised prior to a test at reapproximation of the wound edges, there is a danger that the wound will not be amenable to immediate closure. It is for this reason that preoperative assessment and clinical judgment are key issues for patient selection in abdominoplasty.

Once the paddle has been resected, the flap is temporarily reapproximated to the inferior wound margin using skin staples. A hand is placed under the flap to determine the position of the umbilicus. The superior pole of the umbilicus is marked on the flap at the midline. An incision is made at this point, and the umbilicus is pulled into the defect. Excess fat is removed from the undersurface of the new umbilical site to allow for a smooth contour and to permit the umbilicus to be brought out to the surface. It is then sutured to the fascia at four points to anchor it in place. These sutures are held untied until the flap is reapproximated.

The flap closure begins at the lateral edges of the wound, working toward the midline to prevent bowing at the sides. This is of particular concern because the superior edge is invariably longer than the inferior one, lending itself frequently to the formation of "dog ears" upon wound closure. The defect is closed in

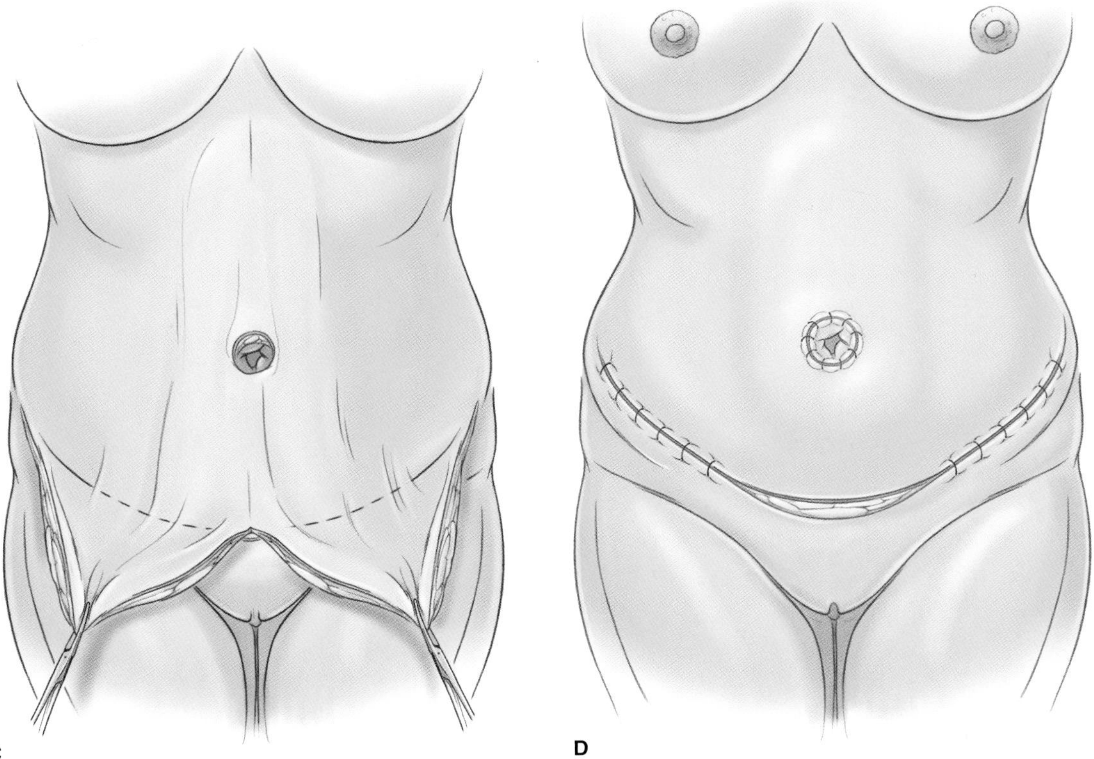

C D

Figure 16–5. (Continued)

several layers, using buried interrupted deep dermal sutures followed by a running subcuticular suture. The staples are removed as the flap is reapproximated, and tension should be minimized to improve healing. Drains are usually placed through stab wounds in the groin while the incision is being closed. The final step in an abdominoplasty is closure around the umbilicus. Using the four previously placed sutures, it is fixed to the abdominal wall. In addition to providing stability for umbilical positioning, this step also helps recreate a depression in the skin and provide a recessed umbilicus. The skin around it is then closed using interrupted deep dermal followed by running subcuticular sutures. Once in place, the umbilicus should rest comfortably in its new position, without evidence of being pulled by the surrounding skin.

There are many useful techniques for optimizing results in abdominoplasty. Several methods have been suggested to address the formation of "dog ears," including variations in the shape of the incision and different angles for excising the excess skin. In some cases, curving the lateral aspect of the wound edges downward can lengthen the inferior margin and compensate for some of the discrepancy. When amputating the excess skin, pulling each side of the flap toward the contralateral side can create more length at the midline compared with the sides, facilitating smooth reapproximation of the outer edges of the wound. Ultimately, while the wound will flatten over time in the postoperative period, efforts should be made to achieve the smoothest contour possible intraoperatively. Liposuction may be used at the end of the case for "fine tuning."

While the raised flap is extensively undermined, the skin inferior to the abdominoplasty wound is generally left intact. As a result, the tissues superior to the incision have flexibility to move and bow, while the tissues that lie inferior are fixed in place. In some patients, this results in the development of a step or a pouch above the incision line. A minimal degree of undermining inferior to the wound margin (at the mons veneris) can help mobilize that skin. This can be helpful both for smoothing the area over the incision and for creating more give at the incision site, facilitating closure. Furthermore, upward retraction of the mons may result in a more aesthetically pleasing form.

During undermining of the abdominoplasty flap, care must be taken to identify and cauterize perforating vessels. If the vessels are transected without being cauterized, they will often retract into the rectus sheath. This can increase the incidence of hematoma formation, and with it the ensuing complications.

Plication of the muscular aponeurosis is also subject to a wide variety of technical considerations (Figure 16–6). While it is most standard to imbricate at the midline, it has been argued that the natural delineation of the rectus muscle focuses on its lateral borders. With this in mind, some surgeons elect to imbricate in two separate vertical lines. The aponeurotic layer is tightened lateral to the midline, recreating the natural silhouette of the abdominal wall. When imbrication is not performed at the midline, the fascia surrounding the umbilical stalk must be tightened as a separate step. Laxity at this position may predispose to hernia formation. The surrounding fascia should be wrapped snuggly around the umbilical stalk, yet with enough give to not compromise blood flow.

Finally, there are a variety of approaches to the final closure of the flap. The abdominoplasty closure has an inherent amount of tension. Closure must be secure and in layers in order to distribute that pressure evenly. An excessive number of tight sutures may compromise blood flow, however, and this can have disastrous results on wound healing. Therefore, it is important in this procedure to achieve a balance between a secure closure and good circulatory perfusion.

D. Complications

Abdominoplasty is a relatively safe procedure, with a low incidence of morbidity and mortality. Most of the morbidity associated with the procedure can be attributed to wound complications, either at the incision site or at the umbilicus. Mortality following abdominoplasty is extremely rare and is usually due to pulmonary embolism.

Pulmonary embolism is the most dangerous complication of abdominoplasty. Its incidence increases with smoking, lack of mobility in the immediate postoperative period, and lack of venous thromboembolism prophylaxis. Increased awareness and prophylactic measures have lowered the incidence of this complication since the initial reports in the 1970s. In a national survey of abdominoplasty-related complications in 2005, it was found that the incidence of mortality has declined, and the use of liposuction as an adjunct to abdominoplasty has not contributed to an increase in morbidity. With regard to technique, there was no correlation between the incidence of complications and degree of experience of the practitioner.

Tension on the wound and inadequate perfusion can lead to breakdown at the surgical site. This occurs most commonly at the

REFERENCES

American Society of Plastic Surgeons. 2009 Report of the 2008 Statistics National Clearinghouse of Plastic Surgery Statistics. Available at: wwww.plasticsurgery.org/Media/stats/2008-US-cosmetic-reconstructive-plastic-surgery-minimally-invasive-statistics.pdf. Accessed August 7, 2009.

Graf R et al. Lipoabdominoplasty: liposuction with reduced undermining and traditional abdominal skin flap resection. *Aesthetic Plast Surg.* 2006 Jan–Feb;30(1):1–8. [PMID: 16404652]

Khan S et al. Do progressive tension sutures really decrease complications in abdominoplasty? *Ann Plast Surg.* 2006 Jan;56(1):14–20. [PMID: 16374089]

Kim J et al. Abdominoplasty, liposuction of the flanks, and obesity: analyzing risk factors for seroma formation. *Plast Reconstr Surg.* 2006 Mar;117(3):773–9. [PMID: 16525264]

Kryger Z et al. The outcome of abdominoplasty performed under conscious sedation: six-year experience in 153 consecutive cases. *Plast Reconstr Surg.* 2004 May;113(6):1807–17. [PMID: 15114149]

Mast BA. Safety and efficacy of outpatient full abdominoplasty. *Ann Plast Surg.* 2005 Mar;54(3):256–9. [PMID: 15725826]

Matarasso A et al. Abdominoplasty and abdominal contour surgery: a national plastic surgery survey. *Plast Reconstr Surg.* 2006 May;117(6):1797–808. [PMID: 16651953]

Matarasso A et al. Abdominal contour procedures: evaluating the options. *Dermatol Clin.* 2005 Jul;23(3):475–93. [PMID: 16039428]

Mayr M et al. Effects of aesthetic abdominoplasty on abdominal wall perfusion: a quantitative evaluation. *Plast Reconstr Surg.* 2004 Nov;114(6):1586–94. [PMID: 15509954]

Michaels BM et al. Outpatient abdominoplasty facilitated by rib blocks. *Plast Reconstr Surg.* 2009 Aug;124(2):635–42. [PMID: 19644285]

Persichetti P et al. Anchor-line abdominoplasty: a comprehensible approach to abdominal wall reconstruction and body contouring. *Plast Reconstr Surg.* 2005 Jul;116(1):289–94. [PMID: 15988280]

Pitanguy I. Evaluation of body contouring surgery today: a 30-year perspective. *Plast Reconstr Surg.* 2000 Apr;105(4):1499–514. [PMID: 10744246]

Pollock H et al. Progressive tension sutures: a technique to reduce local complications in abdominoplasty. *Plast Reconstr Surg.* 2000 Jun;105(7):2583–6. [PMID: 10845315]

Sanger C et al. Impact of significant weight loss on outcome of body-contouring surgery. *Ann Plast Surg.* 2006 Jan;56(1):9–13. [PMID: 16374088]

Shestak KC. Marriage abdominoplasty expands the mini-abdominoplasty concept. *Plast Reconstr Surg.* 1999 Mar;103(3):1020–31. [PMID: 10077098]

von Uchelen JH et al. Complications of abdominoplasty in 86 patients. *Plast Reconstr Surg.* 2001 Jun;107(7):1869–73. [PMID : 11391211]

Yousif NJ et al. Transverse rectus sheath plication in abdominoplasty. *Plast Reconstr Surg.* 2004 Sep 1;114(3):778–84. [PMID: 15318062]

CHAPTER 17

Liposuction

Kevin J. Cross, MD & John E. Sherman, MD, FACS

According to the American Society of Plastic Surgeons, 245,138 liposuction procedures were performed in 2008. Of these, 218,038 were done in women and 27,100 were done in men, making it the third most common cosmetic procedure performed in 2008.

After some controversy regarding whether liposuction could be performed in a non-hospital setting, it has been shown that with proper patient selection and surgical team preparation, liposuction can be safely done in the office or surgical center setting using a choice of purely tumescent anesthesia, sedation, or general anesthesia.

► COMPONENTS & DEVICES

TUMESCENCE DELIVERY

The administration of fluid that acts in both a hemostatic and anesthetic manner prior to lipoaspiration has been one of the fundamental steps in improving the safety profile of liposuction. Large syringes can be attached to an infusion cannula for fluid injection into small surgical sites. However, standard procedure now dictates the use of intravenous infusion devices for larger regions. These can range from a pressure cuff or air-filled bladder that applies positive pressure to a liter bag of solution, with a roll lock or stop-cock to allow the surgeon control of flow, to a motorized, pedal driven pump. The preferred method of tumescent delivery is through a peristaltic pump machine. These devices allow control of speed and rate of delivery in addition to precise on and off control. They may deliver flow upwards of 200 mL/min, but this rate is controlled to ensure maximal patient comfort. Long 27–32 cm cannulae allow infusion over large areas, while shorter 17–20 cm devices offer greater control and precision. Two 3.0 mm diameter cannulae can infuse tumescent solution at rates over 200 mL/min and are useful for large-volume infusion. In smaller cases, such as submental liposuction, better control is afforded by 18–20 gauge spinal needles attached to syringes.

SUCTION-ASSISTED LIPOSUCTION

Suction-assisted liposuction (SAL) evolved from subcutaneous lipectomy techniques that were originally performed using uterine curettes. Schrudde and others found these early techniques to be successful in removing subcutaneous fat, but the high rates of hematoma and lymphatic collections in the resulting dead space lead to a flurry of innovations. Fischer, Kesselring, and Teimourian each developed modifications of suction cannula. In 1978, Illouz described the tunneling lipoplasty technique that has become the current standard from which all further advancements in suction-assisted liposuction have developed.

The negative pressure in suction-assisted liposuction is typically generated from an external mechanical aspirator. Optimal aspiration rates are generally reached at 1 atmosphere of negative pressure (29 inches or 74 cm of mercury) but lower levels are typically preferred when performing liposuction of more delicate regions. For subtle contouring and in areas around the head and neck, manual suction may be performed with the use of a 60 mL syringe. A locking device offers the surgeon complete control of the strength of negative pull through the cannula and ease of maneuverability.

Aspiration is achieved through cannulae that vary in shapes, diameters, and lengths. The shaft portion is made of stainless steel but may be coated with zirconium nitride or polytetrafluoroethylene to reduce friction and enhance glide. Most commonly a blunt or bullet shaped tip is used with one or multiple apertures positioned a few millimeters behind the tip. This orientation protects non-lipomatous tissue from trauma by allowing the tip to lift away dermal and other vital structures of the skin before they are trapped in the suction portals.

Suction cannulae range from 10 cm to 35 cm in length. They should be chosen based on the length needed to cover the entire area of planned treatment to avoid imbalances in aspiration and to allow proper feathering at the edges of the treated areas. Varying the cannula diameter will also aid in contouring.

For large debulking procedures, 4–5 mm Mercedes type cannulae are available. Large caliber cannulae are generally discouraged and should be used with caution because of the ridging and deformation of contour that commonly occurs. Smaller, 2–3 mm Mercedes type cannulae are more often used for feathering and for more refined work in small anatomic regions, or for use in more superficial planes.

In the past three decades, liposuction has evolved from a "fringe" procedure to one of the most common procedures performed by plastic surgeons. Because of this popularity, the results similarly have improved and have evolved to be more predictable with the refinements of technique and instrumentation.

The problem of earlier techniques was that they were dependent on the stamina and strength of the surgeon, and fatigue often preceded poor results, especially if more than one case was performed. Newer modalities have removed the physicality from the procedure, thereby avoiding fatigue and improving results. These improvements included ultrasound liposuction and power-assisted liposuction.

ULTRASOUND-ASSISTED LIPOSUCTION

Although ultrasound-assisted liposuction initially showed great promise, uncertainties mounted regarding its safety profile. Many experts grew significantly concerned over complications related to the heat generated at the cannula tip during the procedure as well as high seroma rates. In addition, the inflated cost of the equipment has encouraged converstion to power-assisted liposuction and other modalities. More recently, however, experience and prudence when using ultrasound-assisted liposuction has led to large studies that have demonstrated its relative safety and cosmetically pleasing results.

To generate high frequency electrical energy, standard electricity is passed through a converter. A piezoelectric crystal located in the hand piece then converts the electrical energy to mechanical vibrations. A titanium probe amplifies and transmits these vibrations at a frequency of 20,000-40,000 Hz, causing fluctuating pressures within the tissues, ultimately leading to cell wall rupture. Fat cells, having the lowest impedance to this form of energy, are most susceptible to the impulses that are transmitted through the subcutaneous tissue, and thus are most affected. Additional energy in the form of heat is produced as a result of the thermal effect of the acoustic wave, by cannula friction, and through conversion of ultrasonic energy waves. Because of this, ultrasound must be performed in a wet, tumescent environment. The exogenously delivered fluid not only acts as a sink for heat dissipation, but also lowers the impedence of fat, allowing better penetration. To avoid tissue coagulation from local heat buildup, the probe must always be kept in motion, and wound protectors and wet towels around the operative field add further protection to the surrounding skin. For short treatments, incision length may be minimized by foregoing the use of the wound protector. In these cases, a continuous drip of physiologic fluid should be maintained on the probe and the entrance site. To further reduce the risk of excessive heat buildup, the wetting solution can be cooled prior to infusion.

Risk of skin trauma and burns as well as peripheral nerve damage appear to be less of a concern with the more recent development of smaller, solid core probes, lower energy output devices, shorter ultrasound times and strict adherence to the principles described above. Solid probes require an added step for lipoaspiration, however, and caution must still be used when considering ultrasound-assisted liposuction in regions where peripheral nerve damage could be catastrophic (ie, the face and extremities).

A recent advancement in ultrasound-assisted liposuction has been the Vaser device. The company claims that a smaller diameter solid probe with a grooved tip region increases the device's ability to fragment solution and improves the depth of penetration of these lasers. After treatment, the released fat is then removed by lipoaspiration in a second step. Recent publications have demonstrated the capability of the Vaser technology in "high definition liposculpturing." High definition liposculpturing is a method of performing liposuction in such a way as to enhance the musculoskeletal shape of the torso and body by "etching" the contour of the underlying muscles and tendinous inscriptions into the overlying tissue. This requires very superficial removal of fat. Published results are impressive, but the added length of time for the two-step procedure, a complication rate above 10%, and the steep learning curve have prevented widespread acceptance of the technique at this time.

POWER-ASSISTED LIPOSUCTION

Originally designed as a rotating blade within an otherwise hollow cannula, power-assisted liposuction has evolved to a system that uses a reciprocating hand piece that is now safer and less traumatic. Options include both electrical and nitrogen powered drive trains, the former being less noise and typically less bulky. These motors can generate reciprocating motion in the hand piece upwards of 8000 strokes/min. Studies show that 40% or more lipoaspirate can be obtained per pass in difficult areas, such as the knees and hips, with the aid of the mechanically driven motion. Some surgeons believe that improved intraoperative and postoperative pain as well as ecchymoses and edema results from the use of these devices, possibly resulting from the need for less passes to achieve the desired results.

Vibroliposuction is a variation of power-assisted liposuction that allows for a reciprocating motion in multiple axes and may afford added benefit over traditional power-assisted liposuction.

External ultrasound-assisted liposuction is accomplished through the transcutaneous application of ultrasonic waves prior to traditional liposuction. After application of ultrasonic gel, either a 3-MHz probe to reach the subdermal fat layer, or a 1-MHz probe for deeper penetration is applied to the skin. Though some suggest that seroma formation occurs with less frequency and that recovery time is shorter as a result of this therapy, results have varied, and thus the benefit to its use is questionable.

LASER-ASSISTED LIPOSUCTION

Many variations of laser-assisted liposuction exist. The probe of the intracannular YAG laser is carried down a hollow cannula. It delivers short pulses of energy that mechanically shears any fat cells that are drawn into the cannula with only marginal elevations in tissue temperature.

A fiberoptic Nd:YAG laser (1064 nm) is thought to selectively target fat cells with a chromophore that is specific for tissue colors in the yellow spectrum. It is delivered through a fiber that is passed along a 1-mm cannula and causes cavitation of fat and lipolysis. The resulting waste product is then removed via suction aspiration, with minimal peripheral damage. On average, 600 j of energy are delivered for each palm-sized area treated.

Compared to suction-assisted liposuction, laser-assisted liposuction has been shown to increase operative times by 30% and can be prohibitively costly to maintain. Furthermore, the removed fat is incapable of being used for lipofilling, and unaspirated emulsified fat has the potential to release fatty acids and triglycerides into the bloodstream, which could have harmful effects on organs such as the liver and kidneys, though animal studies suggest otherwise.

Benefits include a suggested decrease in the amount of blood found in the lipoaspirate as well as reduced postoperative pain. Devices that contain probes emitting in wavelength that are thought to tighten skin are now available in addition to higher energy delivering platforms, opening new possibilities for expanded uses and shorter operative times with the laser liposuction devices.

Low-level "cold" lasers (eg, helium-neon and gallium arsenide diode) transmit transcutaneous energy in the 630–640 nm range. Treatment is thought to encourage proliferation of fibroblasts and keratinocytes, improvement in tissue circulation, and diminution of scars. Additionally, this wavelength range has been shown by electron microscopy to promote transient formation of pores in the cell wall of adipocytes that are large enough to allow fat to escape.

▶ ANESTHESIA

Liposuction should be limited to patients in relatively good health and classified into class I or II (ASA I or ASA II) according to the American Society of Anesthesiologists. An anesthesiologist should be present to provide sedation, pain control, and monitoring. This includes baseline vital signs as well as continuous blood pressure monitoring and cardiac monitoring with a pulse oximeter. Supplemental oxygen should be available if needed, and a plan for management of medical emergencies should be in place.

TUMESCENT SOLUTION

Originally described by Illouz as a hypotonic preparation to help hydrodissect and lyse fat cells, wetting solution was later modified so as to contain lidocaine for pain control and epinephrine for vasoconstriction. Further modifications by Klein and others allowed for safe, large-volume infusions under minimal to no sedation. In addition to reducing pain and blood loss, the increased tumescent volume was thought to prevent hypovolemia through gradual absorption of the infused solution. As larger volume liposuctions were performed, the concern has shifted away from the sequelae of hypovolemia to that of fluid overload. Scattered reports of congestive heart failure following large-volume tumescent liposuction underscore the need to closely monitor fluid delivery. There is no evidence in the literature that ratios of infiltrate to aspirate greater than 1:1 are safer and more beneficial. Today, standard solutions contain normal saline with 0.1% lidocaine, epinephrine 1:1,000,000, and often some amount of sodium bicarbonate.

LIDOCAINE TOXICITY

After liposuction gained popularity, complications and deaths were reported in the lay press as well as the in medical literature. Most mortalities during this time occurred after the patient was discharged from the surgical facility. After lidocaine absorption was studied, it was apparent that an understanding of the metabolism and safe blood levels was essential. Traditionally, the maximum dose of lidocaine injected locally was 7 mg/kg when given with epinephrine. Experience with tumescent solution demonstrated that higher doses can be administered safely into the subcutaneous tissues with little risk of lidocaine toxicity; doses as high as 55 mg/kg are now being reported in the literature. Although some lidocaine is removed during lipoaspiration (approximately 10%–30%) prior to being systemically absorbed, tissue buffering of lidocaine through binding to subcutaneous cells and extracellular matrix affords the greatest limitation to systemic absorption. The 10-fold dilution of lidocaine in tumescent solution (1%–0.1%) means that there is a smaller concentration of lidocaine injected per region of tissue compared with standard local injection, and thus a greater opportunity for the tissue to effectively bind the drug.

This interaction between lidocaine and the surrounding tissue also plays a role in the time at which lidocaine blood levels peak. This has been shown to occur somewhere between 5 and 17 hours after injection and is not related to the rate of tumescent infusion. As these numbers suggest, slow release of protein-bound lidocaine means that peak plasma levels often occur when the patient has been discharged. Using standard tumescent solutions with a maximal lidocaine dose of 35 mg/kg, it is likely that greater than 5% of patients will have levels of the analgesic that peak above 4 mcg/mL, well within the range of symptomatic toxicity. Thus, the surgeon is advised to be familiar with the signs of toxicity at varying plasma lidocaine concentrations. The toxicity begins with numbness of the tongue, lightheadedness, metallic taste, tinnitus, and visual disturbances and progresses to muscle twitching, unconsciousness, and seizures, then coma, respiratory arrest, and cardiovascular depression. Plasma lidocaine levels of less than 5 mcg/mL are unlikely to have cardiovascular toxicities. Levels of 5–10 mcg/mL can cause hypotension by inducing both cardiac suppression and vascular smooth muscle relaxation. Levels of more than 30 mcg/mL are associated with cardiovascular collapse. Anticonvulsants, such as benzodiazepines and barbiturates (diazepam 5–10 mg, thiopental 50–100 mg), are the drugs of choice for seizure control. Phenytoin is not effective and should be avoided. Succinylcholine may also be used to terminate the neuromuscular effects of seizures. Because succinylcholine paralyzes all muscles, the patient requires intubation.

Since it is metabolized by the P450 system in the liver, levels of lidocaine and its major metabolite monoethylglycinexlidide may be potentiated by a host of medications and herbal substitutes. The clinician must note that approximately 5% of the U.S. population takes herbal medications. These medications must be stopped at least 2 weeks prior to surgery.

EPINEPHRINE

The safe dose of epinephrine is 0.7 mg/kg; however, doses as high as 10 mg/kg have been reported without adverse effects. Standard infusion with 1:1,000,000 solution will cause peak epinephrine levels equal to the endogenous levels produced by open abdominal surgery or aortic cross-clamping, however, and occur 1–4 hours after infusion. These levels have been found to be associated with arrhythmias, myocardial infarction, and asystole, offering further emphasis to the need for proper patient selection to avoid such complications. The use of epinephrine not only aids in vasoconstriction and thus results in less blood loss, but it quadruples the length of the anesthetic effect of lidocaine.

▶ PROCEDURES

PATIENT EVALUATION & SELECTION

Careful patient selection is the key to minimizing complications and maximizing results. A careful medical history must start with the search for any contraindications to elective surgery in general, and specifically the use of tumescent solutions. This may include any prior or family history of clotting disorders, any history that potentially puts a patient at increased risk after epinephrine administration (eg, history of pheochromocytoma, hyperthyroidism, severe hypertension, or cardiac disease), and any comorbidities that may be exacerbated by fluid administration (eg, congestive heart failure, chronic obstructive pulmonary disease).

After a thorough medical history is obtained, a weight and nutritional evaluation must be performed. Patients with severe weight fluctuations should not undergo surgery. The patient's weight should remain stable the 6 months preceding surgery. A thorough history should include calculation of the body mass index (BMI), and stability of the patient's weight by recording the patient's weight 6 months and 1 year prior to examination. The patient who is at his or her lowest weight and does not have the ability to maintain this low weight is not a good candidate for liposuction. Both the patient and the surgeon will be disappointed as weight gain ensues. Liposuction reduces the number of fat cells, but the remaining adipocytes can hypertrophy and swell with triglyceride accumulation. The patient will notice a different distribution of fat cells and weight gain in areas where liposuction was not performed.

In a preoperative consultation with the patient, the potential need for revisional surgery should be addressed. A clear policy in writing should be given to the patient concerning the fees, if any, for revisional surgery. This will avoid postoperative conflicts over this important issue.

A thorough history is complemented by preoperative photographic documentation. This will allow the surgeon to view photographs of the patient in the standing position when the patient is supine or prone during surgery, and also will enable the surgeon and patient to compare and review postoperative results.

The patient's preoperative weight must be obtained, and subsequently at all postoperative visits. This way the surgeon and the patient will recognize if untoward aesthetic results are a product of technique or dietary indiscretion. If it is the latter, the weight taken by the nurse and told to the patient will quickly diffuse any dissatisfaction.

Examination of the skin and its elasticity is necessary. Patients who have had large weight loss will not have the same ability to contract the skin after surgery. Similarly, the approach and volume removed for a 60-year-old patient will be different than the amount removed from a 30-year-old patient.

PATIENT PREPARATION

Although large-volume liposuction has been proven to be a relatively safe approach (see below), serial liposuction procedures may be preferable when the volume of aspirate is expected to be greater than 5 L or the total operative time is expected to be greater than 3 hours. Success should be judged not only by results and aesthetic goals, but by the ease of recovery and rapid return of the patient to his or her daily routine. With large fluid shifts accompanying large-volume liposuction, the patient's level of satisfaction with the total procedure significantly decreases.

Prior to the operation, a discussion with the anesthesiologist ensures an understanding about the expected volume of liposuction, the maximum safe dose of tumescence that can be used, and whether there will be a need for positional changes during the case.

A. Preoperative Marking

The patient is marked in a standing position in front of a three-way mirror using topographic relief to outline the areas most bothersome to the patient as well as the regions where feathering will occur (Figure 17–1). Each

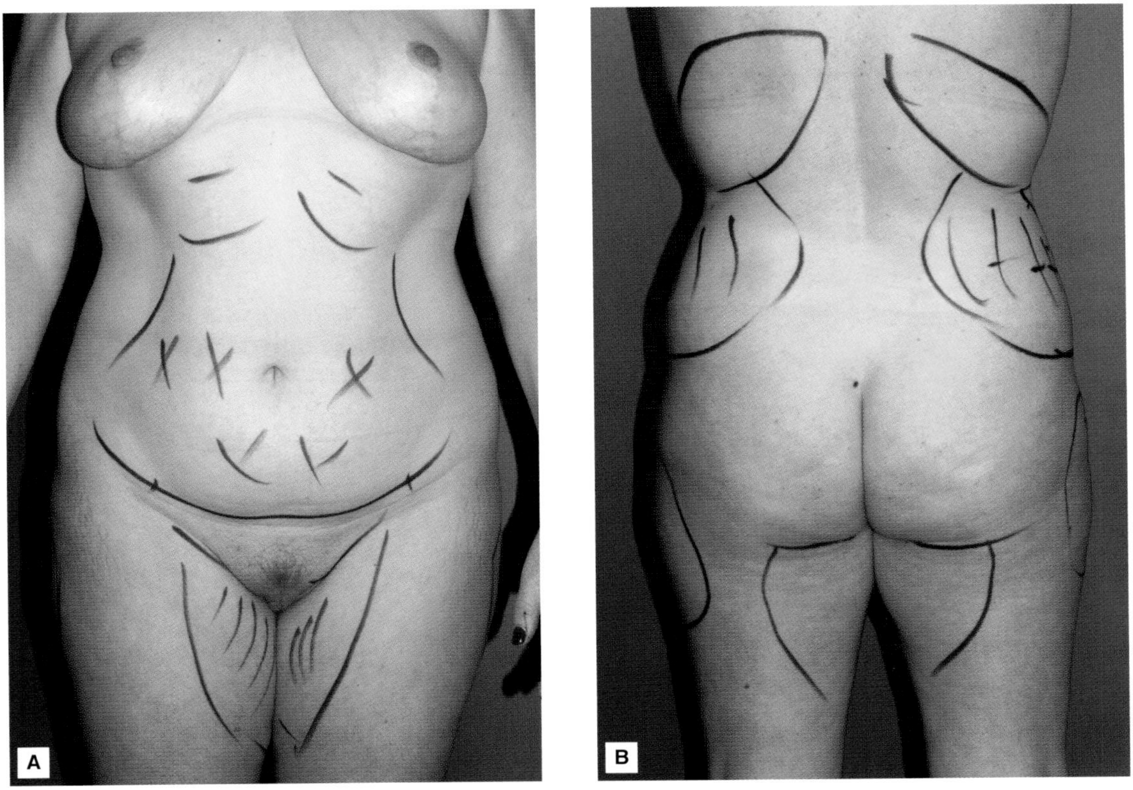

Figure 17–1. Preoperative markings demonstrating areas to be targeted during the liposuction procedure.

UAL Worksheet

Name:	Pre-op Measurements (cm)	Post-op Date	Post-op Date	Post-op Date	Post-op Date	Post-op Date
Thigh Circumference: cm below Asis						
Right:						
Left:						
ARMS: (Mid-Humerus)						
Right:						
Left:						
KNEES: (Top-Patella)						
Right:						
Left:						
Abdomen:						
Costal Margin						
2 cm above umbilicus						
5 cm below umbilicus						
Weight: (lbs.)						

Figure 17–2. Worksheet used to document the circumferential measurements of each part of the body that is addressed during liposuction. These measurements are made preoperatively and at each subsequent postoperative visit. (Used with permission John E. Sherman, MD, FACS.)

planned incision site is shown to the patient. The patient's measurements at given sites are carefully recorded; they are also taken after specific intervals in the postoperative period (Figure 17–2). This will assist in determining the change of the areas that were treated. A perioperative dose of a first-generation cephalosporin (or vancomycin for patients allergic to first-generation cephalosporins) is given prior to skin incision.

B. Positioning

While some surgeons use the lateral decubitus position, most surgeons prefer to approach the back and front using the prone and supine positions, respectively, and in that order. Bolsters are placed cephalad to the trochanteric area and under the chest to avoid distortion of the medial and lateral thighs and waist area (Figure 17–3). There should be no difficulty in obtaining good lateral contour and along the flanks using this technique. For extensive liposuction of multiple sites, the room is warmed, and the patient is prepared with povidone-iodine in a whole body fashion prior to lying on a sterile sheet. Forced air warming drapes are used in the areas that are not exposed during surgery, as well as sequential compression devices placed on the calves.

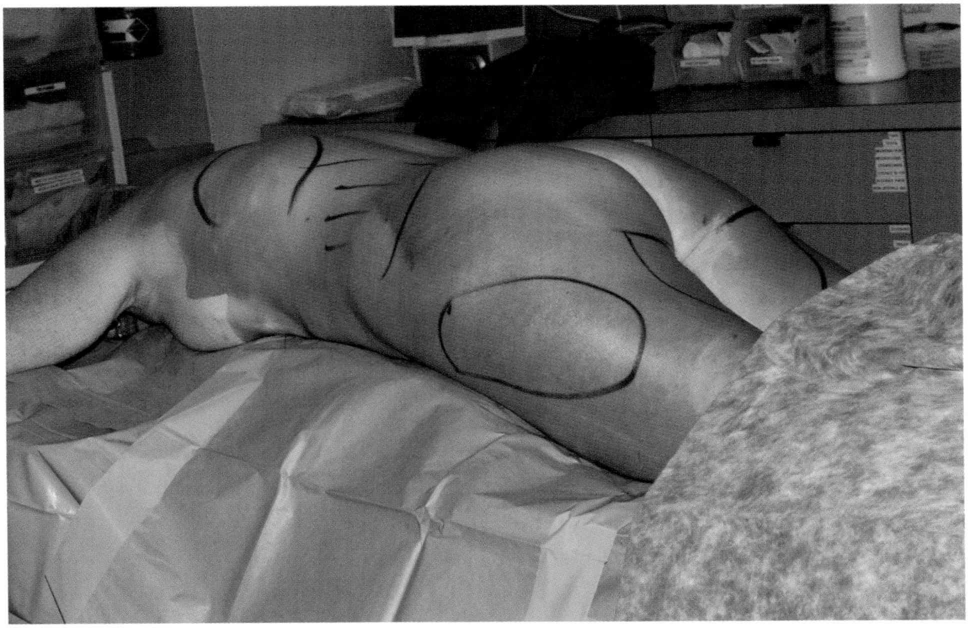

Figure 17–3. Demonstration of the prone positioning used to access the flanks, hips, thighs, and back. Notice that, with the use of bolsters placed cephalad to the trochanteric area and under the chest, there is little distortion to the tissues of the thighs and back, and excellent exposure to the lateral regions in these areas.

TECHNIQUE

Most patients undergo the procedure in a certified free-standing ambulatory surgery facility. A small percentage will have the procedure at the hospital as an outpatient. While this procedure may be performed under general, epidural, and straight tumescent anesthesia, intravenous sedation administered by a board certified anesthesiologist is a common first choice. Prior to the day of surgery, the anesthesiologist speaks with the patient, obtaining a history and allying the patient's concerns.

A. Male Patients

Due to the higher density of the fat in male patients, almost all procedures performed on men involve UAL initially to the breast, abdomen and posterior waist (Figure 17–4). All males undergoing gynecomastia correction are informed prior to surgery of the possible need to use a combined open approach if there is significant breast tissue remaining. Often, this is impossible to determine until the end of the liposuction procedure. A periareolar incision is then made, and an open procedure follows. This occurs in less than 5% of patients and is more frequent in the adolescent.

B. Female Patients

Some moderate liposuction cases can be performed without the use of ultrasound in patients who lack dense fat. They do well with power-assisted liposuction and standard aspiration (Figure 17–5).

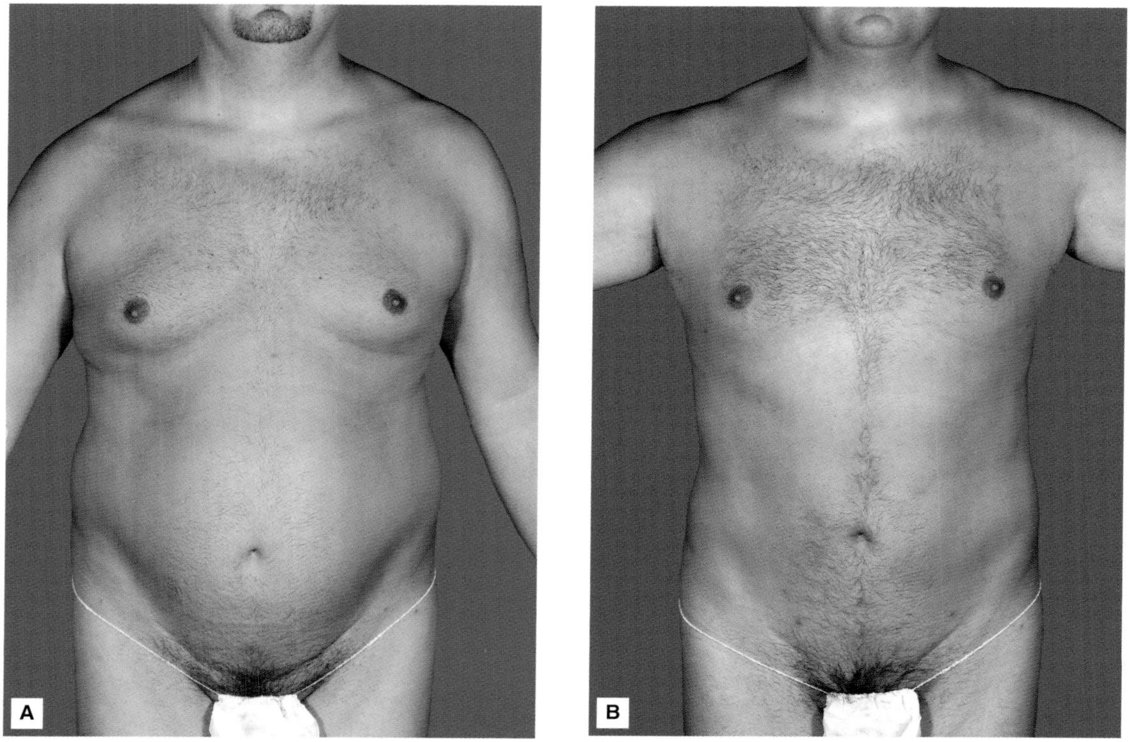

Figure 17–4. Preoperative pictures (A and B) and postoperative results (C and D) after using ultrasound assisted liposuction for the fibrous and densely proportioned fat of the male breast, abdomen, and lower back.

After the patient is positioned as noted above, sedation is administered. Through multiple 2-mm incisions created with a Beaver blade, the tumescent solution is infiltrated to all sites. This allows the epinephrine to take effect. Depending on the site where the procedure is to be performed and the sex of the patient, a triphase procedure is performed. Ultrasound-assisted liposuction is performed first in this triphase approach. Initially, ultrasound-assisted liposuction was the mainstay of the procedure. Now ultrasound-assisted liposuction is performed in a fashion that minimizes overall time of application to minimize postoperative edema. Time allotted to an average abdomen is about 2 minutes via three incisions; to the lateral thigh 90 seconds; and the posterior waist about 90 seconds. Ultrasound-assisted liposuction has no role in treating the following sites: submental region, inner thighs, and lower legs.

In addition to recording the amount of tumescent solution infused and lipoaspirate removed for each region addressed, the time of active ultrasound activity is carefully recorded (Figure 17–6).

The second phase is the use of the Microaire® power-assisted liposuction. This allows for an efficient evacuation of the lipoaspirate from the ultrasound-assisted liposuction, and further contouring. Cannulae are usually

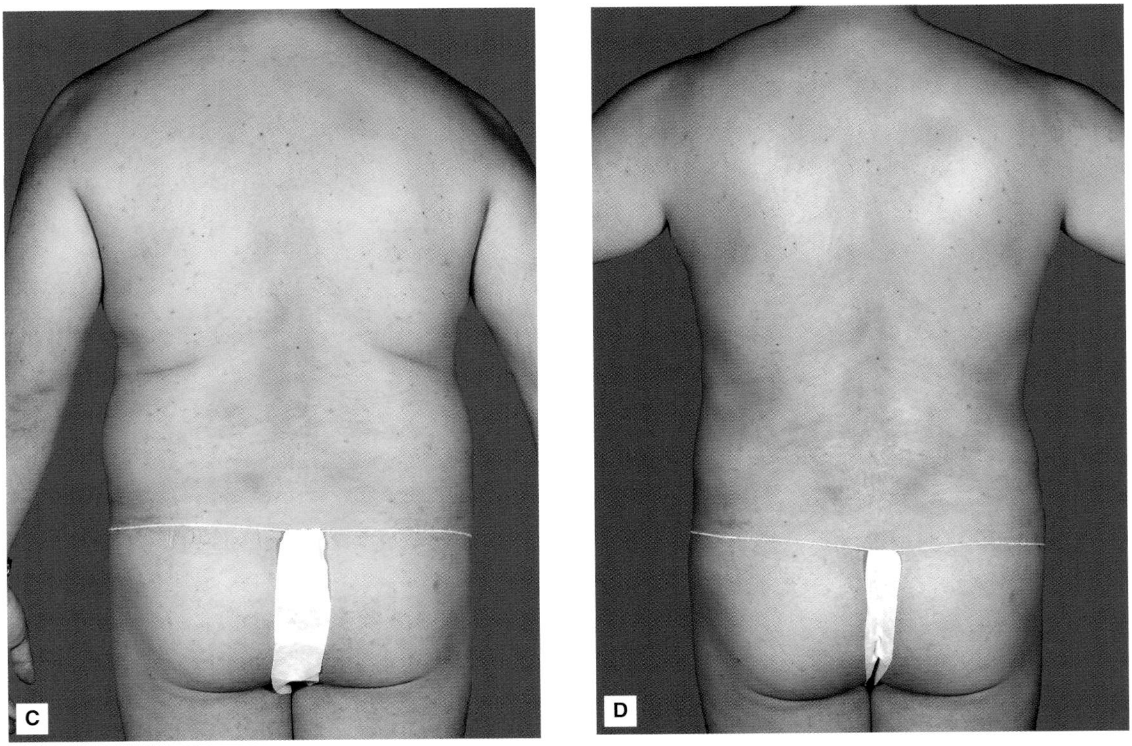

Figure 17–4. (Continued)

no larger than 4 mm. Various types of cannulae are used, depending on the site.

The third phase is the use of standard Grams Mercedes cannulae. Cannulae that are no larger that the 3.7 standard Mercedes tip are used. This allows for feathering of the area, and refinement in the superficial plane.

▶ POSTOPERATIVE CARE

Patients are discharged from the facility after meeting the criteria of the ASA and the American Association for Accreditation of Ambulatory Surgical Facilities (AAAASF). They are given prescriptions for analgesia at the preoperative meeting so that the medications are available immediately after discharge.

At the termination of the procedure, the patient is placed in a compression garment that covers all of the treated areas. They may remove the garment the following day to shower. Garment use is encouraged for 5–7 days following surgery.

Early ambulation is encouraged immediately after discharge and throughout the first night. Oral analgesics are given the first night and immediately tapered the following day. Dosages and class are determined by the need of the patient. Most patients switch to acetaminophen by the first postoperative day. Sutures are removed at 1 week. Patients are then seen at the following intervals: 3 weeks, 6 weeks, and 9 weeks.

Revision surgery, if necessary, is not performed until at least 4 months after the

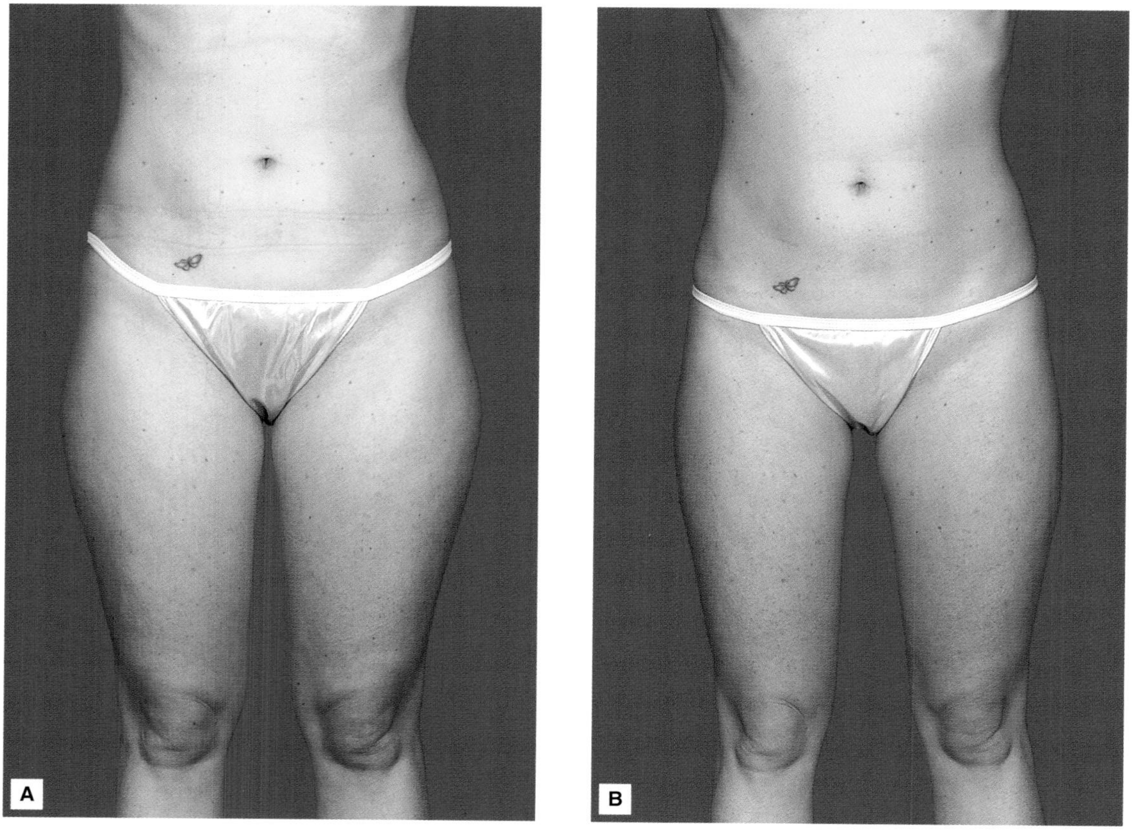

Figure 17–5. Traditional and power assisted liposuction was used in the female with less dense fat on palpation. Preoperative pictures (**A** and **B**) and 6-month postoperative results (**C** and **D**).

procedure. Most of these may be performed under local anesthesia with syringe liposuction; though some require mild sedation.

In larger liposuction procedures, patients are treated with transcutaneous ultrasound therapy twice weekly starting at the second postoperative week, which may help alleviate uncomfortable swelling.

▶ COMPLICATIONS

Complications following liposuction should be classified as either severe and potentially life-threatening or cosmetic. The former is minimized with proper patient selection and preoperative preparation, while the latter is minimized through the use of proper technique.

SEVERE COMPLICATIONS

A. Pulmonary Embolism

Risk of pulmonary embolism (PE) is reduced by screening patients for any prior history of family history of PEs or deep venous

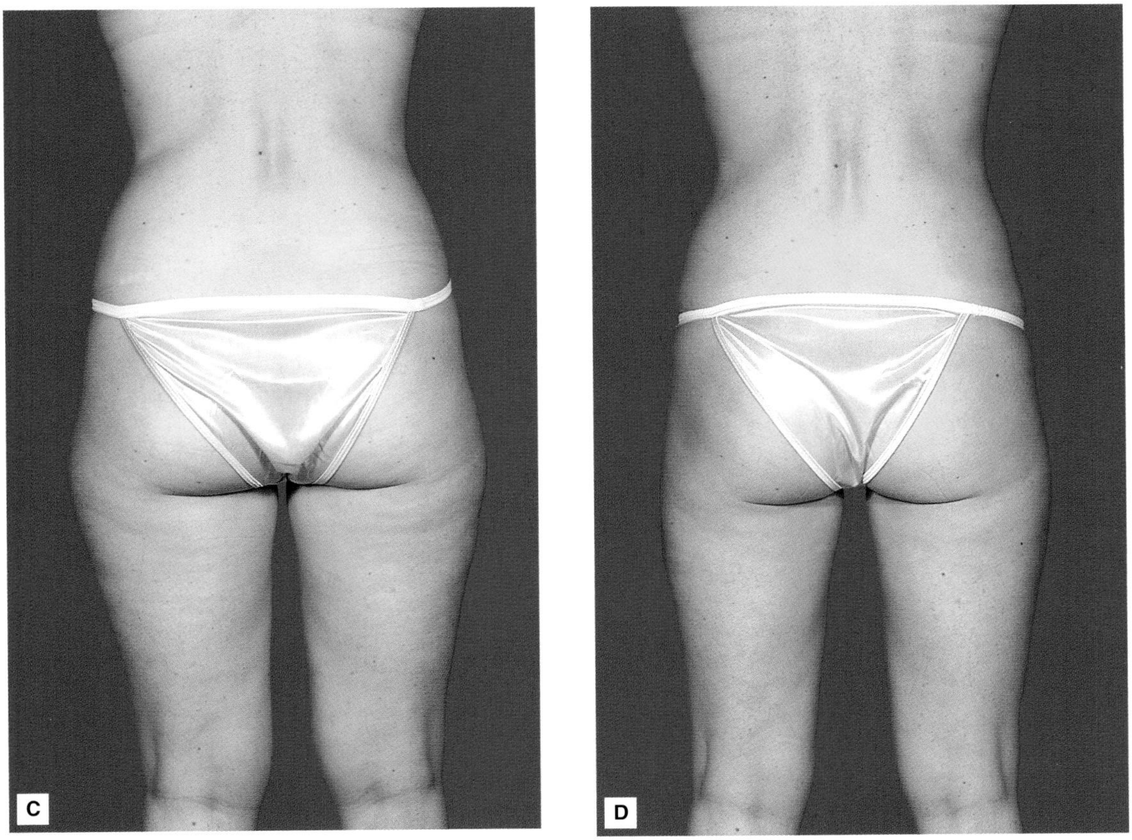

Figure 17–5. (Continued)

thrombosis (DVT). Other risk factors include age greater than 60, obesity, and the use of hormone replacement therapy. Furthermore, if lower extremity examination reveals the presence of significant varicosities, this elective procedure should not be performed.

Intraoperative risk to DVT formation and thus an embolic event is reduced by the routine use of pneumatic compression boots. Although most guidelines recommend using pneumatic compression boots for procedures that are expected to last longer than 1 hour, there is no reason why they should not be mandatory for all cosmetic procedures.

Additional precautions include limiting procedures to 3 hours or less and the use of proper postoperative pain control to allow the patient early active mobility. Rarely, is pharmaceutical DVT prophylaxis necessary if patients are carefully selected and case length minimized. These medications, which include heparin (5000 units two to three times per day) or enoxaparin (20–40 mg/d), are typically indicated for patients at moderate to high risk for an embolic event, such as those with a history of prior DVT, major trauma, or an immobilizing illness.

Fat embolism syndrome is an embolic event related to the direct manipulation of fat and its introduction into the bloodstream. While it may be under recognized, only a few documented cases have been reported, and

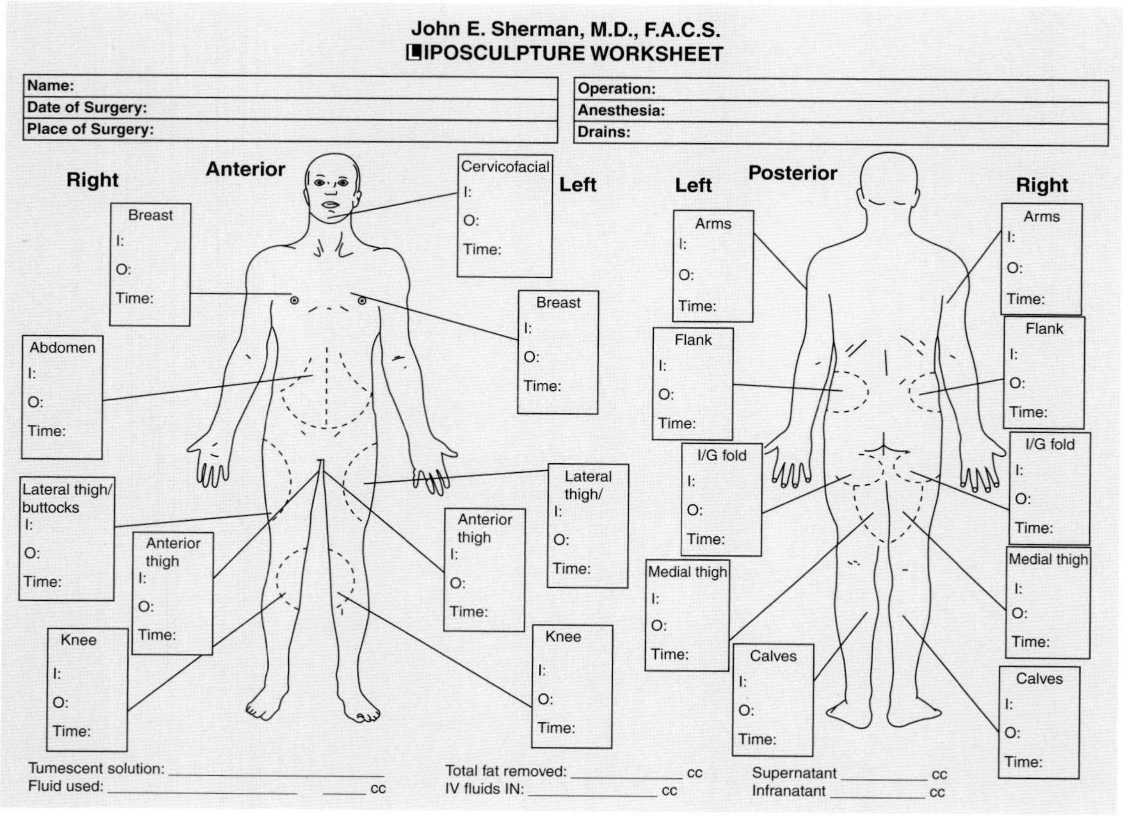

Figure 17–6. Worksheet that allows the operator to record the volume of tumescent solution placed into each region and the amount of lipoaspirate removed. In addition, the amount of ultrasound usage time per body part is accurately monitored and recorded. (Used with permission John E. Sherman, MD, FACS.)

even fewer deaths have been directly related to this event.

B. Tumescent-related Complications

Complications related to lidocaine and epinephrine delivery were addressed earlier, as was the risks of fluid overload. It is important to reemphasize the shift toward the use of less tumescence as well as less resuscitative fluids during routine liposuction. As liposuction volumes increase, the tendency is to over-resuscitate with a combination of tumescent solution and intravenous fluids. Even with an infiltrate-to-aspirate ratio of less than 0.5 and standard maintenance fluids, the patient will get more than enough volume to maintain intravascular pressure and thus organ perfusion.

C. Hemorrhage

Hemorrhage may lead to hematoma and seroma formation, but it is rarely significant enough to place the patient in any real danger.

A rapidly expanding area or hemodynamic instability should raise the possibility of a large vessel laceration and mandates early operative exploration.

Postoperative compression garments, in addition to providing some amount of comfort to the patient, may help small fluid leaks and hollow cavities seal. The trend is to limit their use. The compression garments should be worn continuously for the first week after surgery.

D. Perforation

Visceral or cavity perforations, although exceedingly rare, have been reported in the literature, especially during procedures around the costal margin and pubis. The use of ultrasound-assisted liposuction and power-assisted liposuction, which requires less force to the cannula, should minimize this possibility.

E. Infection

Infection occurs in less than 1% of all cases. The classic signs of infection include erythema, calor, and purulent incision site drainage. Pain out of proportion to the surgical procedure or crepitus on palpation may indicate necrotizing fasciitis and must be worked up and treated aggressively with both laboratory and imaging documentation as well as early surgical debridement. Broad-spectrum antibiotics, whether intravenous or oral, are given depending on the clinical judgment. These antibiotics should be narrowed to sensitivity-specific therapy once culture results are obtained. Reports of rare mycobacterium infections have been documented in the literature, thus cultures should be performed to identify these anaerobic and other less common species.

COSMETIC COMPLICATIONS

Surface irregularities can be caused by repeated passes of the suction cannula through one access port. This may be circumvented with the use of multiple approaches to each area of treatment to create a criss-crossing pattern with the cannula. In addition, prolonged aspiration in any one area should be avoided. Ice packs, compression garments, postoperative massage, and external ultrasound can all be used to promote skin contraction but will not mask irregularities related to overaggressive liposuction. In this case, lipofilling should be used to fill defects.

Depressions or subcisional irregularities are often a result of fibrous adhesions between a region where fat has been removed and the overlying dermis (Figure 17–7). These adhesions can be divided either sharply, with ultrasound or with the use of a V-shaped cannula tip or small ultrasound probe inserted through the old incision site. Following this, fat injection can be used to fill in the defect.

Dermal burns resulting from ultrasound-assisted liposuction were addressed earlier. A similar presentation may appear as a result of trauma to the subdermal vascular plexus with aggressive superficial liposuction. The resultant vasculopathy presents as red to purple lesions in a broad distribution and is resistant to therapy. Conservative management and local skin care should be initiated, although some surgeons advocate various methods of oxygen delivery to the skin, including hyperbaric therapy.

▶ OUTCOMES ASSESSMENT

Preoperatively, the potential need for revision must be addressed. A clear policy in writing should be given to the patient concerning the fees, if any, for revisional surgery. This will avoid postoperative conflicts over this important issue.

Disappointing outcomes most often result from undercorrection or overcorrection of treated areas. These results can be exacerbated by unrealistic patient expectations prior

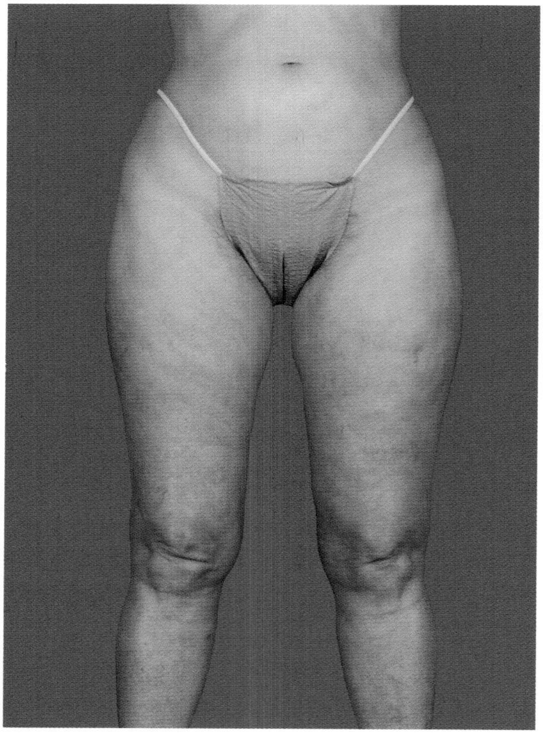

Figure 17–7. This patient was self-referred for a consultation regarding the dimple mark that developed on her left anterior thigh over the first few weeks following thigh and buttock liposuction. Examination revealed a tough patch of scar underlying the skin in this region. Initially, massage therapy was tried unsuccessfully. Sharp release of the scar followed by autologous fat injection was then recommended, but the patient deferred further treatment.

to the surgery or from postoperative weight fluctuations. For this reason, careful preoperative photographic documentation is essential to demonstrate the improvements that were gained as a result of surgery. Postoperative results are photographed at 6 months after surgery.

Disproportional removal of fat is prevented by careful measurement and documentation of aspiration volumes. Constant referral to the preoperative photographs and adherence to the preoperative markings helps the surgeon formulate a mental calculation of the extent of necessary liposuction. Careful operative positioning helps prevent body distortions, and for small deposits of fat, a syringe liposuction may be used.

▶ LARGE-VOLUME LIPOSUCTION

Generally defined as lipoaspiration over 5000 mL, the limits of large-volume removal have been pushed to over 8000 mL in the case of megavolume liposuction and as high as 12,000 mL, which is known as gigantovolume liposuction. Despite the potential for long operative times and huge fluid shifts, the safety of this more aggressive approach to body contouring has been validated in the recent literature. Regardless of its relative safety, however, some surgeons prefer staging operations with smaller volumes of lipoaspiration over multiple procedures. Patients are usually willing to accept this more prudent approach, and understand that the cosmetic result from shorter, more focused cases far outweighs the inconvenience of additional procedures.

Patient selection is crucial for large volume liposuction, and obesity should never be used as an indication for the procedure. Often, general or spinal anesthesia is used to protect the airway or to reduce the dependence on lidocaine, but these approaches may result in vasodilation and further complicate fluid management.

The increased volume of solution needed to adequately tumesce large surface areas must be kept in balance by limiting intravenous fluid administration and reducing the overall use of lidocaine. Urinary output should be carefully monitored with a Foley catheter. Lastly, after carefully positioning the patient and ensuring that all pressure points are well padded, a two-team approach can be considered to keep the operative time to a minimum.

REFERENCES

American Society of Plastic Surgeons. 2009 Report of the 2008 Statistics National Clearinghouse of Plastic Surgery Statistics. Available at: http://www.plasticsurgery.org/Media/Press_Kits/Procedural_Statistics.html. Accessed August 9, 2009.

DiBernardo BE et al. Evaluation of tissue thermal effects from 1064/1320-nm laser-assisted lipolysis and its clinical implications. *J Cosmet Laser Ther.* 2009 Jun;11(2):62–9. [PMID: 19484812]

Fischer G. Liposculpture: the "correct" history of liposuction. Part I. *J Dermatol Surg Oncol.* 1990 Dec;16(12):1087–9. [PMID: 2262614]

Hoyos AE et al. VASER-assisted high-definition liposculpture. *Aesthet Surg J.* 2007 Nov-Dec;27(6):594–604. [PMID: 19341688]

Illouz YG. Complications of liposuction. *Clin Plast Surg.* 2006 Jan;33(1):129–63. [PMID: 16427981]

Jewell ML et al. Clinical application of VASER-assisted lipoplasty: a pilot clinical study. *Aesthet Surg J.* 2002 Mar;22(2):131–46. [PMID: 19331963]

Kesselring UK. Notes on the history of the adoption of liposuction. *Plast Reconstr Surg.* 1997 Feb;99(2):595–6. [PMID: 9030181]

Klein JA. Tumescent technique chronicles. Local anesthesia, liposuction, and beyond. *Dermatol Surg.* 1995 May;21(5):449–57. [PMID: 7743108]

Schrudde J. Lipexheresis (liposuction) for body contouring. *Clin Plast Surg.* 1984 Jul;11(3):445–56. [PMID: 6467805]

Teimourian B. Ultrasound-assisted liposuction. *Plast Reconstr Surg.* 1997 Nov;100(6):1623–5. [PMID: 9385998]

CHAPTER 18

Brachioplasty

Lawrence S. Reed, MD & Joshua B. Hyman, MD

Cosmetic surgery of the upper arm, brachioplasty, has become one of the most common surgical procedures done today. According to the American Society of Plastic Surgeons statistical data, 338 upper arm lifts were done in 2000 and 14,059 upper arm lifts were done in 2008, an increase of 4059%. Although many variations of the procedure exist, the term generally implies the surgical resection of the skin and fat of the upper arm to improve the aesthetic contour of the upper arm. The surgical rejuvenation of the arm is a subject of much debate, which is why numerous procedures and combinations of procedures have been described. Brachioplasty was first introduced in 1954 by Correa-Iturraspe et al and since then has undergone a series of modifications, such as Z-plasties, W-plasties, curving S-incisions, and quadrangular flaps, to improve the appearance of the scar. The goal of any brachioplasty procedure is to approach the ideal, youthful, feminine arm which is lean and tapers smoothly from the axilla to the elbow. Glanz and Gonzalez-Ulloa used the coefficient of Hoyer to quantify the goals of brachioplasty more objectively. They state that the ratio of the distance from the top of the arm to the bottom of the humerus and from the bottom of the humerus to lower arm is 1:1 in a young girl and increases to 1:2.2 by age 70. The goal of surgery is to reapproach the 1:1 distance. Brachioplasty surgery has been plagued by large, often unacceptable, scars to obtain significant improvements in arm contour. Recent advances in brachioplasty surgery include more limited incision approaches combined with aggressive liposuction, which has been successful in some patients.

ANATOMY

A detailed knowledge of the anatomy of the upper arm is a prerequisite for a safe procedure. The entire operation is performed in the skin and deep subcutaneous layer superficial to the deep investing fascia of the arm. Surgeons should be aware of the anatomy of the upper extremity nerves, including the intercostobrachial, medial brachial cutaneous, and medial antebrachial cutaneous sensory nerves. The basilic vein accompanies the antebrachial cutaneous nerves as it emerges through the deep fascia in the lower half of the upper arm. The cephalic vein is generally much more radial and runs superficial to the deep fascia of the arm and should be out of the operative field. The brachial artery and nerve trunks of the brachial plexus are deep to the investing fascia and thus should not be encountered. The lymphatics are concentrated superficial to the investing fascia along the course of the basilic vein.

PATIENT EVALUATION & SELECTION

Women make up 98% of all brachioplasties in 2008 with the majority between the ages of 30 and 50 years old. Only 2% of all brachioplasties done in 2008 were on men. In general, there are two categories of patients who seek brachioplasty surgery: patients with a moderate amount of ptotic skin and subcutaneous fat and patients with a severe amount of excess skin and very little fat after achieving massive weight loss following bariatric surgery. The options for recontouring the upper arms ranges from liposuction to a standard arm lift with the incision extending from axilla to elbow. Teimourian and colleagues described a classification system for upper arm aesthetics and proposed treatment for each (Table 18–1).

PATIENT PREPARATION

A. Standard Brachioplasty

The procedure starts with careful preoperative planning and choosing the correct operation for the patient as explained above. Preoperative markings are made with the patient in the sitting position. The patients arms should be

TABLE 18–1. CLASSIFICATION AND PROPOSED TREATMENT FOR BRACHIOPLASTIES

Category	Description	Treatment
Minimal to moderate subcutaneous fat with minimal skin laxity	Patients have a circumferential increase in fat volume but acceptable skin turgor and elasticity.	Patients may benefit from liposuction procedures only.
Generalized accumulation of subcutaneous fat with moderate skin laxity	Patients may have an increased volume of fatty tissue circumferentially as well as slight but noticeable skin ptosis	Patients may benefit from liposuction alone but most likely will need a minimal incision brachioplasty for acceptable improvement in arm contour
Generalized obesity and extensive skin laxity	Patients have excess fat and a fair amount of loose skin, ptosis	Patients will likely benefit from liposuction as well as a brachioplasty with the incision down the arm for the best results
Minimal subcutaneous fat and extensive skin laxity	Patients (eg, those who have achieve massive weight loss) have marked skin laxity and depletion of subcutaneous fat.	Patients often require incision from axilla to elbow with little or no liposuction.

Source: Teimourian B et al. Rejuvenation of the upper arm. *Plast Reconstr Surg.* 1998 Aug;102(2):545–51.

abducted 90 degrees at the shoulder with the arms flexed 90 degrees.

The biceptal groove is easily identifiable in most patients and should be marked with a dotted line. Then, a solid line should be drawn 1–1.5 cm above this line from axilla to elbow. Then, the excess tissue should be pinched from the solid superior line to gather all excess tissue to the appropriate arm contour. The thickness of the tissue in the pinch needs to be accounted for and the inferior/posterior solid line adjusted accordingly. The markings can vary extensively for patients who necessitate resection of excess tissue along the lateral chest wall and axilla (also known as extended brachioplasty), such as in massive weight loss patients; however, only the standard and minimal incision brachioplasty techniques will be discussed in this text. The solid markings indicate the area of incision and excision and can be elliptical resection or sinusoidal which, according to some surgeons, makes the end scar more aesthetically pleasing. Regardless of the shape of the incision, it is agreed that the end scar placement should be in the biceptal groove and not on the posterior visible aspect of the arm.

The patient should be positioned on the operating table with the arms abducted 90 degrees on arm boards that are appropriately padded. An intravenous line may be placed in the hand and carefully wrapped with sterile 6 ply rolled gauze to maintain sterility in the operative field. The blood pressure cuff needs to be on the lower leg.

After preparing and draping the areas, the surgical site is infiltrated with 300–500 mL of a wetting solution containing 1 L saline with 1 ampule epinephrine and 50 mL 0.5% xylocaine. Even if liposuction is not going to be performed, infiltration of 200 mL of this super wet solution is usually done to decrease bleeding and facilitate dissection. Circumferential brachial liposuction is sometimes needed, and in those cases, the surgeon should infiltrate the entire upper arm circumferentially.

B. Minimal Incision Brachioplasty

Preoperative markings are made with the patient in the standing position. First, with the patient's arms fully adducted, the anterior and posterior shoulders at the visible edges of the axillary crease are marked (Figure 18–1). The final axillary incision line should be contained between these two boundary points to avoid noticeable scarring. The arms are then abducted so that they are perpendicular to the shoulder with elbows flexed (running man position). The final incision line is now marked in the apex of the axillary hollow running transversely from the anterior to the posterior shoulders, stopping 1–1.5 cm short of the previously marked shoulder/axillary crease boundaries (Figure 18–2). This helps avoid extending the final incision line and scarring into visible areas. The longitudinal axis or meridian is now marked from the inner upper arm, bisecting the transverse final incision line, and extending to the midlateral chest. Next, estimate how much axillary tissue must be removed to create an aesthetically pleasing result. First, the skin of the triceps area is moved toward the transverse final incision line, with force adequate to the task, until the arm has a pleasing contour. The advanced skin edge is held against the final transverse incision line and then marked (Figure 18–3A). This normally measures between 6 cm and 9 cm from the axillary crease. This measurement is only an approximate determination, which is later finalized intraoperatively with "tailor-tacking." Next, the skin of the medial axilla/lateral chest is advanced (again, with sufficient force) toward the final transverse incision line. Once more, the leading edge of the advanced skin is marked. This generally measures between 5 cm and 7 cm from the axillary crease. The planned area of excision is completed as a blunt oval by connecting the end points of the longitudinal excision line to the end points of the transverse excision. This generally measures 6–8 cm by 13–18 cm

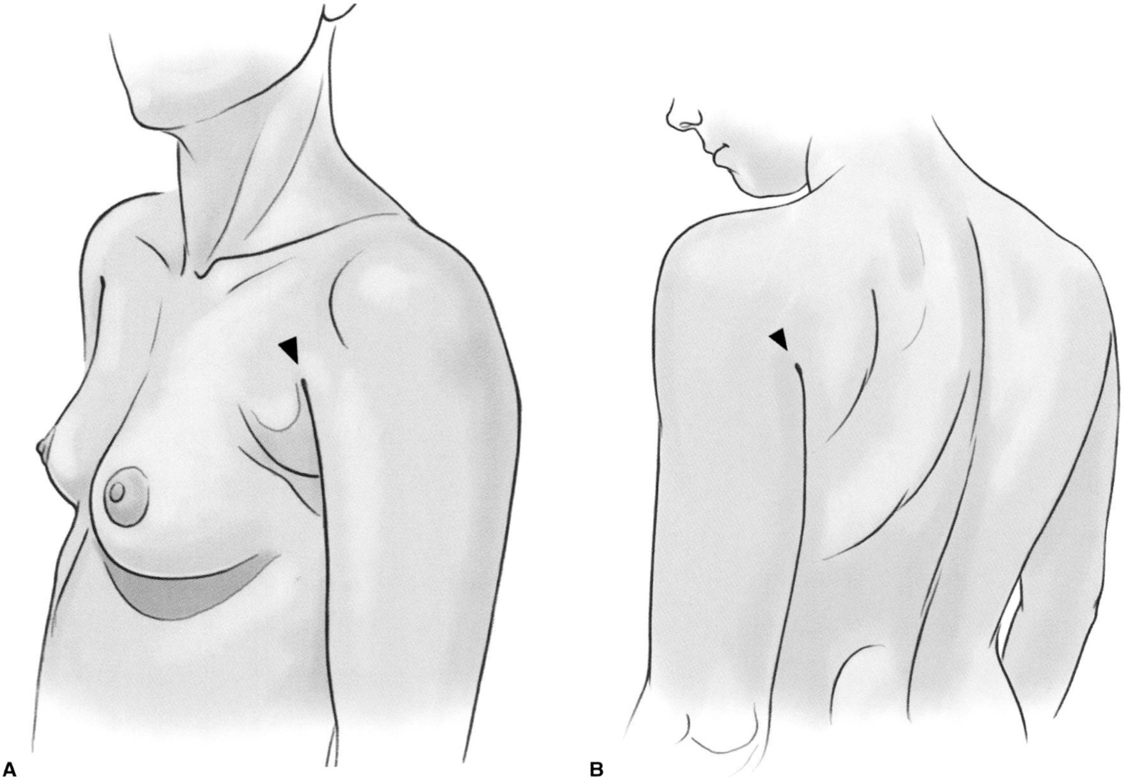

Figure 18–1. Preoperative markings for the minimal incision procedure are made with the patient's arms fully adducted and the visible edges of the axillary crease are marked at the anterior and posterior shoulders.

and almost always includes the entire hair-bearing portion of the axilla (Figure 18–3B). Again, these initial measurements are only an estimate, and a precise determination of the area of resection is finalized intraoperatively. The areas to undergo liposuction are carefully marked after all the other marks are complete. Liposuction is most frequently necessary for the areas overlying the triceps and commonly the anterior and mid-deltoid areas. At times, liposuction of the entire circumferential upper arm is indicated. Other areas to be marked for liposuction are the posterior axillary fullness in the lateral scapular area and anterior axillary fullness, which frequently is more skin than fat.

The patient is positioned on the operating table with the arms abducted to 90 degrees on arm boards. Following anesthesia, the arms are circumferentially prepared with povidone/iodine solution extending into the chest and neck area and appropriate drapes are applied. Tumescent formula solution is infiltrated into the areas undergoing liposuction, and local anesthesia is infiltrated into the areas of resection bilaterally.

TECHNIQUE

A. Standard Brachioplasty

Most brachioplasty procedures are done under general anesthesia. Liposuction, if done, is performed first prior to any incisions. The cannula may be introduced along a mark or within the marks of resection on the anterior medial aspect of the elbow. This tissue will be excised so no additional scars will be created. The cannula, usually 3–4 mm, is introduced around the elbow so that good access to the inferior and posterior arm can be achieved.

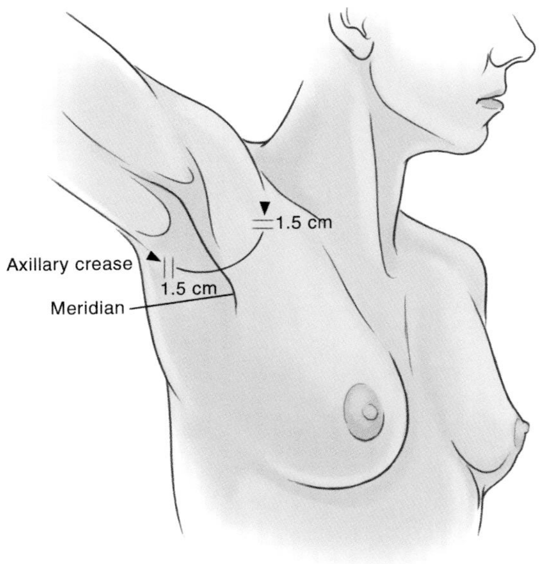

Figure 18–2. The final incision line is marked in the apex of the axillary hollow running transversely from the anterior to the posterior shoulders, stopping 1–1.5 cm short of the previously marked shoulder/ axillary crease boundaries.

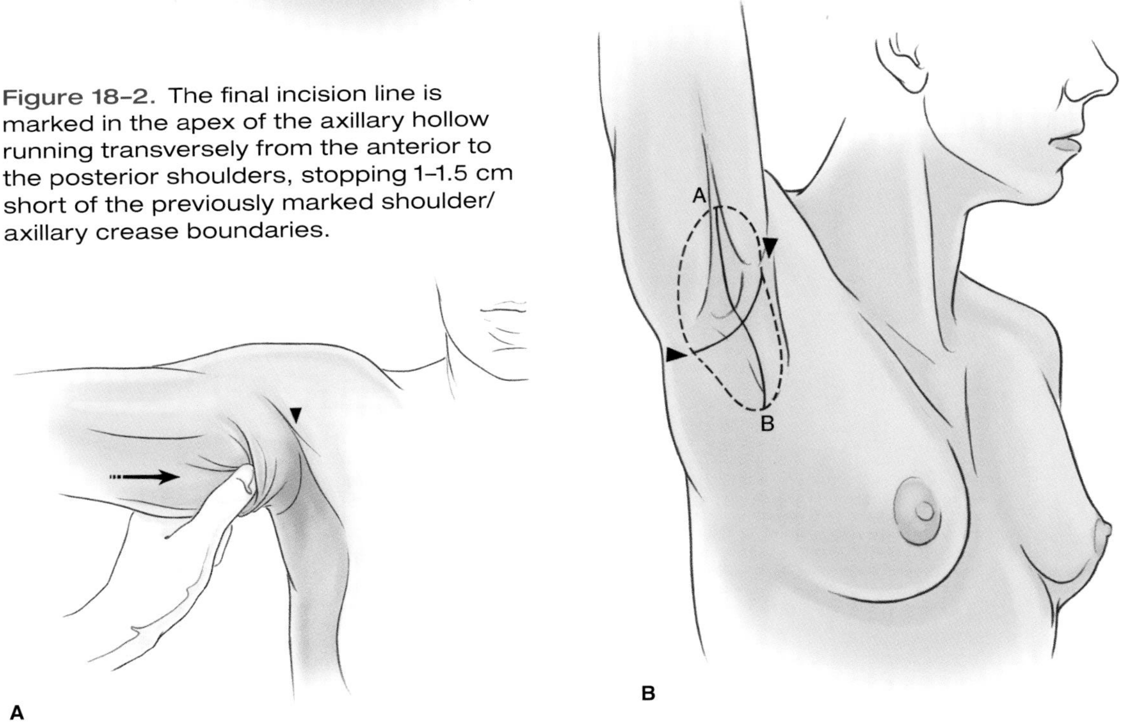

Figure 18–3. A: The advanced skin edge is held against the final transverse incision line and then marked. **B:** The area of excision almost always includes the entire hair-bearing portion of the axilla and is completed as a blunt oval connecting the end points of the longitudinal excision line to the end points of the transverse excision.

However, a second incision is sometimes needed in the posterior lateral proximal elbow region for additional access. Surgeons should not hesitate to use as many access incisions as needed to achieve a good result.

Pascal et al described a brachioplasty technique that emphasizes aggressive liposuction of the upper arm tissue traditionally resected followed by superficial resection of skin only. The benefits of this technique are to preserve all the lymphatic vessels, both the superficial and deep. In addition, no dead space or undermining is involved in this procedure, which eliminates the possibility of effusion and maintains good vascularization of the wound edges.

The incision is made with a number 10 blade along the superior incision first. Hemostasis is obtained with cautery in the usual fashion. It is usually not necessary to suture ligate any vessels during this procedure because the surgeon is careful to avoid going deep to the investing fascia and its underlying vascular structures. The dissection is then done in the middle aspects of the arm to the posterior solid mark or just beyond it. Some fatty tissue should be left on the deep investing fascia. A splitting incision is made in the center of the wound to the appropriate tension. If marking was accurate, the incision will extend to the posterior solid mark. This splitting technique is another way to check the preoperative marks and make sure not too much tissue is resected. A towel clamp is then used to approximate the anterior and posterior marks in the center of the arm incision. The surgeon is now left with an upper and lower triangle of excess skin and subcutaneous tissue. The remaining tissue should be pulled to the appropriate tension and then resected; the surgeon may have to modify or adjust the preoperative markings to obtain the appropriate tension and thus arm contour. The superficial fascia closure is done with 2.0-polydioxanone (PDS) suture. Some surgeons tack these stitches to the underlying axillary fascia. There are many variants and modifications of this technique. Interrupted 3.0 monofilament dissolvable sutures are then used to close the deep dermal layer as well as a subcuticular running closure. If the incision extends into the axilla, some surgeons advocate using a Z-plasty to orient the scar more favorably. In addition, some surgeons do a horizontal incision in the axilla make a T-shaped brachioplasty and do not use a Z-plasty. Drains are usually not used. The wounds are dressed in gauze and commercially available upper arm garments. If drains were used, they should be removed when drainage is less than 30 mL/24 h from each arm.

B. Minimal Incision Brachioplasty

The scar that results from the incision running through the axilla along the inner aspect of the arm to the elbow is understandably not accepted by some patients, which has inspired interest in various "minimal incision" approaches to brachioplasty. The most significant contribution inspiring the minimal incision brachioplasty was made in 1972 by Pollack introducing primary closure after resection for patients with axillary hidradenitis suppurativa (HS). Prior to Pollack's paper, excision of the involved areas was followed either by healing of the axillary defect by secondary intention or, in most cases, skin grafting followed by 3 weeks of airplane splinting.

The minimal incision brachioplasty procedure is most commonly performed under light to moderate sedation using both dilute local anesthesia for the area of excision and a standard tumescent solution for the areas of liposuction. Liposuction of the involved areas of both arms is done first. This not only helps remove the unwanted fat but creates discontinuous undermining, which reduces tension at the final incision line. If liposuction is not required, discontinuous undermining is still done in the triceps area using a 3 mm long liposuction cannula to increase skin mobility. The amount of fat suctioned can vary from as little as 100–150 mL to as much as 500–600 mL.

Attention is then directed to the axillary resection. The first and most important step is to use the "tailor tack" method to close the area of planned resection in order to visualize the final result. There are several advantages to this simulated "final" closure (Figure 18–4). It permits a precise evaluation of the amount of skin that can be safely removed while achieving a good aesthetic result. Any necessary revision of the planned area of resection can be made at this time. In addition, it demonstrates any areas of undesirable rotation of the skin or 'bow-stringing' in areas of excessive tension. Any final changes in the area of excision are made at this time and cross-hatch markings are made before removing the 'tailor-tack' sutures to expedite final closure. The marks are reinforced with staples alternating vertically and horizontally.

The initial incision is made in the lower/posterior aspect of the planned axillary resection. Cutting current is used, and the incision is carried down to a fine, fatty plane above the axillary fascia. Attention is then directed to the upper/superior aspect of the resection. Dissection is again carried down to a fine, fatty plane above the axillary fascia. The entire area to be resected is then carefully removed (en bloc) leaving a fine, fatty plane behind to preserve the superficial lymphatics and to provide a better purchase for the deep sutures. It is important to make note of the critical axillary structures so that sutures are not inadvertently placed in undesired areas. Hemostasis is obtained, although little bleeding is generally encountered. No drains are used. The wound is ready for closure using a multilayered technique. First, the axillary hollow is marked out on the axillary fascia with methylene blue (Figure 18–5). It is important to recreate this anatomic landmark. The wound is closed first with 1 polyglactin suture on a CPX reverse cutting needle. These sutures snug the superficial fascial system to the axillary fascia, re-creating the axillary hollow and effectively closing off the dead space (Figure 18–6). The sutures are tied with the arm adducted to the chest. This is followed by subcuticular closure with 2-0 PDS sutures on a FS 1 needle and placement of subcuticular 3-0 PDS suture on a PS2 needle.

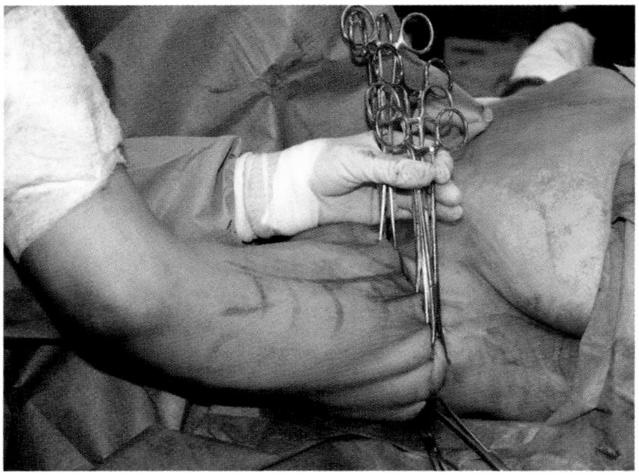

Figure 18–4. The "tailor tack" method simulates the final closure of the resection.

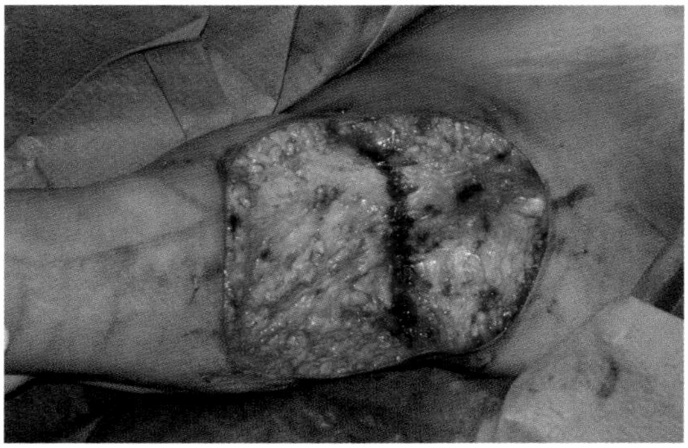

Figure 18–5. Marking the axillary fascia in the axillary hollow with methylene blue is the first step in closing the wound using a multilayered technique.

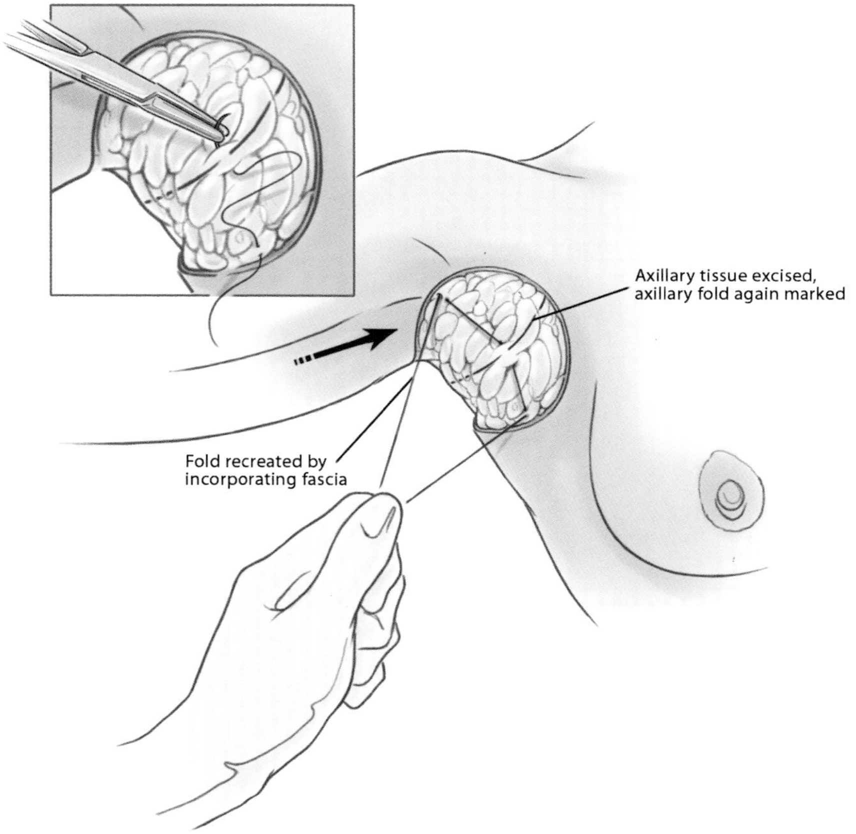

Figure 18–6. Axillary tissue is excised and the axillary fold is marked again. The fold is re-created by incorporating the fascia and purchasing tissue deep to the axillary fold.

At this point, the final transverse incision line has usually increased from an initial transverse diameter of 6–8 cm to 14–19 cm. This will commonly extend visibly in the anterior and posterior shoulder for a distance of 3.5–5 cm. When the incision extends visibly beyond the anterior and posterior boundaries, any noticeable extension should be corrected immediately to the degree possible. The extended visible incision area is first undermined and then defatted to the dermis (Figure 18–7). Liposuction with a fine cannula is of value in this process. A purse-string suture of 2-0 PDS anchored firmly to the axillary fascia or, if necessary, to the closest stable deep 2.0 PDS suture is used to draw the extended incision back into the hidden axillary area (Figure 18–8). This will result in an area of gathered skin normally 1–1.5 cm in diameter (Figure 18–9). This dimpling/bunched appearance from the purse-string suture resolves within 3–4 months in 85% of cases. Persistent dog-ears are revised under local anesthesia usually at 3–6 months. This technique successfully corrects or significantly

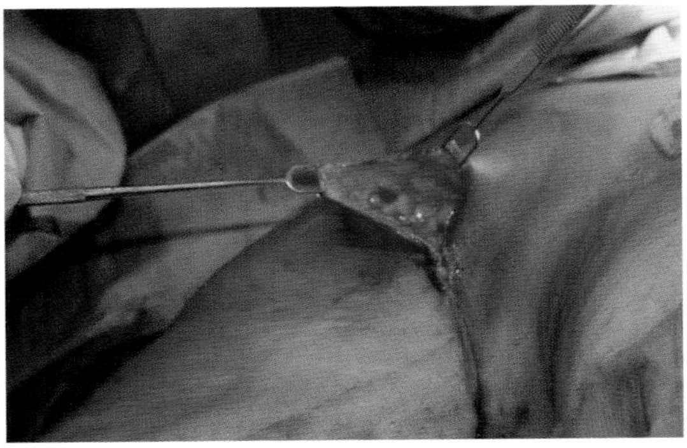

Figure 18–7. The extended visible incision area is undermined and defatted to the dermis.

reduces the area of visible scarring without compromising the final aesthetic result. This technique also corrects the anterior axillary fullness that represents an aesthetic concern for many women. The final transverse incision

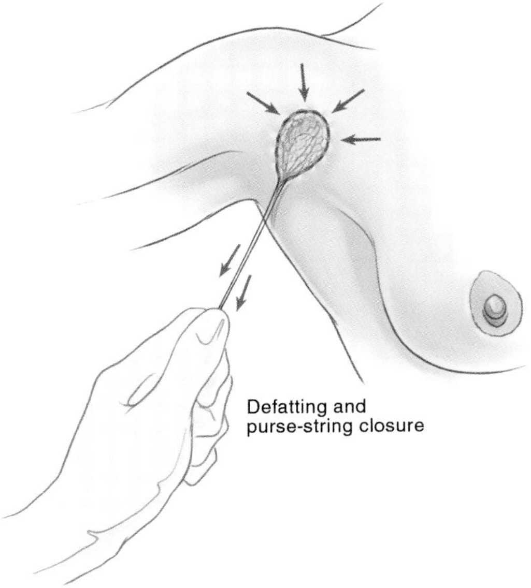

Figure 18–8. A purse-string suture is used to draw the extended incision back into the hidden axillary area.

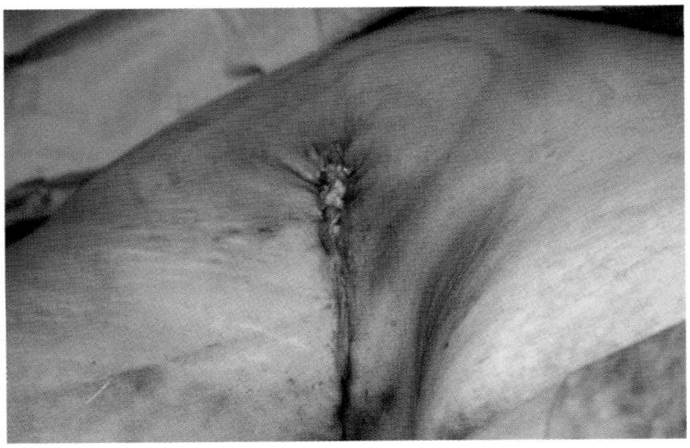

Figure 18–9. The purse-string closure results in an area of gathered skin normally 1–1.5 cm in diameter. The dimpling or bunched appearance from the purse-string suture usually resolves within 3–4 months.

is then closed with a running 3-0 plain gut suture on a PS 2 needle. No JP drains are used in the minimal incision brachioplasty procedure. Finally, a commercially available surgical arm control garment is applied, and the patient is moved to the recovery room.

POSTOPERATIVE CARE

There is surprisingly little discomfort for most patients following minimal incision brachioplasty. Although there are some complaints of pain, they are not frequent. Patients are encouraged to bathe or shower the next day and also to use an alcohol-based hand sanitizer or rubbing alcohol several times a day to keep the wound clean. Patients should not engage in aerobic exercises for the first 2 weeks. Patients are advised not to raise their elbows above shoulder level for the first 4–4.5 weeks and then, with active therapy, slowly extend their arms to the normal position above their heads. This generally takes 6–9 weeks after surgery. Figure 18–10 demonstrates typical postoperative results that can be expected.

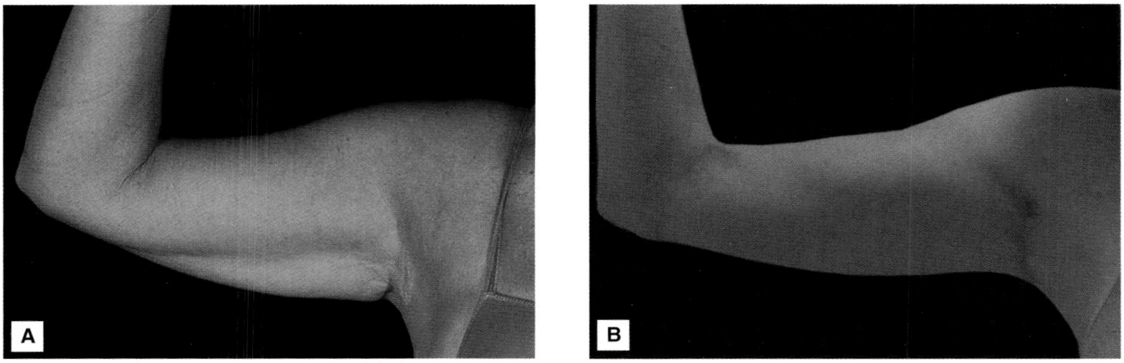

Figure 18–10. Typical postoperative results after minimal incision brachioplasty.

COMPLICATIONS

Complications cited in the literature include edema, wound infection, suture abscess, wound dehiscence, seroma, lymphoceles, severe scarring, and underresection. Knoetgen et al report a 25% complication rate with 95% of the complications of brachioplasty considered minor. These rates of complications are consistent with complication rates of other body contouring procedures. The minor complications of brachioplasty include seroma, hypertrophic scar, cellulitis, wound dehiscence, and subcutaneous abscess.

Major complications occurred in 5% of the patients and consisted entirely of damage to the median antebrachial cutaneous nerve. Seromas can be effectively treated by aspiration or placement of a catheter. The injuries to the median antecubital cutaneous nerves were effectively treated with hand therapy, gabapentin, and antidepressants in some cases. Underresection is unfortunately best addressed with revision surgery. Some additional complications are discussed below.

A. Swelling

Some edema is to be expected after brachioplasty. Excessive early swelling may occur as a result of tissue response to surgery or damage to the lymphatic drainage system. Late swelling can be a result of damage to the underlying venous system. Severe swelling can cause separation of the skin edges or even partial skin/flap loss.

B. Bruising

Some techniques include undermining of the adjacent arm tissue, which can create a space for fluid or blood to collect which may settle out as a bruise. In addition, when liposuction is included in the procedure, the surgeon can expect more bruising.

C. Bleeding

Acute bleeding may indicate damage to an underlying vascular structure and require surgical suture ligation. Slow bleeding may collect under the skin forming a hematoma. Sometimes, serum may also collect forming a seroma. Some surgeons advocate routine use of drains to avoid these issues.

D. Infection

Infection is uncommon; however, the brachioplasty techniques do involve large incisions that almost always extend to or transverse the axilla, which may contribute to a wound infection.

E. Scar

Unacceptable scarring is the most common problem following a brachioplasty. If the scar is placed on the front or back surface of the arm, it is more visible. It is best if the scar is located on the lower surface of the extended arm. In some patients, the scar may become hypertrophic and should be treated accordingly. Hypertrophic scarring may be treated with silicone sheeting and or massage. Keloids are rarely seen in this area but are certainly possible and proper precautions should be taken to obtain a good patient history of poor wound healing.

F. Numbness or Change in Feeling

Damage to superficial nerves in the fat of the upper arm may cause numbness or feeling change, including painful sensations. This is usually temporary in nature.

G. Contour Deformities

Contour deformities may occur anywhere throughout the length of the incision. These deformities are usually in the form of bands, folds, or constrictions as a result of pulling the tissue with inconsistent tension. At each end of the wound "dog ears" may form. Tissue excess at the elbow is frequently unacceptable to the patient and necessitates operative revision.

OUTCOMES ASSESSMENT

The revision rate for brachioplasty surgery is cited to be around 12% in most articles. Revisions are usually performed for residual bulk (fatty tissue) at the elbow, skin redundancy, and patients who lose a lot of weight after brachioplasty.

REFERENCES

Abramson DL. Minibrachioplasty: minimizing scars while maximizing results. *Plast Reconstr Surg.* 2004 Nov;114(6):1631–4. [PMID: 15509962]

Correa-Iturraspe M et al. Brachial dermolipectomy. *Prensa Med Argent.* 1954 Aug 20;41(34):2432–6. [PMID: 13236923]

Knoetgen J 3rd et al. Long-term outcomes and complications associated with brachioplasty: a retrospective review and cadaveric study. *Plast Reconstr Surg.* 2006 Jun;117(7):2219–23. [PMID: 16772920]

Lockwood T. Brachioplasty with superficial fascial system suspension. *Plast Reconstr Surg.* 1995 Sep;96(4):912–20. [PMID: 7652066]

Pascal JF et al. Brachioplasty. *Aesthetic Plast Surg.* 2005 Sep–Oct;29(5):423–9. [PMID: 16151657]

Pollock WJ et al. Axillary hidradenitis suppurativa. A simple and effective surgical technique. *Plast Reconstr Surg.* 1972 Jan;49(1):22–7. [PMID: 4550068]

Reed LS, Hyman JB. Minimal incision brachioplasty: refining ransaxillary arm rejuvenation. *Aesthet Surg J.* 2007 July–Aug;27(4)433–41.[PMID: 19341672]

Richards ME. Minimal-incision brachioplasty: a first-choice option in arm reduction surgery. *Aesthet Surg J.* 2001 Jul;21(4):301–10. [PMID: 19331908]

Richards ME. Reassessing minimal incision brachioplasty. *Aesthet Surg J.* 2005 Mar–Apr;25(2):175–9. [PMID: 19338810]

Teimourian B et al. Rejuvenation of the upper arm. *Plast Reconstr Surg.* 1998 Aug;102(2):545–51. [PMID: 9703097]

CHAPTER 19

Cosmetic Surgery of the Female External Genitalia

John G. Hunter, MD, MMM, FACS & Kevin J. Cross, MD

Long considered a minor aspect of cosmetic surgery, the demand for alterations to the female genitalia is rising. Women seeking cosmetic surgery of their external genitals generally desire to alter the shape or appearance of one of four aspects of their genitalia: the labia minora, labia majora, clitoral hood, or mons pubis. Labia minora reduction is the most common of the four to be requested, constituting the majority of cases. This is reflected in the literature as well, with most publications pertaining to this structure.

▶ ANATOMY

The degree of prominence of the mons pubis is determined by the amount of fibro-fatty tissue present below the dermis and anterior to the pubic symphysis. Extending inferiorly and posteriorly from the mons are the labia majora, which form the lateral boundaries of the vaginal region. Each labium has an outer, pigmented surface that is invested with hair follicles and an inner, nonpigmented, smooth surface with large sebaceous follicles. Anteriorly, the two labia converge to form the anterior labial commissure, while posteriorly, they run parallel to each other and appear to dissipate in the neighboring integument approximately 3 cm from the anus in the perineum. Below the anterior commissure lies the clitoris, which is partially covered by the clitoral hood. This sheath of skin comprises the anterior extent of the labia minora. The clitoris is an erectile structure formed by the two corpora cavernosa muscles, which are connected by a fibrous septum. It has a highly sensitive, spongy erectile tip, the glans. The labia minora are folds of skin that are situated medial to the labia majora (Figure 19–1). Anteriorly, they divide into two portions, the upper division meeting in the midline above the clitoris to form the clitoral hood, or preputium clitoridis, and the lower division terminating in the undersurface of the clitoris as the frenulum of the clitoris or anterior fourchette. Posteriorly, the two sides meet at the bottom aspect of the vaginal orifice to form the frenulum of the labia or posterior fourchette. As with

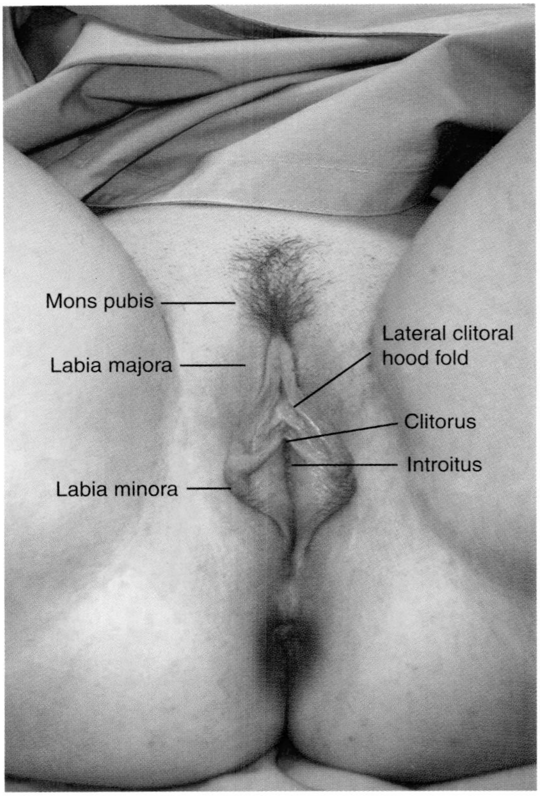

Figure 19–1. Anatomy of the female external genitalia.

the labia majora, the lateral surface of the labia minora is usually more darkly pigmented than the medial surface, which has a mucosa-like appearance.

The principal arterial supply to the perineum is via the internal pudendal artery. This vessel enters the perineum via the lesser sciatic foramen and divides into several branches as it approaches the medial margin of the inferior pubic rami: the perineal artery to the perineum, the posterior labial branches to the labia, and multiple branches to the clitoris and corpus cavernosum. Anteriorly, the labia are supplied by the superficial external pudendal artery. Accompanying this vessel from the main external pudendal is the deep external branch. These two arteries form a rich anastamotic plexus with the internal pudendal blood supply.

Much of the anterior superficial perineum receives its sensory innervation from a combination of the genital branch of the genital-femoral nerve and the ilioinguinal nerve once they pass through the inguinal canal and superficial inguinal ring. These nerves travel inferiomedially toward the vaginal orifice to supply the anterior vulva and mons. The pudendal nerve contributes innervation to the clitoris, labia, and perineum. It exits the pelvis through the greater sciatic foramen and eventually passes anteriorly across the lateral wall of the ischiorectal fossa. At this point, it divides into the dorsal nerves of the clitoris and the perineal nerve. Finally, the posterior cutaneous nerve of the thigh sends a perineal branch toward the posterior perineum and vulva.

▶ INITIAL CONSULTATION

Open conversation is essential to accurately evaluate patients' external genital aesthetic issues. Adequate time must be allowed for the patient to become comfortable enough to freely discuss her concerns. Most women seek surgical evaluation because they either have some discomfort or are embarrassed about genital size or shape. The physician should explain that there is a wide variation in what is considered normal genital size and appearance and that most cases fall within the normal range. Truly abnormally large external genitalia occur rarely.

It is not uncommon for patients to have had past experiences pertaining to their genital appearance that have led to insecurities and diminished libido and self-esteem. Therefore, physician empathy and understanding is required to treat these patients successfully. In the rare cases where the genitalia appear *absolutely* normal to the examiner and the patient has unrealistic expectations or expresses concerns or distress out of proportion to the physical findings, a psychiatric condition should be considered and referral to a psychiatrist may be appropriate.

▶ LABIA MINORA REDUCTION

There is much speculation about the acceptable size of the labia minora and what causes their enlargement. Early literature described the normal size of the labia minora as less than or equal to 5 cm as measured from the midline of the inter-labial sulcus to the distal-most point when the skin is held in mild traction. This does not take into account the anatomic make-up of the surrounding tissues, however; thus, measurements are not of much value. The typical presentation of the labia minora is for them to extend slightly beyond the labia majora. Wrinkling of the labia minora is common, but large, redundant folds may be considered atypical.

ENLARGED LABIA MINORA: ETIOLOGY

Large labia minora should generally be considered the product of normal development. There is no evidence to support the beliefs that early sexual activity and masturbation play a significant role in labial enlargement. Acquired hypertrophy may be caused by activities such as either manual or weighted stretching of the labia. In addition, chronic irritation to the vulvar region, such as may result from long-term urinary incontinence, may produce thickening and gradual enlargement of the minora. Finally, there are scattered case reports of other processes that may cause similar findings. These include infections that block the lymph channels (eg, *Filaria sanguinis hominis*), myelodysplastic disorders that cause swelling and edema of the labia, and treatment with androgenic hormones in childhood. However, in general, acquired hypertrophy of the labia minora is rare.

PATIENT EVALUATION & SELECTION

Examination of the labia minora is conducted with the patient in the lithotomy position. It is critical to ascertain every patient's desired labia size preoperatively. The surgeon should never make assumptions about her preference. A patient's perception of the appearance of her labia minora will largely be based on the relative size of the labia majora. Flat or atrophic labia majora will contribute to the appearance of enlarged labia minora, and the latter may be improved aesthetically by the correction of the former. A combined approach is occasionally used.

Surgery is largely for aesthetic preferences, but functional issues related to labial size do exist. Bilateral labia minora hypertrophy is typical, but asymmetric enlargement is not uncommon. Patients may report dyspareunia secondary to traction of the labia into the introitus during intercourse, or pain during physical activities that put pressure on the protruding tissues (eg, bicycle riding). Occasionally, patients describe concerns with personal hygiene. Rarely, women with urinary retention request the procedure to make the urethra more accessible during self-catheterization.

PATIENT PREPARATION

Preoperative preparations include appropriate positioning and analgesia. Though the use of stirrups and the lithotomy position has been described for labial reduction, the froglike position affords adequate exposure with less distortion of the anatomy. In general, most labia minora and clitoral hood procedures are done in the office under local anesthesia and oral sedation, with the remainder done as an outpatient procedure under local anesthesia and intravenous sedation. Site marking should always be done prior to the injection of local anesthesia. Patients receive a single dose of antibiotics prior to incision. Typically, an oral first-generation cephalosporin or clindamycin (for patients with penicillin allergies) is given. For an average adult patient, 10–20 mg of oral diazepam is given, and topical lidocaine and prilocaine cream (2.5%/2.5%) is applied to the genitalia. A solution of 2% lidocaine with epinephrine and 0.5% bupivacaine is prepared in a 1:1 ratio. The solution is buffered with sodium bicarbonate (in a 9:1 ratio), prior to injection into the premarked incision sites, to decrease discomfort.

TECHNIQUES

Many techniques have been described for the reduction of the labia minora. Each has advantages and disadvantages, and any single technique will not give optimal results in all women. Choice of technique should be based on each patient's anatomic findings and the desired surgical goals. Considerations include the amount of tissue to be removed and the need to preserve sensation and create a scar that will not result in a contracture. Often, there is significant variation in skin pigmentation between the outer edge and inner surface of the labia. If so, the edge should generally be preserved to maintain this difference (Figure 19–2).

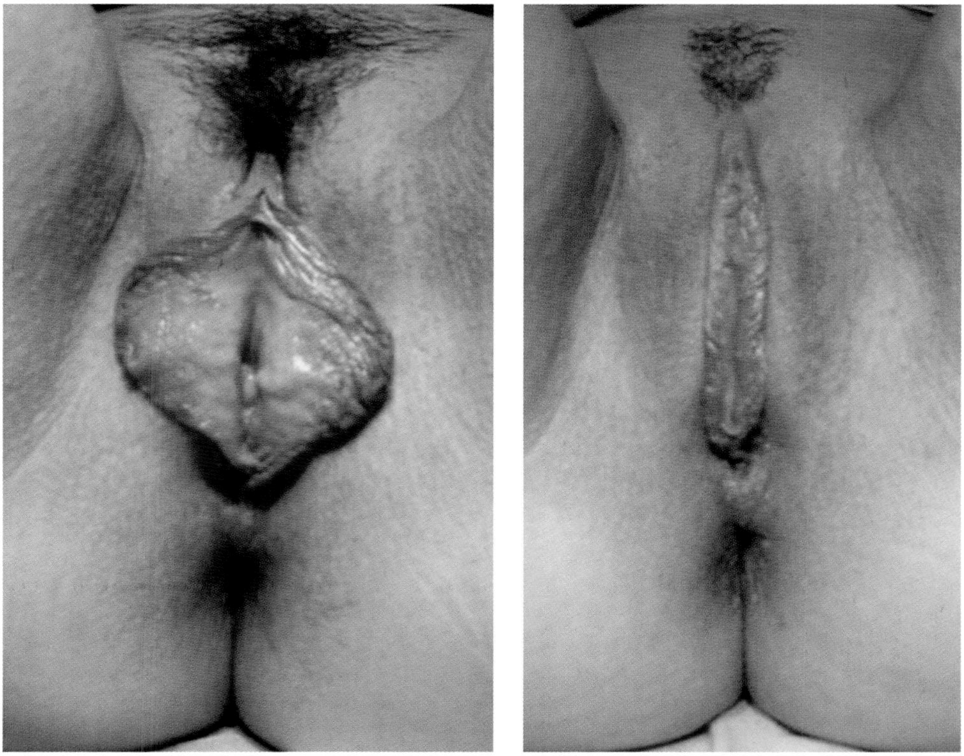

Figure 19–2. Labia minora reduction with preservation of the pigment variation between the inner surface and edge of the tissue.

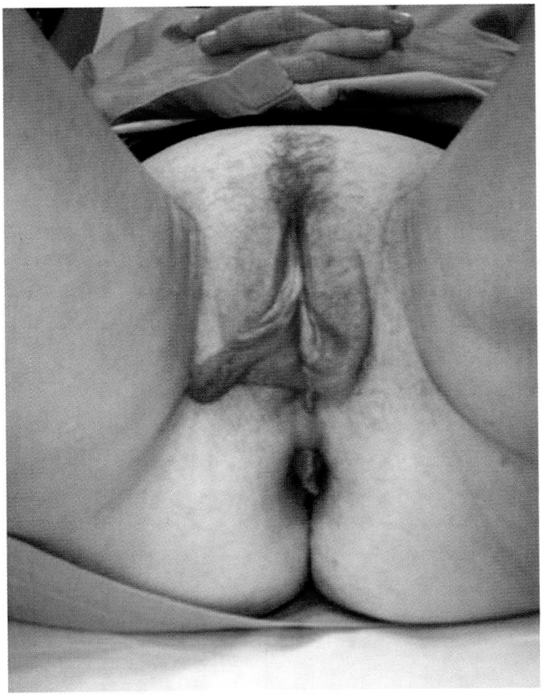

Figure 19–3. Notice the large amount of redundant tissue excised in this unilateral reduction. It is important to maintain between 0.5 cm and 1 cm of width to preserve a natural appearance of the labia, thus a bilateral reduction was not indicated in this case.

Aggressive resections can be performed with good cosmetic results (Figure 19–3), but the surgeon generally should *not* leave the labia less than 1 cm in width (with each labium under gentle traction), as measured from the intralabial sulcus to the anterior-posterior midportion of the labial edge. Resections that leave the labium less than 0.5 cm in width are generally contraindicated. Creating smaller labia may precipitate a sense of disfigurement. While prominent lateral clitoral hood folds and redundant tissue between the introitus and anus must be recognized and appropriately addressed (Figure 19–4), care must be taken to avoid inadvertently tightening the introitus or exposing the clitoris. Toward these goals, three techniques—amputation, wedge resection, and deepithelialization—are suggested for labia minora reduction.

For all techniques, the surgeon should closely follow the incision markings to avoid being misled by the anatomic distortion that will inevitably occur with injection of local anesthesia and edema. A number 15 blade and Colorado tip electrocautery are used to incise tissues and obtain hemostasis. Placement of a traction stitch usually facilitates exposure and resection. Meticulous hemostasis is a must. A close-as-you-go approach can be used effectively, with placement of tacking sutures to reapproximate tissue correctly. This approach is especially helpful when using the amputation technique, as the creation of a large wound, distorted by edema, may lead to inaccurate wound closure. Wound closure is performed using 4.0 polyglycolic acid interrupted sutures, and 5.0 synthetic gut running sutures.

A. The Amputation Technique

For years, classic teaching was that the most appropriate way to treat protuberant labial minora skin was simply to divide the tissue in a straight line and over sew the edges. This amputation technique, still in use today, produces a labial reduction that is technically straightforward with a short operative time and patient satisfaction that is generally high. It is used most appropriately in patients with labia that are enlarged in the direction running from the intra-labial sulcus toward the edge but that have little redundancy in the direction running from the clitoris to the anus. In theory, the resultant labial edge incision might heal with a tender scar or show signs of scar contracture, but this outcome seems to be extremely rare in clinical practice. More commonly, in patients with a distinct difference in color between the lightly colored pink inner labia and the darker labia edge, excision of

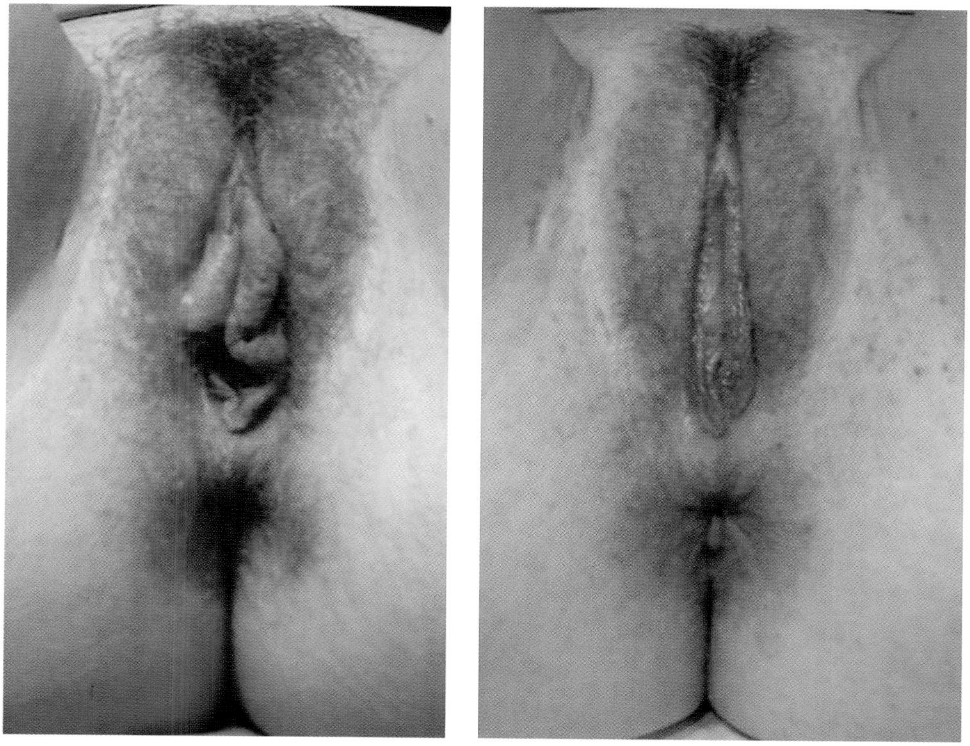

Figure 19–4. Excessively redundant folds of labia majora can be reduced without tightening the vaginal introitus.

the darker native labial edge can result in an unnatural appearance. Thus, the amputation technique is not the most appropriate choice in this setting. Furthermore, this technique carries the highest risk of resecting too large a portion of the labia, so the surgeon must be cautious and prudent when creating skin markings, and must remember not to deviate from these markings once the tissue has been distorted by the injection of local anesthesia.

After sedation and while the labia are under gentle traction, the medial and lateral surfaces are marked so that they run along symmetric paths. The lateral side is marked first in order to ensure that the surgeon preserves a minimum of 1 cm of length from the intra-labial sulcus. The superior and inferior extent of the incision should never violate the fourchettes. While some surgeons advocate placing a hemostatic clamp across the tissue that is to be excised, a close-as-you-go approach is often preferable to maintain hemostasis and facilitate accurate reapproximation.

Some physicians suggest that the scar left after the amputation technique can lead to problems ranging from lack of sensation along the incision to pain, irritation, and scar contracture. Although often stated in publications, there is little actual evidence that these complications are more than rare occurrences. However, modifications on the method have been described. Maas and Hage advocate a running W-shaped incision instead of a linear incision. Once the inner side of the labia is marked, a complimentary W is drawn on the lateral side with the peak of the W on one side corresponding to the trough on the other. Again, care is taken not to extend the incision into the frenulum at the base of the clitoris, and no part of the prepuce or its dorsal hood is resected. Local anesthetic is then injected into the labia to increase the virtual subcutaneous space between the lateral and medial skin layers and the resection is completed. Once the specimen is removed, each resulting triangle composed of skin on one side and subcutaneous tissue on the other can be folded down onto itself so that a straight border is obtained. This technique allows the incision to be distributed across the side walls, thus carrying it away from the labial edge.

B. The Wedge Resection Technique

This technique, made popular by Alter, consists of removing an inverted wedge of tissue from the most prominent portion of the labia followed by reapproximation of the remaining tissue. It has the benefit of preserving the labial edge as well as the native transition in pigmentation and thus is appropriate for patients with a distinct difference in color between the free margins and inner portions of the labia. In addition, it preserves sensation to the free edge of the labia via the intact branches of the superficial perineal nerve. Critics of this technique believe that it can lead to shortening of the labia in the anterior-posterior dimension and a tightening of the introitus if the wedge is too large and carried too close to the labial base, or if scar retraction is severe. This outcome would be a serious, albeit rare, complication that may require vaginal dilation or a difficult surgical revision. In addition, dehiscence of the labial edge, with resultant notching, is possible.

Once appropriate sedation has been given, a V-shaped wedge is drawn, centered over the most protuberant portion of the labia (Figure 19–5). This V can be angled in either an anterior or posterior direction so the resection is contoured to the shape of the labia. For example, if the labia are more protuberant anteriorly, the wedge is created with a more posterior angle so that a portion of the anterior redundancy can be pulled down and distributed over the posterior incision.

A variation of this technique incorporates complimentary 90-degree Z-plasties into each cut edge so that when the tissue is brought together, the incision is offset to prevent significant unidirectional retraction.

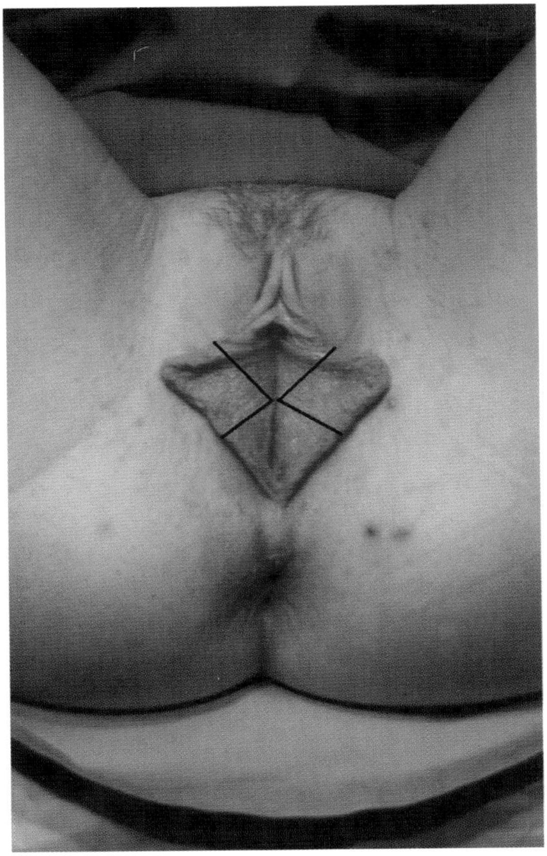

Figure 19–5. Preoperative markings for the wedge technique as described by Alter.

C. The Deepithelialization Technique

The deepithelialization technique is a modification of an older procedure for labial reduction that involved removing a full thickness section of tissue from the central portion of the labia to create a bipedicled flap. This older method was successful in displacing the incision away from the free labial edge and maintained the native color contrast, but essentially denervated the distal flap, potentially reducing sensation. To preserve the nerves running in the subcutaneous tissue, Choi described a technique where the central portion of the medial and lateral surfaces of the labia are deepithelialized, preserving the underlying parenchyma. The margins of the raw surface are then reapproximated with a running fast-absorbing suture (Figure 19–6). When marking the labia, again, it is important not to extend the cutaneous resection to the fourchette and to keep the width of the remaining tissues at least 1 cm after reapproximation.

This technique is generally used less frequently than others. While the free border and sensation remain intact, the labia have a tendency to appear thicker as a result of the retained parenchyma, and the technique does not allow for correction of redundancy in vertical length. Furthermore, postoperative edema seems to be more pronounced and prolonged using this technique. Epidermal inclusion cysts may form if the deepithelialization is not complete.

POSTOPERATIVE CARE

Wounds are typically dressed with an antibiotic ointment and covered with combine pads. Postoperatively, ice packs, minimal ambulation,

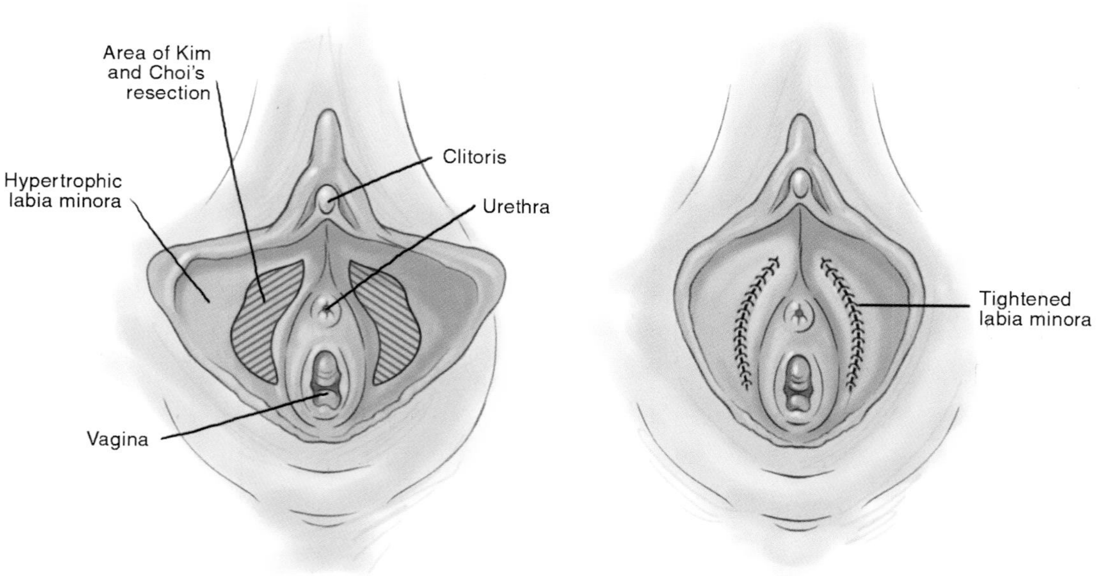

Figure 19–6. The deepithelialization technique first described by Choi. This technique keeps all incisions and resultant scars off of the leading edge of the labia minora.

and opioid pain control is recommended for the first 24–48 hours. Daily showers with tepid water followed by applications of antibiotic ointment and the use of sanitary napkins are recommended for 7 days. Vaginal penetration and the use of tampons are discouraged for at least 4 weeks. Patients are routinely seen in follow-up visits at 7 days, 3 weeks, 6 weeks, and 3 months.

COMPLICATIONS

The most common complication of labia minora reduction surgery is minor wound dehiscence, usually as a consequence of a small hematoma. Surgical treatment is rarely necessary, since wounds usually heal by secondary intention over the course of 7–10 days following conservative management with little or no effect on cosmetic outcome.

Although infection is possible, it is rarely seen. If present, standard procedure for the treatment of a superficial surgical site infection should be followed. As with hematoma formation, treatment of a small abscess collection with opening of the incision and healing via secondary intent should afford acceptable results.

Excessive tightening of the vaginal orifice can occur when a wedge excision of the labia minora is carried too far internally or as a result of excessive scar contracture along the labial rim. A Z-plasty that recruits tissue into the area and lengthens the circumference of the orifice may be necessary if manual massage and gentle dilation by the patient is not successful.

By far, the most dreaded complication is overresection of the labia minora. This mistake may result in the labia majora appearing excessively large in comparison with the absent labia minora. Even worse, as described earlier, it may cause the patient to experience a sense of mutilation. The surgeon is again reminded to leave at least 1 cm of tissue and remain committed to the preoperative markings in order to prevent this from occurring. Once present, while it may be tempting to gain symmetry by reducing the labia majora, be warned that this would be an example of compounding one mistake with another mistake. Other than patient counseling, very little can be done to improve on the original surgical outcome without risking further insult to the region.

OUTCOMES ASSESSMENT

In the only large series published on labia minora reduction surgery, a follow-up questionnaire found that approximately 90% of patients who underwent the amputation technique were satisfied with both the aesthetic and functional results of their surgery. While concerns about scar contracture, decreased sensation, and color mismatch are often discussed in the literature, these appear only rarely to be problems for patients.

REFERENCES

Alter GJ. A new technique for aesthetic labia minora reduction. *Ann Plast Surg.* 1998 Mar; 40(3):287–90. [PMID: 9523614]

Choi HY et al. A new method for aesthetic reduction of labia minora (the deepithelialized reduction labioplasty). *Plast Reconstr Surg.* 2000 Jan;105(1):419–22. [PMID: 10627011]

Maas SM et al. Functional and aesthetic labia minora reduction. *Plast Reconstr Surg.* 2000 Apr;105(4):1453–6. [PMID: 10744241]

Rouzier R et al. Hypertrophy of labia minora: experience with 163 reductions. *Am J Obstet Gynecol.* 2000 Jan;182(1 Pt 1):35–40. [PMID: 10649154]

► LABIA MAJORA ALTERATION

Patients may complain that their labia majora are flat, resulting in a overly visible clitoral hood or labia minora, and may want more coverage of these structures. Some patients feel that their majora are "deflated" or sagging and desire more youthful appearing, "puffy" majora. Other women are embarrassed by prominent, overly puffy majora that show through tight fitting athletic wear and bathing suits. Each of these anatomic variations may be addressed surgically.

LABIA MAJORA REDUCTION

A. Patient Evaluation and Selection

Understanding the patient's concerns and a careful physical examination are crucial when deciding which procedure is appropriate for labia majora alteration. Labia majora concerns require evaluation in both lithotomy and standing positions. Puffiness without skin redundancy can usually be treated with suction-assisted lipectomy. Patients must be made aware that the minora may be exposed or made more visible with defatting of the majora. Although generally effective, this procedure is more difficult than in other parts of the body because of the fibrofatty tissue of the labia majora. In addition, postoperative edema may be significant and may persist for months.

If physical evaluation reveals deflated, sagging majora, two options are available. Autologous fat injection may be performed to restore fullness and a more youthful appearance (see labia majora augmentation) or surgical resection of redundant tissue may be necessary to achieve the woman's desired aesthetic result.

B. Patient Preparation

The same local anesthesia and oral sedation technique used for labia minora reductions is often used for labia majora alteration cases; however, monitored anesthesia care may be preferable for some patients, especially for combined minora and majora cases.

C. Techniques

1. Suction-assisted lipectomy—

Single stab incisions are made within the hair-bearing skin cephalic to each labia majora after infiltration of local anesthesia. Minimal tumescence is used to minimize tissue distortion. A 2.4-mm Mercedes tip cannula is used. Aspirated fat volume rarely exceeds 20 mL per side. Incisions are closed with single 5.0 fast absorbing gut sutures. A sanitary napkin or gauze pad is used for dressing.

2. Surgical resection of redundant tissue—

Excision of labia majora tissue should be done in a crescenteric manner. The resection should be performed in an anterior-posterior orientation, with incisions within the inter-labial sulcus medially and in the hair-bearing majus skin laterally. Excision should generally extend the entire length of the sulcus, with the maximum width determined by the extent of majora redundancy (Figure 19–7). This is determined preoperatively with the patient lying supine with the thighs flat and parted approximately 45 degrees. The extent (width) of resection is determined by "pinching" the planned lateral incision line to the medial incision line. *Resection must not result in pulling the introitus open with the thighs spread.* Incisions should be full thickness to the level of the superficial subcutaneous tissue. Resection should be performed in this plane; deeper dissection will result in unnecessary bleeding.

Robust bleeding may occur; meticulous hemostasis is essential. Incisions are closed in two layers: 4.0 polydioxanone intradermal interrupted sutures, and running 5.0 polypropylene (or 5.0 absorbable gut).

D. Postoperative Care

Postoperative care is the same for surgical resection of redundant tissue as for labia

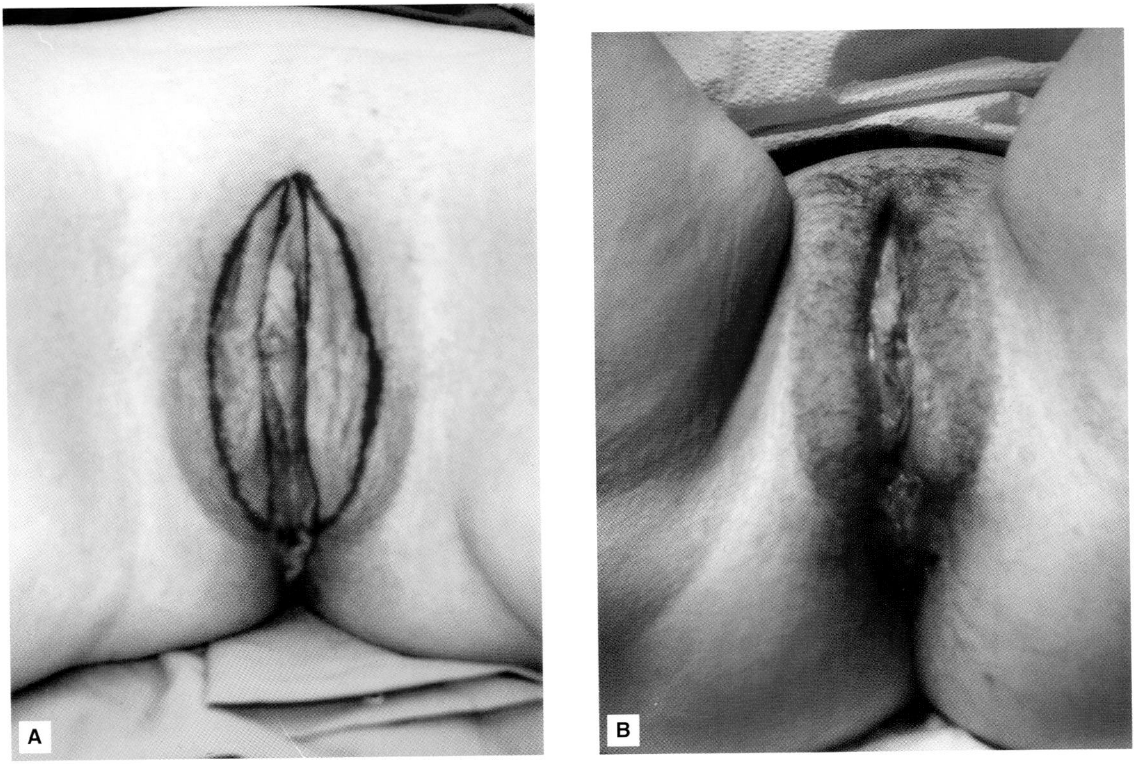

Figure 19–7. Labia majora reduction demonstrating preoperative markings **(A)** and postoperative result **(B)**.

minora reduction. The incisions, if located properly, typically heal so well that the resulting scars are essentially imperceptible.

LABIA MAJORA AUGMENTATION

A. Patient Evaluation and Selection

When the labia majora appear flat or sagging, but without significant skin excess or redundancy, autologous fat grafting is indicated to achieve a fuller appearance (Figure 19–8). This is an office procedure that is done under local anesthesia. Patients should be advised that several grafting procedures may be necessary to achieve the desired effect.

B. Technique

In autologous fat grafting, less than 20 mL of fat generally is injected into each labium. After fat is harvested and prepared, single stab incisions are made cephalic to each majus. Multiple passes are made in the superficial subcutaneous plane using a Coleman fat infiltration cannula, depositing the fat in multiple,

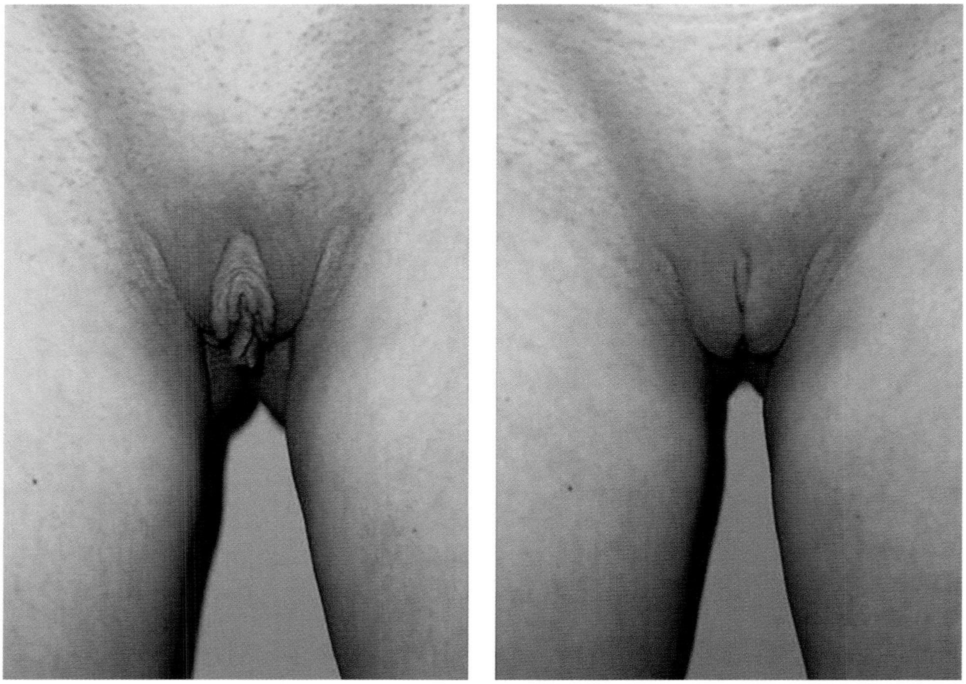

Figure 19–8. Preoperative and 6-month postoperative photographs of autologous fat augmentation of bilateral labia majora after two treatments.

parallel rows as the cannula is withdrawn. This is more effective than injecting large boluses in achieving a lasting result. Deep injection increases bleeding risk, and hematoma formation. Incisions are closed using 5.0 fast absorbing gut sutures. Minimal dressings are needed. Significant edema is common and should be expected.

▶ MONS PUBIS

PATIENT EVALUATION & SELECTION

Isolated mons pubis can usually be evaluated without the lithotomy examination. Contouring the mons pubis is typically achieved using one of three procedures, including suction-assisted lipectomy, a vertical reduction and pexy of the mons, and combined vertical and horizontal "T" reduction and pexy. When the mons pubis appears excessively puffy or protuberant but lacks skin excess or redundancy in the vertical or horizontal directions, suction-assisted lipectomy is appropriate. This procedure is frequently combined with suction-assisted lipectomy of the labia majora. Vertical reduction is most useful in patients in whom the mons (as well as the labia majora) appears to hang and is excessively long. When both vertical and horizontal skin laxity or excess are present, a "T" reduction is generally necessary. The latter two procedures are often combined with a defatting procedure. Defatting may be performed by suction-assisted lipectomy or direct open excision, or both. Open excision usually results in less edema but increases the likelihood of drain placement.

PATIENT PREPARATION

While monitored anesthesia care and local anesthesia are almost always adequate for the vertical reduction technique, on rare occasions, general anesthesia may be necessary. Patients undergoing the T reduction procedure are more likely to request general anesthesia and a thorough discussion with the patient regarding this point is imperative.

TECHNIQUES

A. Suction-Assisted Lipectomy

Suction-assisted lipectomy is performed via a single midline incision, or bilateral lateral incisions, located at or immediately cephalic to the pubic hairline. The mons subcutaneous tissue is fibrofatty in nature, making aspirating somewhat difficult. Power-assisted or ultrasonic suction-assisted lipectomy may therefore be helpful. A 3.0-mm accelerator cannula, or 2.4-mm Mercedes cannula, and moderate tumescence should be used. Adequacy of fat resection is determined using visual inspection and palpation. Incisions are closed using 5.0 fast absorbing gut sutures.

B. Vertical Reduction

The cephalic incision for this procedure is made in a horizontal direction at or slightly within the pubic hair line. The caudal incision is made within the mons itself. Excision is a modified horizontal ellipse (Figure 19–9). A previous Pfannenstiel or abdominoplasty incision scar may be used for the cephalic incision line. The vertical width of excision is planned with the patient standing and readjusted when supine. Defatting is almost always combined with this procedure. If suction-assisted lipectomy is planned, it is performed first, through stab incisions within the island of skin being removed. Open defatting is done en bloc with skin excision. Defatting may, if necessary, extend caudally beneath the remaining mons skin. If the prepuce of the clitoris is approached, the dissection should be in the superficial plane to avoid injuring the sensory nerves to the clitoris. Wounds are closed in two layers with intradermal interrupted 3.0 polydioxanone sutures, followed by running subcuticular 5.0 polypropylene sutures. The postoperative care is notable for the use of a compression bandage or garment. The decision to insert a suction drain is made intraoperatively, based on the extent of defatting or undermining and adequacy of hemostasis. A drain is placed in approximately half the patients.

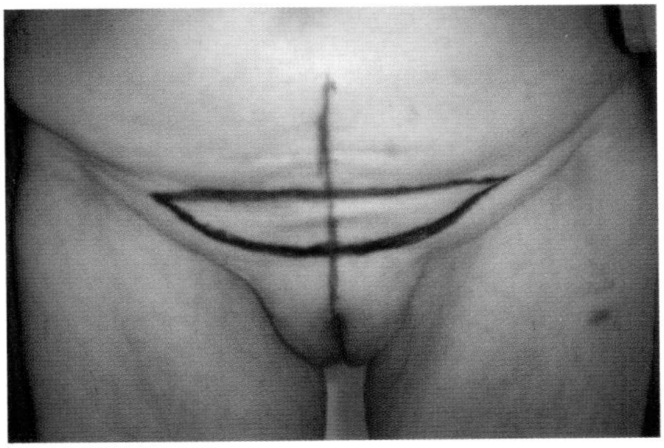

Figure 19–9. Preoperative markings for the vertical mons pubis reduction. The cephalic incision has been placed within the pubic hair region and the caudal incision was placed using a pinch technique with the patient standing. The lateral aspects of the planned incisions converge along a prior Pfannenstiel incision so that the resulting closure will be situated in continuity with this prior scar.

C. "T" Reduction

The horizontal markings (vertical reduction) are done first, and then the vertical markings (horizontal reduction) are made. The midline from umbilicus to the apex of the clitoral prepuce is marked. The extent of horizontal reduction is determined by pinching the mons together from both sides along the midline. The bilateral vertical incision lines are then marked symmetrically on either side of the midline, tapering caudally until they intersect the midline just cephalic to the prepuce apex. The cephalic portion of the vertical incision lines do not taper together, but rather intersect with the caudal horizontal incision marking at 90 degree angles (Figure 19–10).

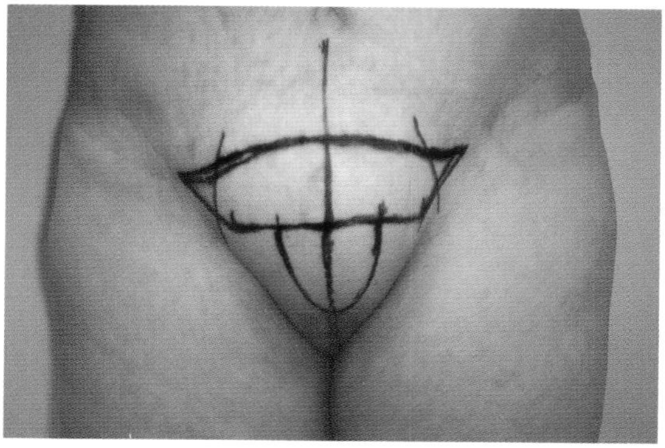

Figure 19–10. Markings for the combined vertical and horizontal mons pubis reduction.

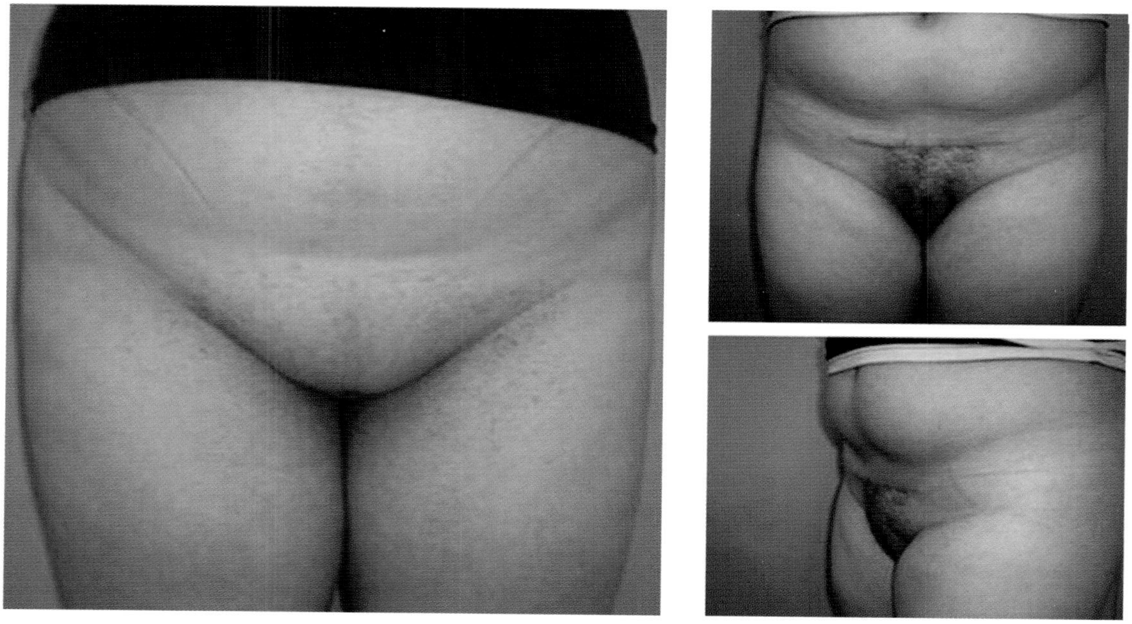

Figure 19–11. Preoperative (left) and postoperative (right above and below) views of the combined vertical and horizontal mons pubis reduction. The vertical component of the scar is well hidden within the pubic region.

The markings are checked with the patient supine and adjusted if needed. The combined procedure is then performed in a similar manner as the vertical reduction. Great care must be taken during the dissection to remain in the superficial subcutaneous plane as the prepuce of the clitoris is approached. Deep dissection in the area where the prepuce attaches to the pubis risks sensory nerve injury. The "T" reduction both shortens and narrows the mons pubis (Figure 19–11). Suction drains are almost always inserted.

REFERENCE

Hunter JG. Considerations in female external genital aesthetic surgery. *Aesthetic Surg J.* 2008 Jan–Feb;28(1):106–7. [PMID: 19083515]

INDEX

Page numbers followed by *f* or *t* indicate figures or tables, respectively.